A novel facial fat grafting technique with a concept of volumetric lifting

군자출판사

SA FI

Sequential
Autologous
Fat
Injection

Author **Kyoung–Jin(Safi) Kang.**
MD PhD & FKCCS

군자출판사

SAF I

1st print : 2017-01-02
1st publication : 2017-01-11

Author : Kyoung-Jin Kang
Publisher : Joo-Yeon Jang
Editor : Eun-Hee Cho
Editorial designer : Seul-Hee Lee
Cover designer : Jae-Uk Kim
Illustration : Koonja illustration dept.

Head office : 338 Hoedong-gil, Paju-si, Gyeonggi-do, Korea, 10881 (Paju book city)
Tel: 82-31-943-1888
Fax: 82-31-955-9545

ISBN 979-11-5955-093-5

List price : US$ 180.00

Author Introduction

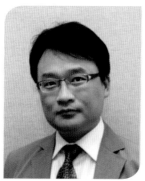

Kyoung-Jin (Safi) Kang
MD PhD & FKCCS

· Sang-San High School, Chonju, Republic of Korea.
· Chon-Buk National University Medical School (MB), Chonju, Republic of Korea.
· Chon-Buk National University Graduate School (MSc and PhD), Chonju, Republic of Korea.
· Assistant of Chon-Buk National University Medical School, Department of Anatomy, Chonju, Republic of Korea.
· Instructor of Chon-Buk National University Medical & Dental School, Department of Anatomy, Chonju, Republic of Korea.
· Researcher of Ministry of Korean Food and Drug Safety, Seoul, Republic of Korea.
· Clinical Internship of Catholic University of Korea, Daejeon ST. Mary Hospital, Republic of Korea.
· Diplomat of International Board of Cosmetic Surgery (IACS certified), London, United Kingdom.
· Ex-Associate Professor of Catholic University of Daegu, Medical School, Republic of Korea.
· Ex-Chief director of Plastic and Reconstructive Surgery of Wallace Memorial Baptist hospital, Busan, Republic of Korea.
· Present Visiting Professor of Young-Nam University Medical School, Daegu, Republic of Korea.
· Founder, 1st president, and Chairman of the directors of KSKCS (Korean Society of Korean Cosmetic Surgery and medicine) and KCCS (Korean College of Cosmetic Surgery), Busan, Republic of Korea.
· Fellow of International College of Surgeons (FICS), Chicago, USA.
· Teaching committee member of Plastic Surgery Fat Group of Chinese Medical Association, R.P. China.
· Managing Editor of Journal of Cosmetic Medicine, Busan, Republic of Korea.
· Director of Seoul Cosmetic Surgery Clinic, Busan, Republic of Korea.

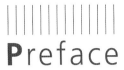

Preface

"Dedicated to my academic advisor of medical school,
the late professor Byoung-Duek Jun,
who had guided me into becoming a human anatomist."

As a cosmetic surgeon who majored in human anatomy, I am very delighted to share my method of SAFI(Sequential Autologous Fat Injection) which considers structure and function, aging process, and influence of gravity on all areas of the face. Various hypotheses and detailed method of SAFI technique are discussed in this book. It is expected to be helpful for doctors who try to perform fat graft for the first time and even for those who are currently practicing fat graft actively. In addition, I hope that the principles of SAFI established from my personal experience in this book are also applicable to any aesthetic augmentation using various man-made fillers.

My first Korean edition of SAFI book had already published in 2011(ISBN978-89-92000-93-4). I would like to introduce that this book is published in English, as an updated version of previous contents and results.

Lastly, the readers' advice and encouragement are always welcomed for further development of facial fat graft technique.

I wish you success in your career of facial fat grafting.

Kyoung-Jin (Safi) Kang
MD PhD & FKCCS

Safi Video Introduction

A novel facial fat grafting technique with a concept of volumetric lifting

1. Table of basic contents (about 52 min.)

1) Preoperative design   (5 minutes 22 seconds)

2) Anesthesia   (3 minutes 38 seconds)

3) Fat harvest   (7 minutes 21 seconds)

4) Fat purification   (3 minutes 2 seconds)

5) SAFI forehead   (7 minutes 47 seconds)

6) SAFI right face   (9 minutes 55 seconds)

7) SAFI left face   (9 minutes 35 seconds)

8) Suture   (1 minute 12 seconds)

9) Baton grip technique   (1 minute 1 second)

All music used in these video clips are downloaded from a website (https://www.youtube.com/audiolibrary/music), which is granted under license of Creative Commons Attribution (https://creativecommons.org/licenses/by/4.0/).

2. How to watch SAFI video?

1) Log in site: Find the title "Video Education" from www.koreancosmeticsurgery.com

2) Sign in using the ID that you are assigned of for e.g. Safi0000.
    Your personal ID is Safi0225.

3) Various Safi videos will be upgraded continuously.

3. Precautions:

1) Safi video can be watched only from your two personal computers.

2) If any user capture images or create video, and then distribute it to other people, the user's ID will be stripped away and the user will be legally responsible for that.

3) If other people sign in using your personal ID, this system will no longer be available.

CONTENTS

Anatomy for facial fat grafting

Facial fat grafting has been applied to recover the volume defect of subcutaneous tissue by congenital anomaly or accidents, and to improve the lack of volume in wrinkled or depressed regions formed by habitual movement and/or aging. And it came out that facial fat grafting can change partial or whole facial contour.

The contours of face are determined by the respective size, quantity, thickness and location of bones, muscles, superficial musculoaponeurotic system (SMAS), and subcutaneous fat and skin. In addition, ligamentous fixation has an important role, which is keeping the facial soft tissue contour by fixing the soft tissues to bone and muscle fascia. These facial tissues have a dynamic feature because the shape, location and properties of each facial tissue are continuously altered by active facial movement and various aging factors.

Therefore, understanding the anatomical structures and their functions, and then realizing how each structures and overall facial contour changed by facial movement or aging process, are very important to most fields of facial cosmetic surgery including facial fat grafting.

1 Facial aesthetic units and skin

1) Facial aesthetic units

As seen in Figure 1, the skin's surface of skin can be divided into several units —by color, texture, thickness and mobility— which are called facial aesthetic units[1, 2]. Each facial aesthetic unit has its' own special

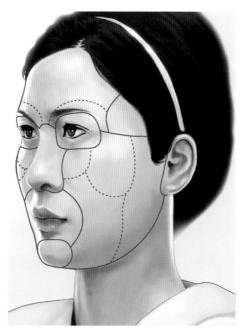

Figure 01 Facial aesthetic units of the forehead, the temples, the cheeks, the nose, the periorbital area, the lips and the chin. The dotted lines express additional areas of variation in skin thickness in the forehead and the cheek.

characteristics according to the presence or absence, and quantitative and qualitative differences of the structural elements of the face such as skin, subcutaneous fat, muscle, bone, and ligamentous fixations.

Moreover, each unit also has various characteristics. For example, in the forehead unit, skin and subcutaneous tissue tend to be relatively thin near the frontal hair line, and become thicker as getting closer to eyebrows and glabella. Additionally, the adjoining boundary region of facial aesthetic units requires careful consideration since they have significantly different or intermediate characteristics. Especially, incisions that cross the unit boundaries should be avoided whenever possible[2].

2) Skin

Skin of face consists of two quite different layers - epidermis and dermis. The dermis is a layer of connective tissue composed mainly of collagen fibers and about 5% elastin. And this layer is divided into two layers, the superficial area adjacent to the epidermis called the papillary region and a deep thicker area known as the reticular dermis. The papillary dermis is a thin layer of loose connective tissue containing thin collagen fibers that are arranged irregularly, reticular and elastic fibers that are arranged in a net shape. The papillary dermis contains rich supply of blood vessels and numerous nerve endings.

The reticular dermis is the thicker and major layer of dermis. This layer contains mainly the collagen fibers, as a form of coarser bundle, and a minority of reticular and elastin fibers. These fibers arranged in parallel with the surface shows a regular direction in arrangement on a particular area, which is called Langer's line[3]. When skin is incised in parallel with Langer's line, the wound can be minimized and less scarring. Amorphous substances filling between fibers and skin appendages are known as glycosaminoglycan, hyaluronic acid, dermatan sulfate, and chondroitin sulfate. Rich blood vessels, nerves, sebaceous glands, sweat glands, hair follicles and erector pili muscles are also located in this layer.

Before fat grafting, measuring the type and thickness of the skin is important to understand the skin elasticity. Since skin elasticity depends on the type and thickness of skin, it is likely to result in different shape of grafted fat and drooping phenomenon by the weight of grafted fat when the volume is increased.

In the facial area, the area with the thickest skin is the chin region, and the thinnest area is the eyelid. The average thickness of each part is estimated as shown in Table 1[4]. In this table, it can be identified that there is a huge difference in skin thickness between lids area and cheek area that are boundary regions.

Table 01 Skin thickness of various regions of the face in post-mortem subjects.

	Epidermis	Dermis	Total(μm)
Forehead	202	969	1171
Glabella	144	324	468
Lids	130	215	345
Cheek	141	909	1050
Nasal tip	111	918	1029
Upper lip	156	1061	1271
Lower lip	113	973	1086
Mental	149	1375	1525
Neck	115	138	253

In general, the type of skin is determined by measuring the degree of skin's hydration and the amount of sebum on the condition of 18°C, 55.5% humidity and 2 hours after cleansing. The criteria for oily, dry and mixed skin are classified in Table 2[5].

Generally, the clinical characteristics of skin types associated with fat grafting are as follows.

Dry skin is a skin condition that involves dryness, sensitivity in irritation, lack of luster and thick dead skin cells caused by decreased function of sebaceous glands or sweat glands and decreased secretion of sebaceous glands-stimulating hormone. A person with dry skin feel tension right after washing his or her face and have other characteristics such as many fine wrinkles, thin skin with less elasticity and lesser subcutaneous fat in general. I personally recommend performing CAL (cell-assisted

Table 02 Classification of skin type.

	Sebum content (µg/cm²) in forehead, nose, cheek and chin	Hydration(AU) in forehead, cheek and chin
Oily Skin	over 70	over 50
Dry skin	less than 69	less than 49
Mixed skin I	less than 69	over 50
Mixed skin II	over 70	less than 49
Measuring apparatus	Corneometer (MPA-580)[6]	Sebumeter (SM815)[7]

lipo-transfer) using adipose-derived stem cells to whom has dry skin with less subcutaneous fat.

Neutral or normal skin with normal function of sebaceous glands and sweat glands is the most ideal skin with good elasticity and ruddy complexion. This is the best skin type for fat grafting because the skin is thicker and contains more developed subcutaneous tissue than the other skin types.

Oily skin is characterized by thick and solid structure with excessive sebum, enlarged pore, and thickened stratum corneum. According to my experience, compared to patients with dry skin, patients with oily skin tend to have higher survival rate of fat. However, there is a tendency that existing acne is worsened or higher incidence of new acne.

Combination or mixed skin is a condition where dry and oily skin exists at the same time caused by unbalanced sebum secretion. Typically, forehead and nose areas present the form of oily skin and surroundings of eyes and cheek present the form of dry skin.

Sensitive skin is a condition that is subjected to be irritated by chemical and mechanical stimulations and psychological factors easily. This skin type looks normal but is significantly dry, itchy and sting in respond to stimulation. Moreover, blood vessels often can be seen and flush or scale also can appear due to thin skin and well-developed neovascularization. I had several patients who have sensitive skin due to frequent laser treatment and chemical resurfacing but their conditions of skin dryness and sensitivity have been improved after fat grafting.

2 Subcutaneous fat layer

Depending on the depth, facial subcutaneous fat layer can be divided into superficial fat and deep fat. The fat above the SMAS layer, the fat is called superficial fat, and beneath the SMAS the fat is called deep fat. Figure 2 shows the recent findings of subcutaneous fat compartments.

Raskin E et al. reported that the basic contour of face almost disappeared in case that facial subcuta-

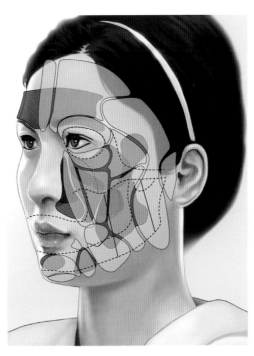

Figure 02 A schematic drawing of the subcutaneous fat compartment which is composed of the superficial fat compartments (yellow colored areas) and the deep fat compartments (gray colored areas). Dashed lines express the rough concour of facial bone, two real lines express the anterior and posterior border of masseter muscle, and a dotted line expresses the zygomaticomaxillary suture.

neous tissue and SMAS of cadaver are removed[8]. It means that subcutaneous fat layer occupies a significant portion of the facial soft tissues, and plays an important role in the formation and maintenance of facial contour.

1) Superficial fat of the face

The superficial fat of the face is densely stuck in the space which is formed by fibrous septa as a form of a small yellow lobule.

The densely populated superficial fat regions are the nasolabial folds, jowl, chin, and anterior neck, etc., and relative rarely and sparsely populated fat regions are the forehead, glabella, temple, orbit, around the mouth, etc[10].

According to the traditional concept, the superficial fat was known so far as a form of homogeneous confluent mass accounting for 57% of the whole facial fat[8]. However, recently Rohrich RJ. et al. reported that superficial fat is not a homogeneous confluent mass, but is partitioned into several independent compartments by the vascularized membranes arising from superficial fascia as shown in Figure 3 and 31 respectively[11]. And then, more concrete structural evidences associated with the aging change of mid-face were noticed by Gierloff M. et al[12,13].

(A) Nasolabial fat

The nasolabial fat abuts on the orbicularis retaining ligament at its superior potion, and overlaps or lies adjacent to the superior jowl fat at its inferior portion. The compartment is bounded laterally by the suborbicularis fat (SOOF) and the medial cheek fat and medially by the maxilla. The lower border of zygomaticus major is adherent to this compartment [11].

(B) Cheek compartment

The superficial fat layer called cheek fat or malar fat is also defined as cheek compartment. It is composed of 3 main compartments: medial, middle, and lateral temporal cheek fat. These boundaries are described as follows11 [11].

① Medial cheek fat

It lies lateral to the nasolabial fold and medial to the middle cheek fat. This compartment is bordered posteriorly by the orbicularis oculi muscle, deep medial cheek fat and buccal fat pad, and superiorly by the orbicularis retaining ligament and inferior orbital fat compartment. The inferior boundary is the Jowl fat and the buccal extension of buccal fat pad. Also, major zygomaticus muscle is attached to the inferior border of this fat compartment.

② Middle cheek fat

It lies between the medial and lateral temporal cheek fat, and is located lateral to the perpendicular line through the lateral orbital rim. Its superior boundary is the inferior and lateral orbital fat. This fat

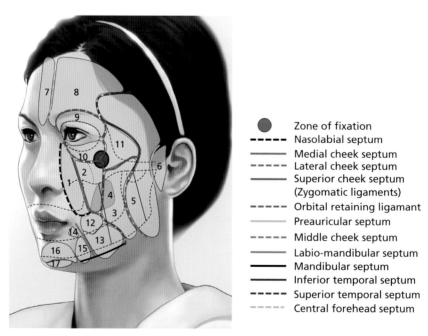

Figure 03 A schematic drawing of the anatomical relationship of the superficial subcutaneous fat compartments and their septums.

compartment is found anterior and superficial to the parotid gland. At the superior portion of this fat, the zygomatic major muscle is adherent. A confluence of septa occurs at this location, zone of fixation as shown in Figure 3, where three compartments meet and fuse into a dense facial network.

③ Lateral temporal cheek fat

It is the most lateral compartment of the cheek, lies immediately superficial to the parotid gland, abuts the pre-auricular fat posteriorly and connects the temporal fat superiorly to the cervical subcutaneous fat inferiorly.

④ Subcutaneous part of the buccal extension of the buccal fat pad

It is a subcutaneous fat protruded from the buccal extension of the buccal fat pad and was first reported by Gierloff M. et al. As shown in Figure 3 and Table 3, the fat abuts the medial cheek fat, the deep medial cheek fat, the middle cheek fat and the jowl fat.

Table 03 Compartments and their subcutaneous fat content.

Compartments	Content of fat
(a) Nasolabial	(1) Nasolabial fat
(B) Cheek	(2) Medial cheek fat (3) Middle cheek fat (4) Superficial part of Buccal extension of the buccal fat (5) Lateral cheek fat
(C) Forehead and temporal	(5) Lateral temporal fat (6) Preauricular fat (7) Central forehead fat (8) Middle forehead fat
(D) Orbital	(9) Superior orbital fat (10) Inferior orbital fat (11) Lateral orbital fat
(E) Jowl	(12) Superior jowl fat (13) Inferior jowl fat
(F) Chin	(14) Lateral lip fat (15) Labiomandibular fat (16) Chin fat (17) Submental fat

Each cheek fat compartment is separated by a fibrous septum. Types and boundaries of the septum formed between each compartment of fat are described in the following Table 4[11].

There are interesting reports that the fibrous septum or its fusion with the superficial fat compartment is closely associated with facial retaining ligaments.

Firstly, the superior portion of the middle cheek fat, where dense adherent zone formed by con-

Table 04 Cheek septums and their locations.

Septum	Locations
1) Medial cheek septum	between the nasolabial fat and the medial cheek fat
2) Middle cheek septum	between the medial cheek fat and middle cheek fat
3) Lateral cheek septum	between the lateral temporal cheek fat and the middle cheek fat
4) Superior cheek septum	between the orbital fats (inferior and lateral) and the middle cheek fat

fluence of adjacent three septum, correspond with the zygomatic retaining ligament(=McGregor's Patch)[13].

Secondly, the dense fascial network formed by fusion of the septum between middle and medial cheek fat also correspond to what has been described as the zygomatic retaining ligamen[14].

Thirdly, it has been reported that the zone where the medial fat abuts the middle cheek corresponds to the location of the parotid-masseteric ligament[14].

Fourthly, the lateral temporal-cheek compartment ends right in front of ear and abuts postauricular fat compartment. At the area beneath the ear, they may simply have a fusion point that is thought as the plastyma-auricular ligament.

To sum up these findings, it is highly suggested that the superficial part of facial retaining ligaments can be is intimately related to the septum of the fat compartment.

(C) Fat compartment of forehead and temple
The subcutaneous fat of the forehead and temple is composed of three compartments as shown in Figure 3, and their boundaries are as follows.

① Central compartment
It is located in the midline region of the forehead. It is located consistently that abuts the middle forehead compartment on both sides and has an inferior border at the nasal dorsum. The lateral boundary, a septal barrier is referred as the central forehead septum.

② Middle forehead fat
It lies on both sides of the central forehead fat. The inferior border is the orbicularis retaining ligament, and the lateral border is corresponds to the superior temporal septum.

③ Temporal fat
It lies between the superior and inferior temporal septum. It abuts the middle forehead fat anteriorly, and is connected to the lateral-temporal cheek fat and cervical fat inferiorly

(D) Orbital fat compartment
The subcutaneous orbital fat compartment is located around the eye, and is composed of three parts

as belows[11].

① Superior and inferior orbital fat

The boundary of superior and inferior orbital fat is the orbicularis retaining ligament, true circumferential membrane that blends into the medial and lateral canthus. However, the superior and inferior orbital compartments are distinct from one another and they are also completely separated. The superior orbital fat lies above the superior orbital limb and the inferior orbital fat lies right below the inferior lid tarsus.

② Lateral orbital fat

The superior border of the lateral orbital fat is the inferior temporal septum and it's the inferior border is the superior cheek septum. The zygomatic major muscle is adherent to this compartment superiorly.

(E) Jowl fat compartment

It is composed of the superior and inferior jowl fat and adheres to the depressor anguli oris muscle. The medial boundary is the lip depressor muscle and the inferior boundary is determined by a membranous fusion of the platysma muscle. These two muscles are fused at the region of the mandibular ligament. This fat is separated from the nasolabial fat, and abuts the upper lip fat and the medial and lateral cheek fat[11].

(F) Chin compartments

① Labiomandibular fat

The labiomandibular fat is located just medial labiomandibular fold and delineated laterally by the inferior jowl fat. It is directly bounded by mandibular retaining ligament, not by inferior jowl fat, in the most inferolateral part of the fat, leaving a gap that forms a retractive depression of prejowl sucus. It is caused by dermal insertions of the mandibular retaining ligament. It is reported through cadaver study that the lateral edge of the fat compartment appeared to be thinner in a prominent labiomandibular fold compared to a not obvious fold and might be secondary to a continuous active movement of depressor anguli oris[12].

② Chin compartment

The chin fat is located almost superiorly to the mentolabial sulcus and is bounded laterally by the labiomandibular fat and inferiorly by the superficial portion of the submentalis fat.

③ Submental fat compartment

Superficial part of the submental fat is located directly under the skin and lies on the infero-central part of the chin compartment as an inferior portion of submental fat. It is not bounded laterally by labiomandibular fat and superiorly by mentolabial sulcus. And it accentuates the shape of the mentum[3].

(G) Preplatysmal fat

The preplatysmal fat is a subcutaneous fat of the jowl and submental area. It has a very important role, which is to make the frontal and lateral contour of the lower face and chin, and neck.

The suggestion of highly compartmentalized subcutaneous fat has significant meaning as followings.

First, it is possible to explain the phenomenon such as atrophy and sagging of some areas of the face, which could not be explained by previous concepts that the subcutaneous fat migration or displacement as a confluent or composite mass is migrated or displaced by aging and the influence of gravity.

Second, each fat compartment goes through independent aging process and aging of one compartment affects other compartments. So it will lead to better understanding of the possibility of cascade effect as a cause of aging. These findings are considered to greatly impact the choice of appropriate facial filler injection technique in the future.

2) Deep fat of the face

The deep fat of the face is less abundant and accounts for about 44% of total fat in the facial fat[8]. Unlike the superficial fat, it is discontinuous and partitioned as an independent structure which is en-

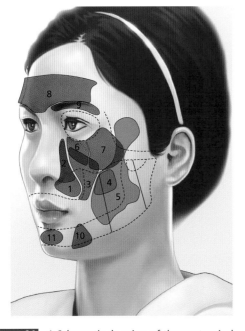

Compartments	Content of fat
(A) Cheek	(1) Medial of deep medial cheek fat (2) Ristow's fat (space) (3) Lateral part of deep medical cheek fat (4) Deep part of Buccal extension of the buccal fat (5) Buccal fat pad (6) Medial SOOF (7) Lateral SOOF
(B) Forehead	(8) Galeal fat pad (9) Brow fat pad
(D) Chin	(10) Deep lateral lip(Prejowl) fat (11) Deep submental fat

Figure 04 A Schematic drawing of the anatomical relationship of the deep facial fat compartments.

veloped by non-vascularized fascia as shown in Figure 4. It distributed in larger white lobules divided by a sparse network of thin fibrous septa.

The deep fat is densest in the temporal fat pad, brow fat pad, galeal fat pad, orbital fat, suborbicularis oculi fat (SOOF), deep medial fat, deep lateral fat, buccal fat pad of Bichat, and subplatysmal fat pad. However, the deep fat is sparse in the lateral cheek and lateral neck regions and almost absent in the upper forehead, upper temporal, glabella, mental and perioral regions.

Recently, the volume change of the deep fat is becoming more interesting, since it is known as an important factor that affects facial contour change by decreasing the anterior projection and sagging. In addition, we can also recognize very dynamic contour change of the face according to presence of deep fats, suggesting that the deep fats support the superficial fat compartments and effect the aging process of each superficial compartment proceeds independently[16].

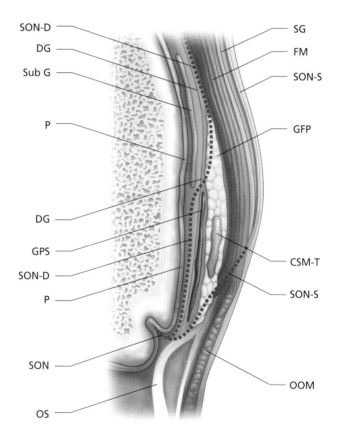

Figure 05 Cross section view of the forehead. All of the forehead soft tissue is shown[18].
P: Periosteum, DG: Deep galea, Sub G: Subgaleal, GPS: Galeal plane space, GFP : Galeal fat pad, SON-D: Supra-orbital nerve deep branch, SON-S: Supraorbital nerve superficial branch, OOM: orbicularis oculi muscle, SON: Supra-orbital nerve, CSM-T: Transverse fiber of corrugator supercilii muscle, SG: Superficial galea, FM: Frontalis muscle, BFP: Brow fat pad, and OS: Orbital septum.

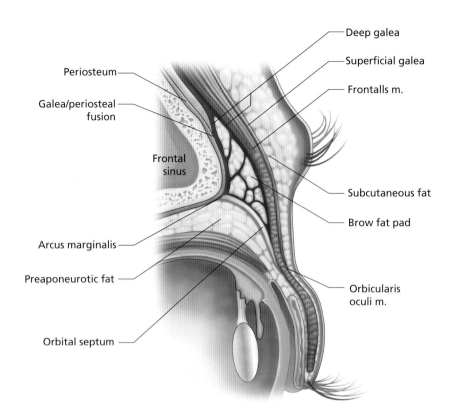

Deep galea

Superficial galea

Frontalls m.

Periosteum

Galea/periosteal
fusion

Frontal
sinus

Subcutaneous fat

Brow fat pad

Arcus marginalis

Preaponeurotic fat

Orbicularis
oculi m.

Orbital septum

Figure 06 A schematic drawing of the brow fat pad and surrounding structures.

(1) Deep fat of forehead

① Galeal fat pad

The galeal fat pad is a deep subcutaneous fat located between periosteum and deep galea lining the posterior surface of frontalis muscle, as shown in Figure 5. This fat pad provides fullness in the lower half of the forehead, and contains the transverse head of corrugator supercilii muscle. In case of people who use frontalis and corrugator supercilii muscle excessively, the fullness of their fat pad tends to decrease earlier.

② Brow fat pad

As seen in Figure 5 and 6, as the deep galea of forehead lies on the galea fat pad, as it approaches the eyebrows, it splits into two layers above the eyebrows. One layer forms the suborbicularis oculi muscle fascia, and the other fuse to the periosteum of superior orbital rimb and contributes to the formation of arcuate marginalis. The fat located between these two layers is called the brow fat pad[18]. It is placed in the same plane with subgaleal space of the forehead which contains the galeal fat pad. In conjunction with the subgaleal space, this extensive fat layer allows the muscles to slide around the convex bony forehead. The brow fat pad also allows the eyebrows to undergo sufficient excursion, so that the eyes are protected by brow descent and better visualization by brow elevation. It continues downward into the upper eyelid and forms submuscular fibroadipose connective tissue layer, anterior to the orbital septum[19]. This fat pad is named retro-orbicularis oculi fat (ROOF) by Siegel RJ. due to its location[20].

2) Deep fat of mid-face

The deep fat of mid-face has three components: the suborbicularis oculi fat, suborbicularis oris fat, buccal extension of buccal fat pad and deep medial cheek fat.

① Suborbicularis oculi fat (SOOF)

The suborbicularis oculi fat (SOOF) is a layer of periorbital fat that lies deep to the lower lid orbicularis muscle and superficial to the preperiosteal fat of zygoma[21]. As shown in Figure 4, this fat abuts the deep medial cheek fat medially and is divided into two parts: the medial and the lateral part.

The medial SOOF lies between the medial limbus and the lateral canthus. The lateral SOOF starts at the lateral canthus and ends at the lateral orbital thickening[22]. The inferior portion of the medial SOOF overlaps the lateral part of the deep medial cheek fat. And the fat is covered by the nasolabial and medial cheek fat. The lateral part of the fat is located underneath the lateral orbital compartment and the middle cheek fat. It lies above the prominence of the zygoma but does not reach above the superior margin of the zygomatic arch. It abuts the buccal fat pad inferiorly. The SOOF is finely lobulated and distinctly yellow in contrast to the preperiosteal fat. The multiple radiating branches of the zygomatico-facial nerve and vessels, and the motor branches tothe orbicularis oculi are distributed within the thin layer of SOOF[23].

② Suborbicularis oris fat

The suborbicularis oris fat is located posterior to the orbicularis oris muscle. It also lies immediately posterior to the wet-dry border of the lip, an area defined by the insertion of the orbicularis oris muscle. Most ideal augmentation of the lip is known to increase the volume of this fat layer at the vermilion-cutaneous junction[24].

③ Deep medial cheek fat

The deep medial cheek fat is located deep to the superficial cheek fat (medial and middle) compartments and medial to zygomaticus major muscle, and lies on the periosteum of maxillar bone as shown in Figure 2 and 4 [16].

The deep medial fat is divided into two parts, the medial and the lateral compartment as shown in Figure 2 and 4.

The triangular shaped medial part of the deep medial cheek fat is located underneath the nasolabial fat compartment and extends further medially. Thus, the most medial part of the medial cheek fat is located medial to nasolabial fold. The lateral boundary is the suborbicularis oculi muscle and the lateral part of the deep medial cheek. The medial part of the deep medial cheek fat does not lie immediately on the periosteum of the maxilla. It is bordered posteriorly by another small, triangular fat compartment located in Ristow's space. This space is regarded as a potential site for rejuvenation, which has high possibility to improve midface projection through the injection of autologous fat or artificial fillers.

The lateral part of the deep medial cheek fat is located beneath the superficial medial cheek fat. Its cranial extension abuts the SOOF. The lateral boundary is the buccal fat pad. In contrast to the medial part, the fat lies directly on the maxilla.

The deep medial fat surrounds the levator anguli oris muscle and is mainly supplied by the infraorbital artery. In particular, it is well known that this artery may be injured (laceration or occlusion) during facial trauma and orbitomaxillary fractures. Disruption of the main blood supply to this fat may lead to a diminished anterior cheek projection.

④ **Deep part of buccal extension of the buccal fat pad**

It is a protruded portion of the buccal extension of the buccal fat as shown in Figure 2 and 4. The fat abuts the deep medial cheek fat, the middle cheek fat, the SOOF and the fat of the premasseter space. This fat stays in the profound facial spaces and its appearance is distinct, resembling orbital fat, and is easily differentiated from the subcutaneous fat of the cheek. It is located in the interspace of the temporalis muscle, masseter muscle, buccinators muscle and zygomatic muscles. It was known to be divided into three extensions —body and temporal extension, pterygoid extension and buccal extension[25].

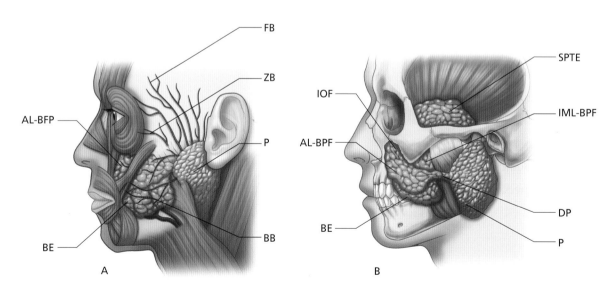

Figure 07 Different shape and location of buccal fat pad in a child (A) and an adult (B). The anterior lobe of buccal fat pad (AL-BFP), buccal extension (BE), frontal branches of the facial nerve(FB),buccal branches of facial nerve (BB) (BB), infraorbital foramen (IOF), zygomatic branches (ZB), parotid gland (P), intermediate lobe of buccal fat pad (IML-BFP), and superficial part of the temporal extension (SPTE).

Table 05 Zhang's classification of the buccal fat pad.

	Previous classification	Zhang's classification
Constitution	1 body	3 lobes 1) Anterior lobe 2) Intermediate lobe 3) Posterior lobe (include 4 extensions)
Constitution	3 extensions 1) Buccal extension 2) Pterygoid extension 3) Temporal extension	4 extensions 1) buccal extension 2) pterygoid extension 3) pterygopalatine extension 4) temporal process (superficial and profound)
Classificatory criterion	According to the external appearance	According to the structure of the lobar envelopes, the formation of the ligaments and the source of the nutritional vessels
Function	1) Fill the masticatory spaces, which is good for mastication and sucking. 2) Contour of cheek	1) Filling and slippage 2) Protection and cushion. 3) Changing of the buccal fat pad volume in different periods of life 4) Mechanism of deepening the nasolabial folds by anterior lobe in child. 5) Mechanism of buccal chubbiness 6) Free or islanded buccal fat pad flaps 7) Rhytidectomy of the nasolabial fold 8) Partial resection of the buccal process

Recently, it has been reported that it is composed of three lobes and four extensions by Zhang HM et al[25]. as shown in Table 5 and Figure 7. Among these, the anterior and intermediate lobe, and the buccal extension of the posterior lobe have great importance in facial cheek contour.

The anterior lobe of the buccal fat pad is triangular shape and located below the zygoma, extending to the front of the buccinator, maxilla, and the deep space of the quadrate muscle of the upper lip and major zygomatic muscle as shown in Figure 7. Because the infraorbital vessels and nerves are packed in this deep fat, deep facial neurovascular bundles can be protected from from injury caused by the extrusion of muscle contraction or the outer force impulsion. The volume of the lobe is rich in children, less rich in adults, and tends to increase in volume by aging.

The intermediate lobe lies in the space around the posterior lobe, lateral maxilla and anterior lobe. It is a membrane-like structure with thin fat tissue in adults and a large mass in children.

Buccal extension of the posterior lobe is the most superficial segment and imparts fullness to the cheek. It enters the cheek below the parotid duct and extends along the anterior border of the masseter. It overlies the main portion of the buccinators muscle as it crossed the cheek. Its anterior limit is marked by the facial vessels, which are in the same plane as the buccal fat pad[26]. This extension joins with buccinator membrane by the buccinators ligament. The parotid duct lies superficial to the fat pad, and then penetrates the fat pad and buccinator to enter the oral cavity opposite the maxillary second molar.

The size of buccal extension can affect the buccal appearance. The buccal protrusions are larger in children because this extension often extends backward and lies on the surface of the masseter muscle, but, the reverse occurs in adults and finally becomes almost invisible due to the involution by aging as shown in Figure 7. However, the buccal chubbiness appears often in adults. Usually, the cause is the antero-inferior protrusion of the buccal extension of the buccal fat pad. It is known that the causes are the weakness of the ligaments, relaxation of deep fascia, and the rupture of the buccal fat pad capsules due to the external trauma. For example, it was reported that the buccal extension drops or prolapses into the mouth or maxillary sinus by trauma[27,28], and it also pseudo-herniate into the facial subcutaneous layer resulting in submalar hollow and jowl expansion by aging[29].

Resection and suction for the buccal fat pad removal are often practiced in order to reduce the cheek prominence. Hwang K et al. reported by cadaver dissection study that the buccal branch of facial nerve passes through buccal extension of the buccal fat pad in 5 of the 19 specimens (26.3%). Therefore, there is a 26.3% chance of injury to the buccal branch during total removal of buccal fat pad[30].

3) Deep fat of the lower face and neck

(1) Deep submentalis fat
The deep submentalis fat is located between periosteum and mentalis muscle, which is clearly distinguished from the suboricularis oris fat of lower lip. The reduction of volume in the submental fat increases the concavity of the labiomental angle and deepens the mentolabial sulcus.

(2) Subplatysmal fat
Subcutaneous fat deep to the platysma muscle is the subplatysmal fat, which is more fibrosis than preplatysma fat, and has well-developed blood vessels.

▋3 Superficial musculoaponeurotic system (SMAS)

1) Definition
SMAS represents the fibro-fatty and muscular network that is running between dermis and facial motor nerves[31]. SMAS surrounds facial muscles and divides the subcutaneous fat into two layers: superficial and deep fat. In the superficial compartment, fat lobules are enclosed by fibrous septa running from the SMAS to the dermis. And in the deep compartment, the fat is abundant and lies between the deep facial muscles, and is not divided by fibrous septa. SMAS is composed of several layers that

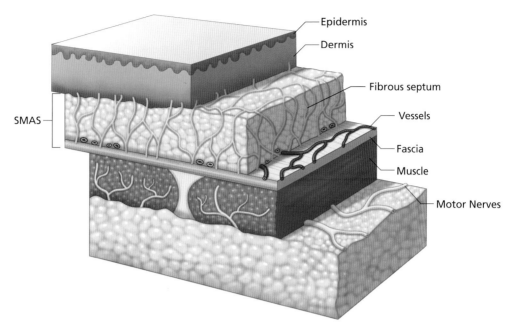

Epidermis

Dermis

Fibrous septum

Vessels

SMAS

Fascia

Muscle

Motor Nerves

Figure 08 Cross section of the superficial musculoaponeurotic system (SMAS) in face.

invest superficial mimetic musculature and major neurovascular structures. Actually, the facial nerve initially deep to the peripheral SMAS but pierces the central SMAS to innervate the facial muscles.

As seen in Figure 8, the movement of facial muscles is directly transmitted to the skin since SMAS and the dermis are connected with the fibrous septa. SMAS acts as a distributor and amplifier of facial muscular activities. Its structures and movement are the major cause of the facial expression and wrinkles. The connection between SMAS and dermis is tightest in the forehead, temple, and anterior region of jaw, with progressive loosening on the mid-face, cheek, and neck regions.

2) Regional features

The composition and thickness of SMAS are significantly different depending on the location. Typically, the SMAS is thickest and mostly uniform in the parotid-masseteric region. It tends to be quite substantive and quite thick in the temporoparietal region, and less substantive in the region of the masseteric muscle and buccal fat pad. In the malar region, it becomes thinnest and fused with the epimysium of the upper lip elevator muscles. In the scalp, the SMAS is represented by the fibrous gala aponeurotica. In the temporal region, the SMAS, where it is called the superficial temporal fascia or the temporoparietal fascia, they are synonymous. In the lower face, the platysma muscle is also included in the SMAS.

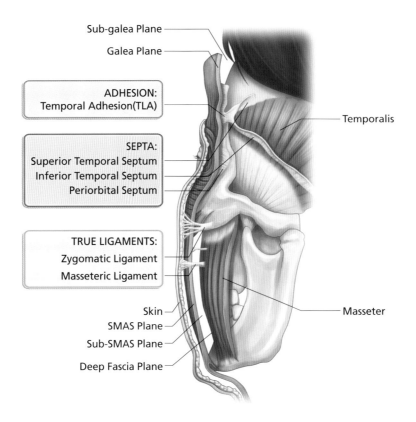

Sub-galea Plane

Galea Plane

ADHESION:
Temporal Adhesion(TLA)

Temporalis

SEPTA:
Superior Temporal Septum
Inferior Temporal Septum
Periorbital Septum

TRUE LIGAMENTS:
Zygomatic Ligament
Masseteric Ligament

Skin

Masseter

SMAS Plane

Sub-SMAS Plane

Deep Fascia Plane

Figure 09 Facial layers and 3 forms of ligament fixation of the face. The major tissue planes from deep to superficial include the deep fascia/pericranium, the subSMAS plane, the SMAS/galea, subcutaneous tissue, and the skin. The diagram shows the three morphologic forms of ligaments that pass through the subSMAS plane to the superficial tissues.

4 Ligamentous fixation

Facial ligamentous fixation indicate special structures that maintain soft tissue contours by restricting or fixing the movement of facial soft tissue exist between the periosteum or the deep fascia and the dermis. As shown in Figure 9, the structures are classified according to three morphological forms: retaining ligament, septum (=membranous septal reflection), and ligamentous adhesion. The following is a brief description of each of the structures [32].

1) Retaining ligament

Retaining ligaments are ligamentous structures that arise from the periosteum or the deep fascia, attach to the undersurface of the SMAS, where they divide into numerous branches in a tree-like fashion and then attach to the dermis via the reticular cutis of subcutaneous fascial system[33].

True type retaining ligament connects the periosteum and the dermis tightly, and false type retaining ligament connects the layers of soft tissue between the fascia and the dermis. In addition, in whole regions of face, fibrous septa developed between the dermis and the superficial fascia is also called the fasciculo-cutaneous retaining ligament.

(1) True retaining ligament

True retaining ligaments are located mainly in sutural interface or its surroundings. These short, stout, and tight ligaments are originated from the periosteum and are strongly connected to the dermis. In the subcutaneous portion, those appears as a part of the subcutaneous septa that divides the subcutaneous fat into compartments. True ligaments found in the medial mid-face and lower face limit the movement of all the attached structures strictly.

As shown in Figure 10[14,33], orbital ligament, zygomatic ligament, mandibular ligament and buccal-maxillary ligament are typical true retaining ligaments of face. The zygomatic ligament termed as Mc-Gregor's patch is the solid bundle-shaped white ligaments as shown in Figure 11. It has been reported

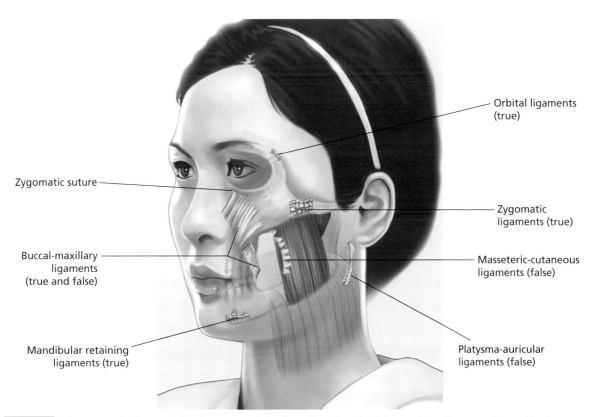

Figure 10 The true and false retaining ligaments of the face. Note that the false retaining ligaments located in the anterior, middle and, posterior cheek regions, but, the true ligaments are in the superolateral (orbital, zygomatic, and buccal-maxillary) and inferior(mandibular) regions.

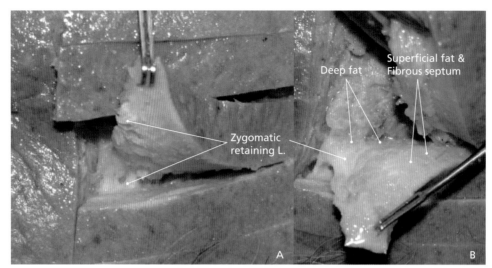

Figure 11 The zygomatic retaining ligaments and the malar fat in cadaver dissection. Two strong whitish columns of the zygomatic ligaments are seen (A). The thick zygomatic ligament is surrounded by the large lobules of the deep malar fat, and the spaces between ligament and next to ligament or its branch are also filled with that of the deep malar fat (B). The small lobules of the superficial fat are tightly woven into fibrous septa that connect SMAS to the dermis.

that its origin is from a variety of locations. Generally, these ligaments originates from the periosteum of the posterior 1/2 of zygomatic body and antero-lateral 1/3 of zygomatic arch, postero-lateral to the origin site of the zygomaticus minor muscle. They are also found at 4.2~4.8 cm anterior to the tragus in male and 3.9~4.5cm in female[34] and are attached in the skin as an anchoring point. A small zygomatic branch of facial nerve courses deep and inferior to this ligament and a branch of the transverse facial artery passes through the center of it. The importance of zygomatic ligaments lies in their ability to suspend malar soft tissues over the zygomatic eminence. But, with aging, reduction of soft tissues in the malar region and an attenuation of the ligaments lead to an antero-inferior migration of the malar soft tissue and increase the volume of soft tissues lateral to the nasolabial folds. Consequently, nasolabial folds have become more prominent.

The orbital ligament is attached to the center of zygomatico-frontal suture. The mandibular ligament arises from the periosteum of anterior 1/3 of the inferior mandibular border, extending through the anterior fibers of the platysma, anterior to the origin of the depressor anguli oris muscle, and attaches the skin anterior to the jowl. It securely fixes the anterior skin to the underlying bone, preventing gravitational sagging, while the mobile skin just posteriorly tends to sag and form jowls.

The buccal-maxillary retaining ligament is composed of thick and dense fibroelastic tissues. It arises from the periosteal surface along the zygomatico-maxillary suture and attaches to the skin of the nasolabial folds. The ligament is situated adjacent to the nasolabial folds and support the soft tissues of the anterior cheek.

(2) False retaining ligament

The false retaining ligaments are bunches of filamentous connective tissues that connect the facial fascia to the dermis. There are 3 typical false retaining ligaments in the cheek: platysma-auricular ligament, masseteric cutaneous ligament, and false bucco-maxillary ligament.

The platysma-auricular ligament is a thick fascial aponeurosis that is tightly adhere to the postero-superior border of the platysma, the lobule of the ear to the SMAS, and skin overlying the angle of the mandible.

The masseteric cutaneous ligament is a thin and narrow septum-like epimysium fibers and identified superiorly in the malar area where they mingle with the zygomatic ligaments. These fibers are extend along the entire anterior border of the masseter muscle as far inferiorly as the mandibular border and insert into the overlying dermis of the middle cheek of the face.

The importance of these ligaments consist in their support for the soft tissues of the cheek superiorly above the mandibular border. An attenuation of the ligaments leads to an inferior migration of cheek soft tissues below the mandibular border and largely responsible for the formation of jowls, the submalar hollows and prominent labio-mandibular folds in elderly patients.

The buccal–maxillary ligaments arise from the fibrofascial sheath covering the upper buccal mucosa and extend supero-laterally in an oblique direction into the SOOF and anterior cheek. They densely adherent to the deep fat and the dermis of 1 to 2 cm lateral to the nasolabial folds and support the soft tissue of anterior cheek. They are the weakest retaining ligaments, hence the anterior cheek is more susceptible to sagging with aging.

2) Septum

A fibrous wall passing between the deep fascia and the undersurface of the SMAS is called as septum (= membranous septal reflection). This fibrous wall arranged linear to deep fascia and permits mobility only in perpendicular direction.

(1) Peri-orbital septum (orbicularis retaining ligament)

Hargiss JL. described firstly about the fascia traveling from the inferior orbital rim to the cheek skin as peri-orbital septum (PS) in 1963[35]. After that, it had been called different names such as suborbicularis fascia, septum separate orbital parts from nose and cheek, and orbitomalar ligament. In 2002, Muzaffar et al. named the orbicularis retaining ligament as currently accepted nomenclature, according to its origin from the bone and insertion to muscle[36].

Orbicularis retaining ligament needs to be addressed in more details, because it plays important roles in maintaining the soft tissue contour and aging process of the eyelids and the mid-face. It arises from arcus marginalis and spans the entire circumference of the orbits from the medial and lateral canthus as shown in Figure 12[37]. It attaches to the posterior fascia of orbicularis oculi muscle, where separating it into the preseptal and periorbital portion, and fix orbicularis oculi muscle on orbital rim. Internal to the orbital rim, it continues as the orbital septum; external to the orbital rim, it continues as the fibrous periosteum.

At the superolateral orbital rim, the orbital retaining ligament attaches to the deep galea, which lining the posterior fascia of the frontalis and orbicualris oculi muscle, and provides an indirect bony origin for both the forntalis and the orbicularis oculi muscle and plays a significant role in restraining the brow and upper eyelid soft tissues.

① Superior orbicularis retaining ligament

The superior orbicularis retaining ligament has a origin on 2 to 3 mm superior to rim edge as shown in Figure 12. Medially, it is short and taut, and support the medial part of the eyebrow against downward movement of the brow depressor muscles. However, the lateral orbicularis retaining ligament is more lax and redundant and greater in length, and the frontalis muscle is also not attached directly to

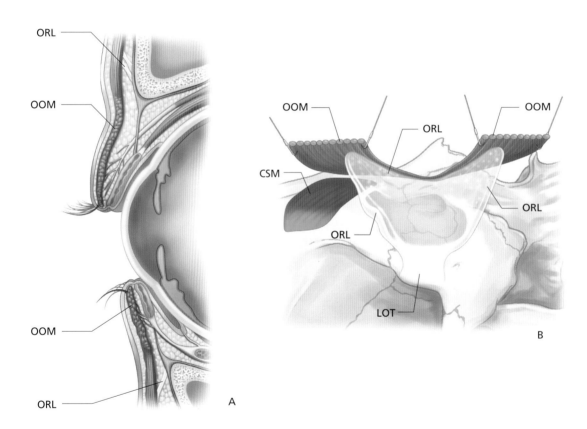

Figure 12 A schematic cross-sectional drawing of the relationship of the orbital septum, the orbicularis retaining ligament and orbicularis oculi muscle (A), A schematic 3-dimentional drawing of the relationship of orbicularis retaining ligament, orbicularis oculi muscle, and lateral orbiral thickening (B). orbital septum (OS), orbicularis oculi muscle (OOM), orbicularis retaining ligaments (ORL), corrugator supercilii muscle (CSM), lateral orbital thickening (LOT).

the lateral brow. These interesting anatomical features may explain why lateral hooding of eye brow occurs readily with aging compared to the medial hooding.

② Inferior orbicularis retaining ligament

The inferior orbicularis retaining ligament has a variable length at different positions along the inferior orbital rim as shown in Figure 12. Medially it is closely attached to the orbital rim but is negligible length. The length of this attachment increases to maximum towards the center (10-14mm distance from the orbital rim to the orbicularis and 1.5-5mm in thickness) and then diminishes laterally until it becomes negligible at the lateral orbital thickening. The characteristic feature of the retaining ligament creates a V-shaped deformity as shown in Figure 12B.

As shown in Figure 13, the inferior orbicularis retaining ligament is a bilaminar membrane enclosing a layer of fat, its thickness is dependent on the amount of fat within the bilaminar membrane[36]. The cephalic membrane is derived from a reflection of the septum orbitale in the orbital side, whereas the caudal membrane is derived from a continuation of the membrane covering the preperiosteal fat over the zygoma. These two membranes are directly attached to the periosteum of the orbital rim and form a bilaminar structure, and leads to the posterior surface of orbicularis oculi muscle. The thickness of the ligament varies in accordance with the thickness of the intervening fat layer[38].

(2) Temporal septum

There are superior temporal septum (STS) and inferior temporal septum (ITS) in temporal region[32].

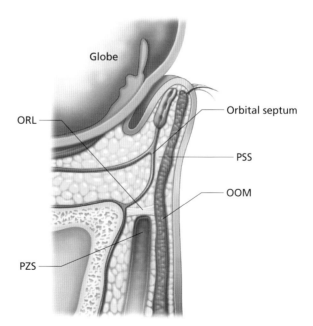

Figure 13 A schematic drawing of the inferior orbicularis retaining ligament (ORL), which indirectly attaches the orbicularis oculi muscle (OOM) at the junction of its pars palpebrarum and pars orbitalis to the periosteum of the orbital rim and, consequently, separates the prezygomatic space (PZS) from the preseptal space (PSS).

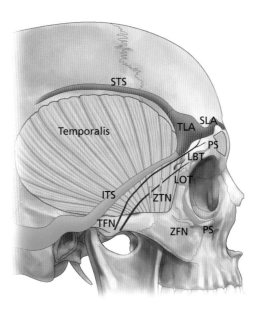

Figure 14 Periorbital and temporal ligamentous fixations with major neurovascular. Temporal ligamentous adhesion (TLA), supraorbital ligamentous adhesion (SLA), superior temporal septum (STS), inferior temporal septum (ITS), orbital retaining ligament (ORL), lateral brow thickening of ORL (LBT), lateral orbital thickening of ORL (LOT), sentinel vessel (SV), temporal branches of facial nerve (TFN), zygomaticotemporal nerve (ZTN), zygomaticofacial nerve (ZFN).

① Superior temporal septum

The superior temporal septum arises from the periosteum along the superior temporal line of the skull and is fused into the line of junction between the superficial temporal fascia and the galea. As shown in Figure 14, it more closely resembles a septum posteriorly, but it becomes a broad adhesion at its anterior termination 30 mm from the supraorbital rim. Its expanded end is the temporal ligamentous adhesion.

② Inferior temporal septum

The inferior temporal septum comprises criss-crossed fibers that reflect from the deep temporal fascia to their insertion into the deepest layers of the superficial temporal fascia. This septum takes an oblique course along a line extending from the lateral corner of the temporal ligament towards the external acoustic meatus, and divides the temple into the upper and lower temporal compartments.

The upper temporal compartment is the potential space above the inferior temporal septum. It is composed of areolar tissue and has no specific structures crossing beneath the superficial temporal fascia. Therefore it is easy and safe for dissection. But, within the lower temporal compartment, the planes are more adherent because of numerous fine, fibrous adhesions contained within a variable amount of adipose tissue. The triangular lower compartment contains the temporal branches of the facial nerve. Above the level of the inferior temporal septum, the deep temporal fascia divides into its deep and superficial layers.

3) Ligamentous adhesion

A low-density area of fibrous or fibro-fatty adhesion between the deep fascia (or periosteum) and the superficial fascia is called a ligamentous adhesion. The role of the adhesion is to restrict mobility in all directions between two layers. Aside from the preauricular and parotid regions, adhesion are found only in the forehead and temporal regions.

(1) Temporal ligamentous adhesion

The temporal ligamentous adhesion (TLA)[32], as shown in Figure 14, arises from the frontal bone of the periosteum as an expansion at the anterior end of the superior temporal septum and insert into the superficial temporal fascia on the deep surface of the frontalis muscle. The temporal ligamentous adhesion supports the region immediately superior to the eyebrow at the junction of its middle and lateral thirds.

(2) Supraorbital ligamentous adhesion

The supraorbital ligamentous adhesion (SLA) arises from the frontal bone above the orbital rim, extending between the temporal ligamentous adhesion and the origin of the corrugators muscle and insert into the deep galea which encloses a fat pad and the lower frontalis muscle. The ligament is condensed around the branches of the supraorbital nerve and the corrugators muscle origin. The adhesion allowed minimal mobility, and therefore retained the deep tissues of the lower brow.

(3) Lateral orbital thickening

The lateral orbital thickening (LOT) is formed by the condensation of the expanded lateral end of the orbital retaining ligament and extends onto the deep temporal fascia. This thickening is a fibrous fusion between the orbicualris fascia of the peripheral part of orbicularis oculi and the underlying periosteum or deep temporal fascia[40]. The lateral orbital thickenings are seen as thickened fibrous tissues on the orbital rim and the posterior aspect of the orbicularis oculi muscle as shown in Figure 15. Aging changes of the orbital thickening are associated with a reduction of its area. The smaller lateral brow thickening (LBT) arises from the bony crest on the lateral supraorbital rim. Both of these thickening are inserted into and retain the deep surface of the orbicualris oculi muscle fascia.

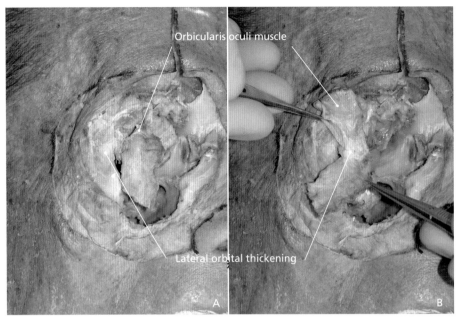

Figure 15 Lateral orbital thickening (LOT). The lateral canthus is analysed. The orbicularis oculi muscle (OOM) is bluntly detached from the lateral orbital rim. The thickened fibrous tissue on the bone is called the "lateral orbital thickening". The LOT supports the OOM from behind (A). The posterior aspect of the OOM and the remaining LOT (white fibrotic tissue) can be seen. These figures are provided by Dr. Hirohiko Kakizaki (Professor of Aichi Medical University, Japan) (B).

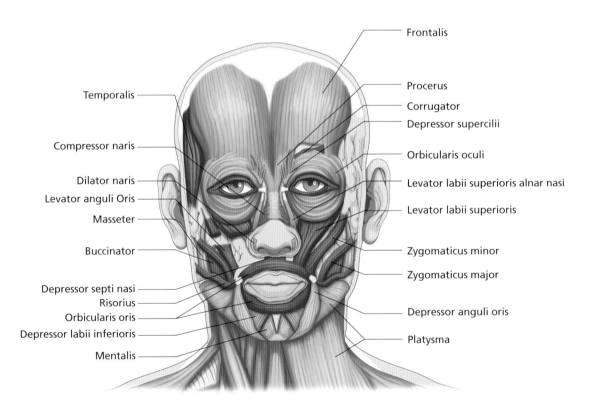

Figure 16 The anterior view of the facial expression muscles.

5 Muscle of face

The facial mimetic muscles are densely arranged adjacent to the skin between superficial fat and deep fat layer of the face as shown in Figure 16.

Figure 17 shows the characteristic wrinkles of face by facial expression. It can be estimated that active movements of facial expression muscles have influences, on the aging features such as wrinkles and depressions, to some extent.

1) The muscles of the forehead and peri-ocular area

Most muscles of the forehead and periocular region are closely associated with the movements of eyebrows and eyelids. The muscles may be grouped in relation to the depth that they exist. The fron-

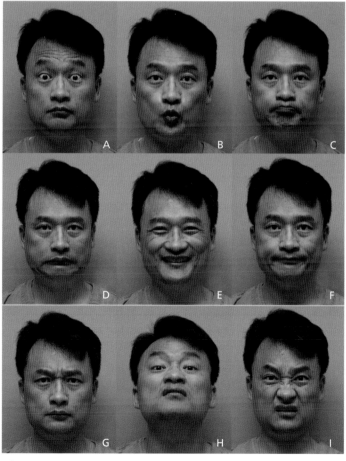

Figure 17 Various facial expression muscles and their typical wrinkles in action. These muscles are sphincters and dilators of the orifices of the head. The facial muscles are attached to and move the skin of the face, producing various facial expressions.

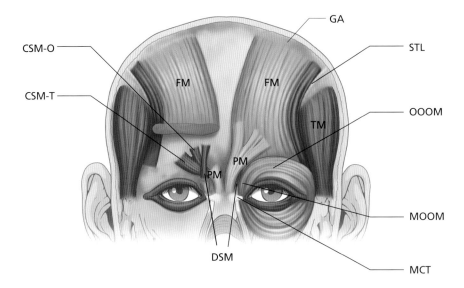

Figure 18 A schematic drawing of facial expression muscles of the forehead, temporal, and peri-ocular area.
FM: Frontal muscle, DSM: Depressor supercilii muscle, CSM-O: Oblique fiber of corrugator supercilii muscle.
CSM-F: Transverse fiber of corrugator supercilii muscle, PM: Procerus muscle, OOOM: orbital part of orbicularis oculi muscle. MOOM: medial part of orbicularis oculi muscle, MCT: Medical canthal tendon, STL: Superior
temporal line, and GA: Galea aponeurosis.

talis, procerus and orbicularis oculi exist in the superficial layer, the depressor supercilii exist in the middle layer, and the corrugator supercilii exist in the deepest layer as shown in Figure 18[17]. Most muscles arise from the bone or fascia and insert into the skin directly. They play an important role in facial expression and aging phenomenon in these regions.

(1) Frontalis muscle

Frontalis muscle, anterior part of the occipitofrontalis, is a unique muscle that has no bony attachments at its origin site. The frontalis muscle originates on the galea aponeurotica near the coronal suture, and inserts on the superciliary ridge of the frontal bone and skin of the medial 2/3 of the eyebrows, and the root of the nose. Medial fibers are interdigitating with procerus; intermediate and lateral fibers with orbicularis oculi and corrugator supercilii. The galea aponeurotica, a broad and intermediate tendinous sheet, is located between the frontalis and occipitalis and unite them. In addition, the subgaleal space under the galeal aponeurotica is formed by loose areolar connective tissue and provides the free sliding movement for the frontal and occipital muscles.

As shown in Figure 19, when the frontalis contracts normally, the special action of the frontalis raises the eyebrows and the skin over the root of the nose, and at the same time draws the galeal aponeurotica forward, throwing the integument of the forehead into transverse wrinkles, as in the expression of surprise; if the action is exaggerated like a secondary contraction, the eyebrows are still further

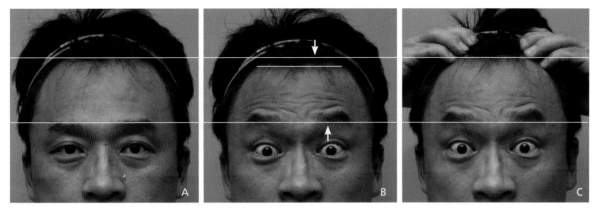

Figure 19 Primary and secondary contraction of frontalis muscle and narrowing of the forehead. Resting state, no contraction of frontalis muscle (A), Primary and secondary contraction: the eyebrow is elevated and the frontal hairline is descended simultaneously due to the secondary contraction of the upper part of frontalis muscle (B), and Secondary contraction can be limited by pulling the scalp toward crown of the head or putting pressure on the frontal scalp with fingers (C). Some of the transverse wrinkles were decreased due to the loss of the secondary contraction.

raised, the skin of the forehead thrown into deeper transverse wrinkles. As a result, the vertical width of the forehead becomes narrow. This repetitive movement compresses the skin, subcutaneous fat, and galeal fat pad of the lower half of the forehead. It is one of the main contributors to the transverse lines and the depressions of the same site.

Also, when the patients who have eyelid ptosis tend to try lifting their eyelid higher to see better, at this very moment, the frontalis muscle can lift the eyebrow directly and the eyelid in a secondary fashion. It can compensate for eyelid levator muscle to a certain degree. It is called a brow compensation phenomenon. So, transverse wrinkles and depressions of forehead always appear in eyelid ptosis patients. This feature can also be seen in patients who have a habit of lifting their eyebrows without having eyelid ptosis. Therefore, when we want to do fat grafting, we must confirm whether the patient has eyelid ptosis or the habit of lifting eyebrows.

Approximately 3.5cm superior to the superior orbital rim, medial superficial branch of the supraorbital nerve penetrates the frontalis muscle and runs upwards following the surface of this muscle. Under the frontalis muscle, lateral deep branch pierces the deep galeal plane to enter the galeal fat pad space and runs superiorly and laterally between periostem and galea as shown in Figure 20. The frontal branch of facial nerve enters the lateral border of this muscle and divides into two branches; the upper and the lower.

(2) Procerus muscle

The procerus muscle is an antagonist of transverse nasalis muscle. It originates from aponeurosis of the transverse nasalis, periosteum of the nasal bone, and perichondrium of the upper lateral cartilage

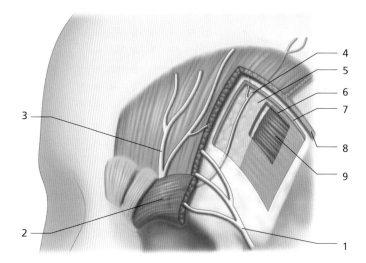

Figure 20 Relationships between the nevers and anatomical planes.

1: temporal branch of the facial nerve, 2: supraorbital nerve, 3: medial branch of the supraorbital nerve, 4: lateral branch of the supraorbital nerve, 5: periosteum, 6: deep temporal fascia, contiguous with the medial periosteum to the temporal crest, 7: layers I and II of the superficial temporal fascia, which contimue in the medial subplane, 8: I layer of the superficial temporal fascia, which contimues medially as the aponeurotic galea, and 9: temporalis muscle.

of nose. It attaches to the skin between the two eyebrows and upper part of the lateral nasal cartilage. This muscle belongs to the nasal muscle according to a precise anatomical classification[40]. It helps to pull the skin between the eyebrows downwards, which assists in flaring the nostril. It can also contribute to an expression of anger. Its contraction can produce transverse wrinkles.

(3) Orbicularis oculi muscle

The orbicularis oculi muscle is a broad, oval sheet of muscle which surrounds the orbit and occupies the eyelids. As shown in Figure 21, its peripheral orbital portion spreads upwards onto the forehead, 3-4 cm lateral to lateral canthus, and downwards to the cheek; its palpebral portion constitutes the voluntary muscle of the eyelids[41].

The orbital portion has bony origins from the medial part of the inferior orbital rim, the frontal bone and a tendinous origin from medial palpebral ligament, and attached to the lateral palpebral raphe.

Also, the muscle is divided into pretarsal, preseptal and orbital part as shown in Figure 22. In the preseptal part, there is an indentation parallel to the muscle fiber over medial 1/3 of inferior orbital rim. It is caused by the thin skin, with scant subcutaneous, adherent to the orbicularis oculi muscle that is attached to the orbital rim. The indentation is thought to be related to the formation of the tear trough and its deformity [42].

The major role of this muscle is an eye sphincter. The upper lateral portion of this muscle acts as a

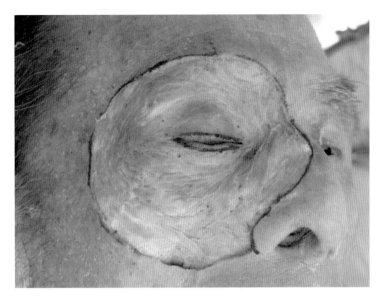

Figure 21 Anatomical illustration in a preserved cadaver dissection showing the full extension of the orbicularis oculi muscle. This figure is provided by Dr. Hirohiko Kakizaki (Professor of Aichi Medical University, Japan).

depressor of lateral 1/3 of eyebrows and worsens the lateral crow's feet, the lateral canthal depression and the temporal hollow. The medial part of this muscle is involved in the formation of the medial crow feet by vertical contraction. Also, this muscle elevates lower eyelids when blink reflex and is dominated by zygomatic branch of facial nerve.

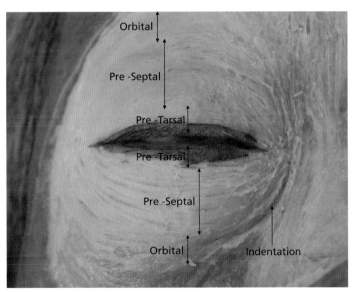

Figure 22 Anatomical illustration in a preserved cadaver showing the orbicularis oculi muscle which is composed of the pretarsal, preseptal and orbital part, and showing the depression in the preseptal muscle where the tear trough deformity forms. This figure is provided by Dr. Hirohiko Kakizaki (Professor of Aichi Medical University, Japan).

(4) Depressor supercilii muscle

Depressor supercilii muscle arises from nasal process of the frontal bone that is located around 1cm upper to the medial canthal ligament and attached to the skin of the medial head of eyebrow. The zygomatic branch of facial nerve dominates this muscle.

(5) Corrugator supercilii muscle

Corrugator supercilii muscle has two origins. The lower one is the supraorbital ridge which extends along the supraorbital notch; the upper one is the junction of bony glabella and forehead. The muscle has two heads. The oblique head is attached to the dermis under the medial half of the eyebrow. The transverse head passes through the galeal fat pad, and is attached to the dermis just superior to the middle third of the eyebrow as shown in Figure 5 and 18. The muscle draws the tail of eyebrow down, and pulls the head of eyebrow upward and inward. When the muscle contracts, a small, crescent-shaped dimple appears above the middle of the eyebrow, and typical glabella frown lines appear at the inner end of the eyebrow. The transverse head is supplied by the frontal branch of facial nerve, and the oblique head is supplied by the buccal branch of facial nerve.

2) Muscle of perioral region

Several muscles alter the shape of the mouth and lip. The shape of the mouth and lips is controlled by a complex three-dimensional group of muscular slips. The classification of the muscles of perioral region is shown in Table 6 and Figure 23.

(1) Levator labii superioris alaeque nasi

The levator labii superioris alaeque nasi lies in the sulcus between the nose and cheek. Arising from the upper part of the frontal process of maxilla, it descends and divides into two slips that attach to the lower lateral alar cartilage of nose and the skin of the lateral half of the upper lip. It dilates the nostril and elevates the upper lip. It also draws the superomedial segment of the nasolabial folds upward.

Table 06 Functional classification of the perioral muscles.

Lip elevator	Levator labii superiors alaeque nasi Levator labii superioris Zygomaticus major and minor Levator angular oris Risorius
Lip depressor	Mentalis Depressor labi inferiors Depressor anguli oris
Sphinctor	Buccinator Orbicularis oris

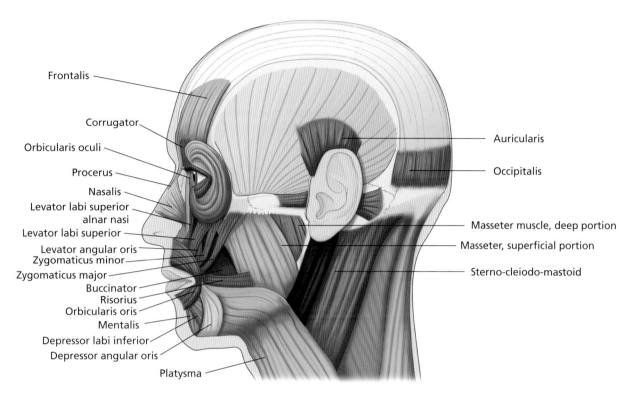

Frontalis

Corrugator

Orbicularis oculi

Procerus

Nasalis

Levator labi superior alnar nasi

Levator labi superior

Levator angular oris

Zygomaticus minor

Zygomaticus major

Buccinator

Risorius

Orbicularis oris

Mentalis

Depressor labi inferior

Depressor angular oris

Platysma

Auricularis

Occipitalis

Masseter muscle, deep portion

Masseter, superficial portion

Sterno-cleiodo-mastoid

Figure 23 Lateral view of the facial expression muscle.

(2) Levator labii superioris

The levator labii superioris arise from the inferior orbital rim of the maxilla and the zygomatic bone just above the infraorbital foramen. It descends to insert into the lateral half of the upper lips between the levator labii superioris alaeque nasi and levator angular oris muscle. It raises and everts the upper lips. It also helps the zygomaticus minor to deepen the middle segment of the nasolabial folds.

(3) Zygomaticus minor

The zygomaticus minor arises from the lateral aspect of the malar bone just posterior to the zygomatico-maxillary suture and extends downward and medialward to the upper lip just medial to the angle of the mouth. It lies superficial to the levator labii superioris. It elevates of the upper lip and turns up the corner of the mouth. It also involves in the formation of the lateral segment of the nasolabial folds.

(4) Zygomaticus major

The zygomaticus major arises from the zygomatic bone anterior to the zygomatico-temporal suture. Descending obliquely, the muscle crosses the masseter muscle and reaches the oral commissure, where the fibers partially attaches to the skin and partly blends with orbicularis oris. On the basis of the Frankfort horizontal line, on average, the zygomaticus major arises from 1.40 cm and 1.50 cm inferior to the line at 1 cm lateral to and at the lateral canthus, respectively. But, in 15 percent of cases, it is identified 1 cm or less from the line[43]. It turns the angle of the mouth upward, carries it outward, and deepens the lateral segment of the nasolabial folds, as in smiling and laughing.

(5) Levator angular oris

The levator angular oris is thick and rounded and lies deep to the levator labii superioris and zygomaticus minor muscle. It arises from the canine fossa of the maxilla just below the infraorbital foramen. Its fibers descend, inclining lateralward, to the angle of the mouth. The muscle elevates and depresses the angles of mouth, at the same time, drawing it medialward, finally deepens the nasolabial folds more. It is innervated by a buccal branch of the facial nerve.

(6) Risorius

The risorius arises from the platysma and fascia of the masseter. It attaches to the fascia covering the parotid gland, runs transversely and attaches to the skin and mucosa of oral commissure, and draws the corner of the mouth laterally, as in expressions of mirth. The muscle may be absent.

(7) Mentalis

Mentalis muscle is a small conical muscle arises from the mandible below the incisor teeth and attaches to the skin of the chin. It draws up the skin of the chin and thus assists in protrusion of the lower lip during the expression of doubt. The mandibular branch of the facial nerve innervates this muscle.

(8) Depressor labi inferiors

The depressor labii inferiors is small and quadrilateral. Its fibers arise from the mandible above its oblique line and medial to the mental foramen. Its fiber are directed upward and medial ward and attach to the skin of the lower lip, more medial fibers decussating with those of the opposite side. The muscle draws the lower lip downward and slightly lateralward, as in frowning. Posterior fibers of the platysma assist with this movement. The mandibular branch of the facial nerve innervates this muscle.

(9) Depressor anguli oris

The depressor anguli oris lying below the angle of the mouth, is triangular in shape. Its fibers arise from the oblique line of the mandible and, passing upward, converge at the angle of the mouth. They blend with orbicularis oris and attach to the skin where the labio-mandibular folds begin. The muscle is responsible for the labio-mandibular crease. This muscle is innervated by buccal and mandibular branches of the facial nerve.

(10) Buccinator

The buccinator lies on a deeper plane than other perioral muscles. It is quadrilateral in shape, and it arises from the alveolar portion of the maxilla, the mandible lateral to the molar teeth, the pterygomandiular raphe, pass toward the angle of mouth, and forms the deep stratum of the orbicularis oris and end chiefly in the mucosa of the lips. The buccal fat pad lies superficial to the buccinator muscle at the anterior border of the masseter muscle. The parotid gland duct penetrates the buccinators muscle. The muscle compresses the cheek, draws corners of the mouth laterally, and forces the lip against the teeth. It assists in whistling and in blowing wind instruments. A buccal branch of the facial nerve is its innervation.

(11) Orbicularis oris

The orbicularis oris is the sphincter of mouth composed of numerous interlacing muscular fibers surrounding the orifice of the mouth. There are two functional components in the orbicularis oris muscle. The extrinsic bundle is the retractor, which is associated with facial expression, whereas the intrinsic bundle is the constrictor of the mouth. The deeper layer of orbicularis derived from the buccinator muscle fibers and intrinsic bundles within the substance of the lips. The muscle is responsible for sphincter action, flattening of the lips against the alveolar arch, and protrusion. This muscle is innervated by buccal branch of the facial nerve.

3) Muscles of mastication and lower face

(1) Masseter muscle

The thick quadrangular masseter muscle overlies the angle of the mandible and is composed of two parts: superficial and deep portion.

The superficial portion is the lager and thicker, arises from anterior two third of the inferior margin of zygomatic arch and the zygomatic process of maxilla, and descend posteriorly and inferiorly. The smaller deep portion arises from the posterior one third of the lower border of zygomatic arch and forms the entire medial surface of it. The smaller deep portion descends anteriorly and inferiorly and attach to the lateral surface of the coronoid process, ramus, and angle of the mandible. The masseter is separated by the buccal fat pad from the buccinators muscle anteriorly and is crossed by the parotid duct; it is partly overlapped by the parotid gland. The nerve to the masseter muscle is a branch of the mandibular division of the trigeminal nerve.

The triangular lateral cheek depression, below the posterior one third of the lower border of the zygomatic arch is mainly caused by the absence of the superficial portion of the master muscle. The superior boundary is the lower border of the zygomatic arch, the anterior boundary is the posterior border of the superficial masseter muscle, and the postero-inferior boundary is the ramus of mandible and the parotid gland. The floor is formed by the deep portion of the masseter muscle.

(2) Platysma

The platysma is a broad, thin sheet of muscle that originate from the superficial fascia of the pectoralis and deltoid muscle, and attaches to the inferior border of the mandible and into the subcutaneous tissues of the lower face, the orbicularis oris muscle, and the angle of the mouth. The muscle depresses the mandible and draws the corner of the mouth inferiorly, as in grimace.

6 Facial blood vessel

The common complications associated with the facial blood vessels following fat grafting are bleeding, occlusion and embolism. The bleeding occurs mainly in temporal region, sometimes even around

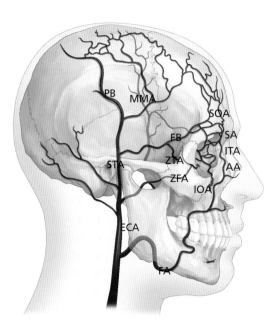

Figure 24 Blood supply of the face.
AA: angular artery, ECA: external carotid artery, FA: facial artery, FB: frontal(anterior) branch of the superficial temporal artery, IOA: infraorbital artery, ITA: infratrochlear artery, LPA: lateral palpebral artery, MPA: medial palpebral artery, MMA: middle meningeal artery, PB: parietal (posterior) branch of the superficial temporal artery, SA: supratrochlear artery, SOA: supraorbital artery, STA: superficial temporal artery, ZFA: zygomaticofacial artery, and ZTA: zygomaticotemporal artery.

the eyes, and lips. Occlusion and embolism occur frequently in glabella, nasolabial folds, nose and temporal region. In this part, important features of facial blood vessels related to fat grafting will be described.

1) Artery

The blood vessels in the face and forehead are extremely well-developed; these vessels arise from the carotid arterial system as shown in Figure 24[17]. Among these, the branches of external carotid artery, the facial, the maxillary, the transverse facial, the superficial temporal, the zygomatico-orbital and the middle meningeal artery, supply the superficial layer of face. Also, the supratrochlear artery and the supraorbital artery that arise from the ophthalmic division of the internal carotid artery supply the forehead and the scalp, and the palpebral artery from the ophthalmic division supply the eyelids.

When fat grafting is performed, some precautions that are related to arterial blood vessel are as follows:

Firstly, bleeding of temporal region which is supplied by superficial temporal artery can be frequently occurred. I would like to describe superficial temporal artery and frontal branch of facial nerve together because these two structures are run closely at the same region as shown in Figure 25[44].

The superficial temporal artery (a, Figure 25) divides into the anterior frontal branch and the posterior parietal branch above the zygomatic arch. Depending on whether the bifurcation point is superior

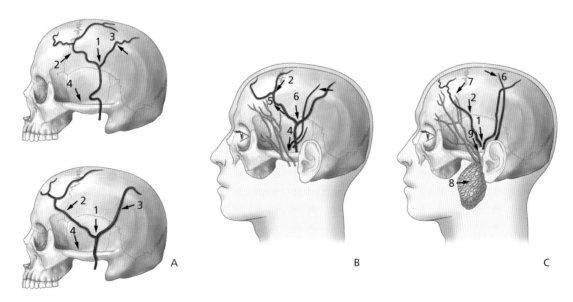

Figure 25 Bifurcation point of the superficial temporal artery and its relationship with the frontal branch of the facial nerve. 1: Bifurcation point of the superficial temporal artery (STA), 2: Anterior frontal branch of the STA, 3: Posterior parietal branch of the STA, 4: Superior margin of the zygomatic arch, 5: Temporal branch of the facial nerve, 6: Auricular temporal nerve, 7: Terminal branch of the temporal branch, 8: Parotid gland, and 9: Frontal branch of the facial nerve.

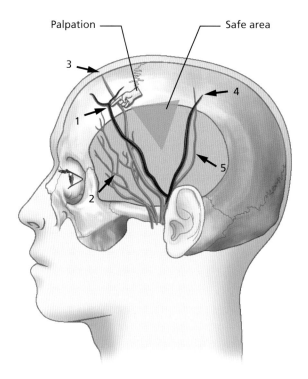

Figure 26 A schematic illustration of safe area of temporal scalp in principle.
1: Preoperative palpation of the pulse of the frontal branch, 2: It helps to mark its course and to aid in predicting the course of the temporal branch, 3: The oblique and longitudinal incisions, or any practical incisions superior to the frontal branch, might be made behind the temporal hairline, 4: Parietal branch of the superficial temporal artery, and 5: Auricular temporal nerve.

or inferior to the horizontal line of the superior orbital rim, it can be classified as high- bifurcation type (about 64%) or low-bifurcation type (about 36%). As the bifurcation point rises, obliquely running frontal branch becomes horizontal. In the high- bifurcation type (b, Figure 25), the temporal branch and its terminal twigs of facial nerve run deeper into the superficial temporal fascia and distribute in the area inferior and deeper to the frontal branch of superficial temporal artery. And, in the low-bifucation type (C, Figure 25), one or more terminal twigs of the temporal branch interweave with the frontal branch above the horizontal plane of the upper orbital rim and terminate below the frontal eminence.

The temporal branch of facial nerve locates within a triangular area formed by the lower aspect of the zygomatic arch, the frontal branch of superficial temporal artery, and the vertical line where it crosses the highest point of the frontal eminence. This temple is a well-defined danger zone, where the temporal branch of the facial nerve and the superficial temporal artery and vein lie vulnerable to injury.

Figure 26 shows the safe area in temporal region and explains its identification[44]. Fat grafting of temporal hollow is commonly performed. Even though it can be popularly performed, it is recom-

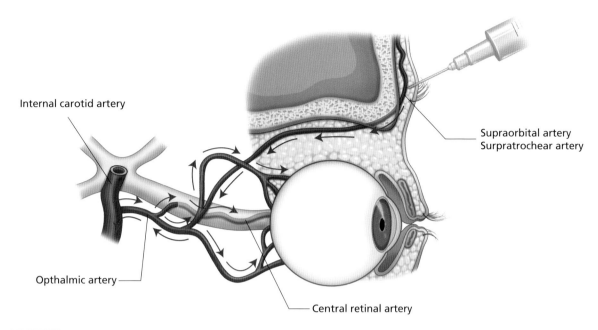

Internal carotid artery

Supraorbital artery
Surpratrochear artery

Opthalmic artery

Central retinal artery

Figure 27 Possible mechanism of blindness by cosmetic filler injection in the glabella. Schematic representation of retro-grade flow in the ophthalmic artery (in blue) and anterograde flow in the central retinal artery (in red).

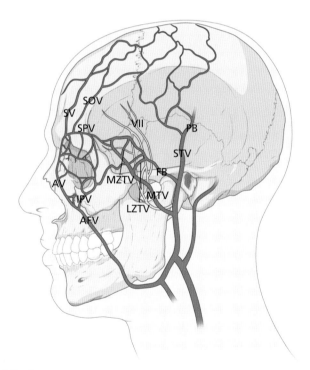

Figure 28 Venous drainage of the face.

AV: angular vein, FB: frontal(anterioi) branch of the superficial temporal vein, IPV: inferior palpebral vein, LZTV: lateral zygomaticotemporal vein, MZTV: medial zygomaticotemporal vein (sentinel vein), MTV: middle temporal vein, PB: parietal (posterior) branch of the superficial temporal vein, SV: supratrochlear vein, SOV: supraorbital vein, STV: superficial temporal vein, SPV: superior palpebral vein, and VII: rami of the temporal branch of the facial nerve.

mended for beginners to have extreme attention because of relative high risk of bleeding and hematoma, and vascular occlusion. When fat grafting, beware of the nerves and blood vessels to avoid damage by following these points: perform with a minimal strength, do not force to insert or move the cannula, do not inject excessive volume at one time, avoid hypercorrection, and inject fat only when drawing back the cannula.

Secondly, the most delicate blood vessels that require attention when fat is injected into glabella are the supratrochlear and supraorbital artery.

It is well known that when fat is injected into these artery, the fat can follow retrograde flow to ophthalmic artery or internal carotid artery and then follow anterograde flow to central retinal artery by high arterial pressure, causing a loss of sight [45,46, 47] as shown in Figure 27. It is not overemphasized on the importance of prevention of this arterial occlusion when fat is injected into the glabella region. Besides, surgeons have to be careful that this phenomenon can also occur as a sign of irritation, vasospasm of posterior ciliary artery, and anterior ischemic optic neuropathy during botulinum toxin injection[48].

2) Vein

Venous system of face is shown in Figure 28. Supratrochlear and suprorbital vein are in charge of venous drainage from forehead and frontal scalp; they form the angular vein and become the facial vein at the infraorbital margin. In addition, these veins are connected with the superior ophthalmic vein via the nasofrontal vein, and then connect with cavernous sinus of dura mater. This facial vein runs downward and backward along the inside of the orbit and nose with the facial artery, passes below the zygomaticus major muscle, crosses mandible, united with the anterior ramus of retromandibular vein, and leads to the internal jugular vein.

The venous system of temporal region is composed of frontal and parietal branch of superficial temporal vein, and middle temporal vein. The retromandibular vein is formed by the confluence of superficial temporal vein and maxillary vein.

Like Figure 28, the zygomatico-temporal veins are formed by junction of frontal branch of the superficial temporal vein and the middle temporal vein in temporal fossa. The medial one of these is called sentinel vein or medial zygomatico-temporal vein. This vein is thicker than the lateral one, located on superior and lateral 1.5 cm from lateral canthus in the supine position. Since the frontal branch of the facial nerve runs 1 cm above this sentinel vein, this vein is an important marker that displays predictable location of frontal branch of facial nerve. Lateral zygomatico-temporal vein is close to zygomatico-temporal nerve. If the cannula is moved forcefully during fat grafting, these nerves and blood vessels can be damaged, so requires attention.

As shown in Figure 29[49], blood of nose, upper lip, and inside of medial canthus is drained downward via a facial vein in standing position. However, there are no valves in angular vein, facial vein,

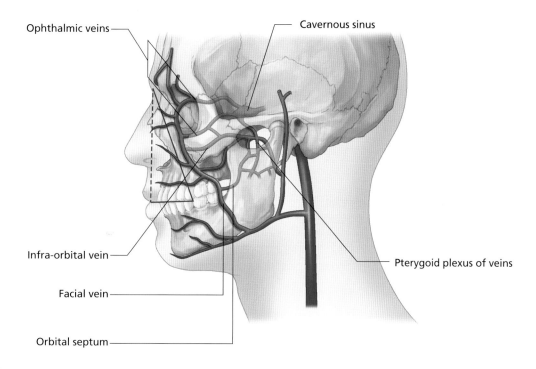

Ophthalmic veins

Cavernous sinus

Infra-orbital vein

Facial vein

Orbital septum

Pterygoid plexus of veins

Figure 29 Venous system and drainage of the danger's triangle of the face. The dangerous triangle of the face consists of the area from the corners of the mouth to the bridge of the nose, including the nose and maxilla (red triangle area).

and ophthalmic vein; so, the blood can flow backward and enter cavernous sinus through the superior and inferior ophthalmic vein. It is possible (although very rare), surgeons need to be aware that any infection which is clinically related to facial vein can be spread to the intracranial venous system, and concerned facial region is called 'danger triangle of the face'.

3) Vascular distribution of subcutaneous fat layer

Figure 30 shows the cutaneous vascular plexus and their anastomosis[50]. Subcutaneous vascular plexus and fascial plexus are interchanged with each other as perpendicular form, but not with subdermal plexus. Therefore, preservation of subdermal vascular plexus is very important to liposuction and face lift surgery because the excessive destruction of this vascular plexus directly causes skin necrosis. In addition, surgeons should be careful that excessive amounts of filler injection into the dermis or subdermis also can cause skin necrosis by high pressure on the vascular plexus.

Many doctors have found perforating arteries within connective tissue column that connects superficial fascia with skin in the subcutaneous layer through their face lift surgery. Recently, it is confirmed that several perforating arteries pass through fibrous septa which is between adjacent subcutaneous fat compartments. Also, it has been agreed that each fat compartment has distinct vascular boundaries by

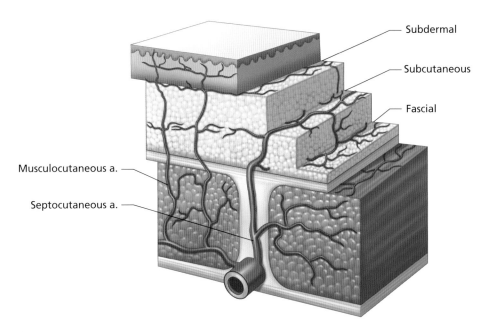

Subdermal

Subcutaneous

Fascial

Musculocutaneous a.

Septocutaneous a.

Figure 30 Cutaneous vascular plexus. The cutaneous vascular plexus form a stacked series of interconnected vascular tissue planes that derive their blood supply from septo-cutaneous and musculocutaneous arteries. The fascial, subcutaneous, and subdermal (cutaneous) layers are shown.

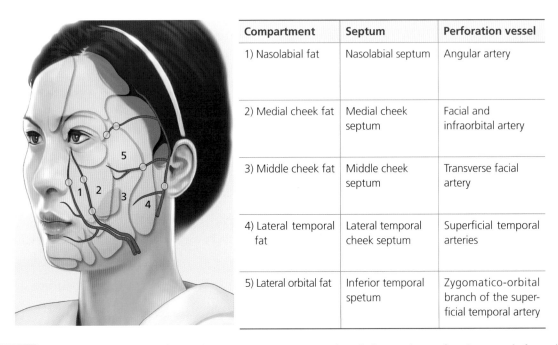

Compartment	Septum	Perforation vessel
1) Nasolabial fat	Nasolabial septum	Angular artery
2) Medial cheek fat	Medial cheek septum	Facial and infraorbital artery
3) Middle cheek fat	Middle cheek septum	Transverse facial artery
4) Lateral temporal fat	Lateral temporal cheek septum	Superficial temporal arteries
5) Lateral orbital fat	Inferior temporal spetum	Zygomatico-orbital branch of the superficial temporal artery

Figure 31 An schematic drawing of the subcutaneous compartments in relation to the perforating vessels from the source arteries.

the perforating arteries even though anatomical variation of facial arteries is possible to occur. **Figure 31** shows a brief explanation of the subcutaneous compartments and their fibrous septum, the course of facial artery and its branches, and the perforating vessels that supply the skin travel between adjacent compartments through fibrous septa on their way to the skin[51].

7 Facial nerve

Functionally, the nerve of the face is largely composed of sensory and motor nerve.

1) Sensory nerve

As shown in **Figure 32**, the sensation of face and scalp is mainly dominated by the trigeminal nerve and the cervical spinal nerve[52].

(1) Opthalmic division

The frontal nerve – the biggest nerve of ophthalmic division—comes into the orbit via the superior orbital fissure. This nerve is divided into two branches: supraorbital and supratrochlear within the

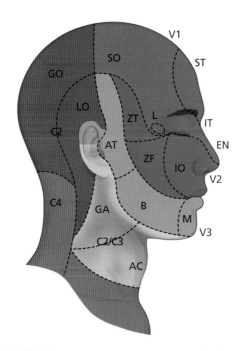

1) Branch of trigeminal nerve

(1) Opthalmic division (V1)= pupple
   supraorbital (SO)
   supratrochlear (ST)
   infratrochlear (IT)
   lacrimal (L)
   external nasal br of ant ethmoid(EN)
(2) Maxillar division (V2)= blue(ZT)
   zygomaticofacial (ZF)
   infraorbital (IO)
(3) Mandibular division (V3)= green
   auricular temporal (AT)
   buccal (B)
   mental (M)

2) Branch of cervical spinal nerve(C2=red, C3=orange)

   Greater occipital (GO)
   Lesser occipital (LO)
   Ant cutaneous (AC)
   Greater auricular (GA(C2,3)= yellow

Figure 32 Sensory nerve innervation and its branches in face and neck.

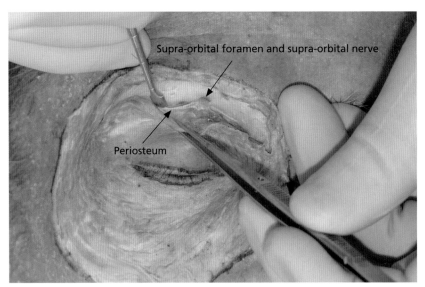

Supra-orbital foramen and supra-orbital nerve

Periosteum

Figure 33 The superior orbital foramen and nerve. The periosteum is detached from the frontal bone with an elevator to the arcus marginalis. The superior orbital notch or foramen, through which the superior orbital nerve passes, can be identified. This figure is provided by Dr. Hirohiko Kakizaki (Professor of Aichi Medical University, Japan).

orbit. As shown in Figure 33, the supraorbital nerve emerges from the superior orbital notch or foramen. The medial superficial branch innervates the lateral part and the front of the forehead scalp, and the lateral deep branch supply the vertex of scalp. This nerve emerges from the obvious notch that is located on the supraorbital margin or foramen that is located in the superior part of the supraorbital margin. The supratrochlear nerve is located at 0.9-1.0 cm medially from this nerve in general.

Infratrochlear nerve is a branch of nasociliary nerve of ophthalmic division; it runs along the inner wall of orbit in the lower part of superior oblique muscle, passes below the trochlear, and then leaves the orbit. Supratrochlear nerve passes along the inner side of orbit above the trochlear of superior oblique muscle and ascend to the supero-medial part of orbital rim. It innervates the center of forehead and the upper eyelid.

(2) Maxillar division

The zygomatic nerve of maxillar division enters the orbit through the inferior orbital fissure. It passes along the lateral orbital margin and divides into two branches: zygomaticotemporal and zygomaticfacial nerve.

The zygomatico-temporal nerve passes along the lateral wall of orbit, emerges from the temporal fossa through zygomaticotemporal foramen, traverses between temporal bone and temporalis muscle, and then penetrates deep temporal fascia 2 cm above the zygomatic arch and 2 cm away from the lateral orbit; also, it innervates the skin of temporal region.

The zygomatico-facial nerve passes along the infero-lateral angle of orbit, emerges upon the face

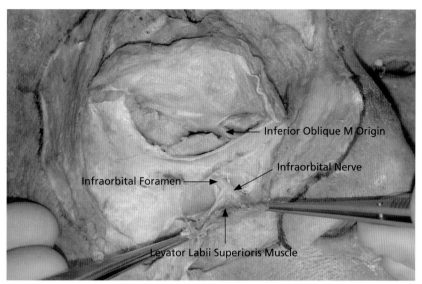

Figure 34 After dissecting the area under the OOM, the levator labii superioris muscle can be visualized. After incising the origin of the levator labii superioris muscle and reflecting it downward, the infraorbital nerve is seen rising from the infraorbital foramen. The position of the infraorbital foramen is generally around 25 to 28 mm from the central facial line and 6 to 9 mm from the inferior orbital rim. The inferior oblique muscle origin is around on the vertical line through the lateral margin of the ala nasi. This figure is provided by Dr. Hirohiko Kakizaki (Professor of Aichi Medical University, Japan).

through the zygomaticofacial foramen in the zygomatic bone, and perforates orbicularis oculi to reach the skin of inferior malar region.

Infraorbital nerve, arisen from the zygomatic nerve, enters the orbit through the inferior orbital fissure and passes along the infraorbital groove. It passes through the infraorbital foramen as seen in Figure 34 and, it innervates the skin of cheek and the upper lip.

(3) Mandibular division

The buccal branch is a principle cutaneous nerve of the cheek. It emerges from deep to the ramus of the mandible and enters the subcutaneous tissue at the anterior border of the masseter muscle. Some of its branches are distributed to the skin and subcutaneous tissues of the cheek; others perforate the underlying buccinators muscle, and they are sensory to the mucous membrane of the cheek and gums. Over the buccinators muscle, the buccal branches of the mandibular nerve communicate with buccal branches of the facial nerve, but only latter nerve innervates the muscle.

Auriculotemporal nerve emerges from the infratemporal fossa at a point between the condyle of the mandible and the external acoustic meatus. Turning upward across the root of the zygomatic arch, it is found posterior to the superficial temporal artery which is accompanied into the scalp. It innervates to the skin of temporal region, ear, external ear, and tympanic membrane.

Mental nerve as a large cutaneous branch of the inferior alveolar nerve arises in the mandibular canal and emerges from the mental foramen which is located midway between the alveolar and basal borders of the mandible and below the second premolar tooth. The mental nerve is divided under the depressor angular oris muscle into three branches; one descends to the skin of the chin and others supply the skin, mucous membrane of the lower lip, and inferior labial gingiva.

(4) Cutaneous branches of the cervical spinal nerve

The cutaneous branches of the cervical spinal nerves that innervates the face and temporal scalp are the greater auricular nerve (C2-3) and the lesser occipital nerve (C2).

The greater auricular nerve, after perforating the deep cervical fascia located at the mid-section of the posterior border of sternocleidomastoid muscle (SCM), turns onto above the muscle and crosses it obliquely in a course towards the auricle and the parotid gland. One branch of this nerve runs 0.5-1 cm parallel and posterior to the external jugular vein over the upper half of the SCM. It is located approximately 6.5 cm inferior to the external auditory meatus. This nerve is damaged easily during face lift surgery because platysma fibers become attenuated with little overlying subcutaneous tissue in this location over the SCM. It is divided into two branches; the anterior branch is distributed to the skin of the face over the parotid gland, and the posterior branch supplies the skin over the mastoid process and on the back of the auricula.

2) Motor nerve

Motor innervation of the face is supplied by the trigeminal and facial nerve. The trigeminal nerve supplies the motor to the muscles of mastication (masseter, temporalis, medial and lateral pterygoid muscle). The facial nerve emerges from the skull through the stylo-mastoid foramen. Almost immediately, it enters into the parotid gland, runs superficially, and is separated into superficial and deep trunk; then, it gives rise to its five branches: temporal or frontal, zygomatic, buccal, marginal mandibular, and cervical. Among them, the temporal branch and the marginal mandibular branch are terminal branches which have no anastomose with adjacent branches. When these nerves are damaged during the procedure, it leads to permanent neuropathy.

(1) Frontal nerve

The branch divisions of frontal nerve emerge from the upper border of parotid gland, which are divided into 2~4 branches, pass obliquely the middle of zygomatic arch and temporal region. Then, they enter the lateral border of frontalis muscle which is located just within 2 cm above the lateral eyebrows[53,54].

All divisions of the frontal branches are located in the regions accounting for 50 % of the length of the inferior aspect and 62 % of the length of the superior aspect of the zygomatic arch such as hatched area shown in Figure 35, when the nerve passes the zygomatic arch[54,55].

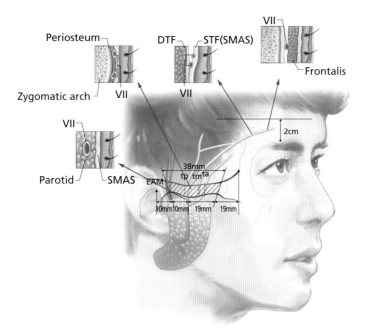

Figure 35 Course, level, and landmarks of the frontal branch of the facial nerve. The posterior (tp), middle (tm), and anterior(ta) divisions of the temporal branch crossed the lower aspect of the zygomatic arch a median distance of 3 mm posterior, 4 mm anterior, and 12 mm anterior to the articular eminence (E). The initial EMA represents external acoustic meatus.

(2) Marginal mandibular nerve

Marginal mandibular nerve is a branch of the facial nerve. Muscles supplied by this nerve are responsible for facial symmetry around the lips and mouth, pleasant expressions and phonation. There-

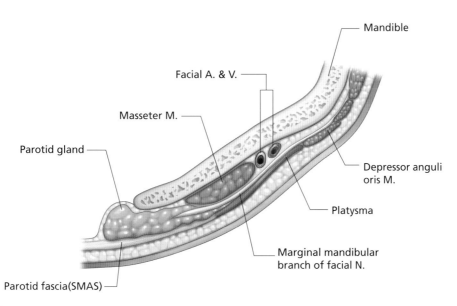

Figure 36 The marginal branch of the facial nerve and its level and course.

fore, an injury to this nerve during a surgical procedure can distort the expression of the smile as well as other facial expressions. As shown in Figure 36[56], it emerges from the anterior border of parotid gland near its apex and course forward over the masseter muscle and the mandible adjacent to the margin of the lower jaw. During the whole course, this nerve lies constantly in a deep to the SMAS and platysma muscle.

This nerve shows multiple anatomic variation and branching pattern, therefore it often gets injured by surgeons in operative procedures in the submandibular region due to lack of accurate knowledge of variations in the course, branches and relations. At the level of the angle of mandible, there are several kinds of branching pattern: a single division in 21%, 2 major branches in 67%, 3 major branches in 9%, and 4 major branches in 3%[57]. But, this nerve is found superficial to the facial artery and facial vein, thus the facial artery can be used as an important landmark in locating the marginal mandibular nerve during surgical procedures.

Also, the intersection point of this nerve with facial artery, whether above or below the inferior border of the mandible, was widely different to each research. It is endangered by incisions along the inferior margin or by liposuction from the submandibular triangle.

Therefore, surgeons should be careful within the distance of 2 cm below the mandibular margin at all times because the average distance of this branch farthest from mandibular margins is 1.2 cm, and only in 6% can be seen at distance of 1.5 cm. These branches were even found 3 to 4 cm below the mandibular border in individuals with lax and atrophic tissues[58].

When the mandibular nerve passes through the mandibular notch, it courses superficial to the facial artery at approximately one-third of the distance from the masseteric tuberosity to the mental midline (11.3 ± 0.54 cm), runs continuously deep to the platysma above the mandible, enters the depressor anguli oris muscle, and then innervates the depressor labii inferiors and the mentalis muscle. Also, according to vertical measurement at some landmarks along the inferior border of the mandible, this nerve is appeared average at 10.7 mm superior to a point 2 cm anterior to the facial artery[59].

The facial danger zone is known as an area which is located 2 cm posterior to the oral commissure and 2 cm around the area. This circular area is susceptible to injury during jowl liposuction and deep plane face lift surgery plan face lift surgery because the platysma and the SMAS are thin, and facial vessel crosses in this zone.

8 Facial bone

Facial skeleton is the most fundamental structure that determines the shape of face and continually

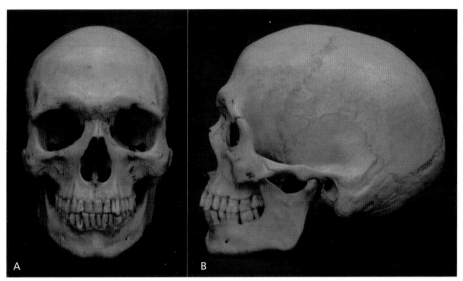

Figure 37 Frontal (A) and lateral (B) view of an adult skull.

changes from infancy to old age. Especially, the loss of the bone density by aging affects the facial contour; for example, the loss of the bone density of maxilla and frontal bone causes sagging of forehead and face; and that of the mandible also causes large jowl and sagging of neckline. The facial skeleton is shown in Figure 37.

1) The frontal bone

The slight prominences of the forehead on each side, 3 cm superior to the superciliary arches, are called frontal eminences. These are of unequal size, more protruded in women and children. Bony ridge, just superior to and parallel with each supraorbital margin, is the superciliary arch. This arch is more pronounced in males. Between these arches there is a gently rounded, median elevation called the glabella.

Over most of the frontal bone, periosteum is loosely adherent. But, it is densely attached to bone over a transverse band in approximately 2.5 cm width just superior to the orbital rims and a zone in approximately 6 mm width just medial to the temporal fusion line[60].

Supraorbital foramen or notch is located in the junction of the medial one third of the supraorbital margin, corresponding with a vertical line from medial limbus of the cornea. In most cases, the supraorbital foramen is located within 5-10 mm superior to supraorbital margin. Another frontal notch, where the supratrochlear nerve and vessel transmit, located medially 0.9-1 cm away from supraorbital foramen in approximately 50%.

2) The zygomatic bone

The prominences of the cheeks for anterolateral orbital rims and much of the infraorbital margins of the orbits are formed by the zygomatic bones (cheek bones, malar bones). The zygomatic bone has sutural connections with the maxilla and the frontal bones such as zygomatico-temporal suture, zygomatico-frontal suture, and zygomatico-maxillary suture. On the lateral aspect of the zygomatic bone near the infraorbital margin is a small hole for the nerve and vessels, both referred as the zygomatico-facial foramen.

The size and shape of the zygomatic bone are very important factors to determine the mid-facial contour. For example, congenital malar hypoplasia or malar hyperplasia has large influence on facial contour, soft tissue foundation, and aging process. Additionally, the thickness of soft tissue that covers the zygoma is also important in facial contour. Thus, the contour sometimes can be improved by liposuction in case of large-looking cheek due to the soft tissue hypertrophy with normal bone size and by fat grafting or implantation in case of small-looking cheek due to the lack of soft tissue or the small bone.

3) The maxillary bone (Maxillae)

In the front part of face, maxillary bone forms entire upper jaw, inner surface, and floor of orbit.

As shown in Figure 38, the maxilla bone (upper jaw) is laterally connected with zygomatic bone

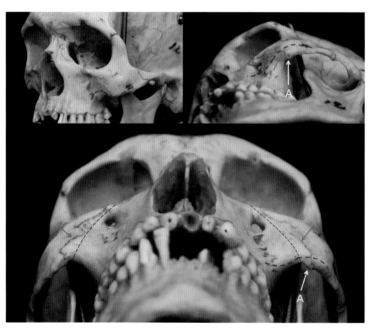

Figure 38 Oblique and basal views of an adult skull. Note that the smooth transition between the zygomatic bone and the maxillary bone is from convex (red dotted lines) to concave surface (blue dotted lines). The junction of the two surfaces (black dotted lines) is located inside the maxillary bone and the zygomatico-maxillary suture (green arrows) are located on the convex surface of the two bones. Anterior inferior prominence of the maxilla bone (A).

by zygomatico-maxillay suture. In most cases, smooth transition between the zygomatic and maxilla bone is from convex to concave surface. In addition, the junction of transition surface is located inside the maxilla bone, and zygomatico-maxillary suture is located on the convex surface of this bone. This characteristics act as an important factor for the mid-face facial contour, especially for the formation of the mid-cheek furrow.

Anterior inferior prominence of the maxilla bone is the lowest part of this bone, located on a downward vertical line from lateral orbital margin as shown in A of Figure 38.

Below the infraorbital margin (IOM) of the orbit and over the canine fossa, there is the infraorbital foramen (IOF)-an opening in the maxilla bone- transmitting the infraorbiral neurovascular bundles. The IOF-IOM distance is variable from 6.10 to 10.9 mm[61]. The levator labii superioris muscle that arises from inferior margin of the orbit over the infraorbital foramen. And the the levator anguli oris muscle arises from the canine fossa of the maxilla just below the infraorbital foramen.

The maxilla bone, with the zygomatic bone, is a major structure which forms the mid-face. Particularly, the degree of development of the maxilla bone is closely related to the aging process and the contour of the mid-face. For example, maxillary retrusion is formed frequently by idiopathic underdevelopment of the maxilla bone in nature, but likely to be associated with congenital deformities. The characteristic of the appearance is one of a flattened or dished in mid-facial region. It also causes the facial shape for creating the illusion of protuberance of the lower jaw. Therefore, healthy young individuals with maxillary retrusion have two features in soft tissue that are usually seen in much older individuals: a prominent nasolabial fold and a vertically inclined nasolabial crease at their early age. In a similar pattern, infants who have the craniofacial proportions of aged individuals frequently display the triad of a prominent nasolabial fold, malar mound, and a nasojugal fold; but, very interestingly, these features tend to self-correct during the aging process as youth is achieved. These findings are intrinsically intriguing; so it is suggested that the skeletal remodeling has a substantial effect on the overlying facial soft tissues during the aging process[62,63].

4) The mandible

The mandible is the strongest and largest bone among the facial bones, which forms the skeleton of the lower jaw. The mental foramen is located 1 cm below the second premolar (bicuspid) tooth midway between the alveolar and basal margin of the bone, and generally corresponds with vertical line from the medial limbus of the cornea. It transmits the mental nerve and blood vessels in the face.

01. Gonalez-Ulloa Flores ES. Senility of the face. Basic study to understand its caused and effects. Plast Resconstr Surg. 1965;36:239-246.

02. Wayne F Larrabee, Jr, Kathleen H Makielski, and Jenifer L Henderson. Surgical anatomy of the face. 2nd Edition, Lippincott Williams and Wilkins. 2004:p46.

03. Gierloff M, Stöhring C, Buder T, Wiltfang J.The subcutaneous fat compartments in relation to aesthetically important facial folds and rhytides. J Plast Reconstr Aesthet Surg. 2012 Oct;65(10):1292-7. doi: 10.1016/j.bjps.2012.04.047. Epub 2012 May 31

03. Song LS. Histologic study of arrangement patterns of dermis fibers to facial Langer's lines and Kraissla's lines. Zhonghua Kou Qiang Yi Xue Za Zhi. 28(4):212-5, 255. 1993

04. Lee JJ, Chun IK, Kim Y. A study of skin thickness in Korean, The Korean J Dermatol. 24:4:4690-479.1986.

05. Bae HS, Choi SI, Ahn HS. Nutritional and antioxidant status by skin types among female adults. Nutr Res Pract. 4(3):215-221,2010.

06. U. Heinrich, U. Koop, et al. Multicentre comparison of skin hydration in terms of physical-, physiological- and product-dependent parameters by the capacitance method (Corneometer CM 825), International Journal of Cosmetic Science, 25, 45-51,2003,

07. Soh BH. The application of non-invasive skin bioengineering devices for measuring the skin physiology(I). Korean Edu J Aesthetics. 1:177-184.2003

08. Raskin E LaTrenta GS. Why do we age in our cheeks ? Asethetic Surg J 2007;27:19-28.

09. Donofrio LM. Fat distribution: a morphologic study of the aging face. Dermatol Surg 2000;26:1107-1112.

10. Gregory Stephen LaTrenta. Atlas of Aesthetic Face and Neck Surgery. Philadepphia, Saunders, 2004: Pp6.

11. Rohrich RJ Pessa JE. The fat compartments of the face: anatomy and clinical implications for cosmetic surgery. Plast Reconstr Surg. 2007;119: 2219-2227.

12. Gierloff M, Stöhring C, Buder T, Gassling V, Açil Y, Wiltfang J. Aging changes of the midfacial fat compartments: a computed tomographic study. Plast Reconstr Surg. 2012 Jan;129(1):263-73. doi: 10.1097/ PRS.0b013e3182362b96.

13. Furnas DW. The retaining ligaments of the cheek. Plast Reconst Surg 1989:83(1):11-16.

14. Stuzin JM, Baker TJ, Gordon HL. The relationship of the superficial and deep facial fascias: Relevance to rhytidectomy and aging. Plast Reconstr Surg 1992: 89: 441-449.

15. Rohrich RJ, Pessa JE. The fat compartments of the face: anatomy and clinical implications for cosmetic surgery. Plast Reconstr Surg 2007;119: 2219-2227;discussion 2228-2231.

16. Rohrich RJ, Pessa JE, Ristow B. The youthful cheek and the deep medial fat compartment. Plast Reconstr Surg. 2008 Jun;121(6):2107-12. doi: 10.1097/PRS.0b013e31817123c6.

17. Knize DM. The forehead and temporal fossa, Anatomy and technique. Lippincott Williams & Wilkins, Philadelphia, PA 19106. USA. 2001.

18. Daniel RK, Landon B.Endoscopic forehead lift: anatomic basis. Aesthet Surg J. 1997 Mar-Apr;17(2):97-104.

19. Lemke BN and Staior OG. The anatomy of eyebrow ptosis. Arch Ophthalmol 1982;100:981-986.

20. Siegel RJ. Advanced blepharoplasty. Aesthetic Plast Surg. 1984:347-70.

21. Aiache AE, Ramirez OM. The sub-orbicularis oculi fat pads: An anatomic and clinical study. Plast Reconstr Surg. 1995;95:37-42.

22. Rohrich RJ, Arbique GM, Wong C, et al. The anatomy of suborbicularis fat: implications for periorbital rejuvenation. Plast Reconstr Surg 2009;124:946-951.

23. Bryan C Mendelson, Arshad R Muzaffar, and William P Adams Jr. Surgical anatomy of the midcheek and malar mounds. Plast Reconstr Surg. 2002:110:885-896(Pp.890).

24. Rohrich RJ and Pessa JE. The anatomy and clinical implications of perioral submuscular fat. Plast Reconstr Surg. 2009;124: 266-271.

25. Zhang HM, Yan YP, Qi KM, Wang JQ, Liu ZF. Anatomical structure of the buccal fat pad and its clinical adaptations. Plast Reconstr Surg. 109(7):2509-2518; discussion 2519-2520. 2002.

26. Stuzin JM, Wagstrom L, Kawamoto HK, Baker TJ, Wolfe SA. The anatomy and clinical application of buccal fat pad. Plast Reconstr Surg. 1990; 85(1):29-37.

27. Browne WG. Herniation of buccal fat pad. Oral Surg

1970;29: Pp181.

28. Marano PD Smart EA and Kolodny SC. Traumatic herniatin of buccal fat pad into maxillary sinus: Report of a case. J Oral Surg 1970;28:Pp531.

29. Matarasso A.Pseudoherniation of the buccal fat pad: a new clinical syndrome. Plast Reconstr Surg. 2003 Nov;112(6):1716-8; discussion 1719-20.

30. Hwang K, Cho HJ, Battuvshin D, Chung IH, Hwang SH. Interrelated buccal fat pad with facial buccal branches and parotid duct. J Craniofac Surg. 2005 Jul;16(4):658-60.

31. Har-Shai Y, Bodner SR, Egozy-Golan D, Lindenbaum ES, Ben-Izhak O, Mitz V, Hirshowitz B. Mechanical properties and microstructure of the superficial musculoaponeurotic system. Plast Reconstr Surg. 1996 Jul;98(1):59-70; discussion 71-3.

32. Moss CJ, Mendelson BC, Taylor GI. Surgical anatomy of the ligamentous attachments in the temple and periorbital regions. Plast Reconstr Surg. 105: 1475-1490, 2000.

33. Gregory Stephen LaTrenta : Atlas of Aesthetic Face and Neck Surgery. Philadelphia, Saunders, 2004: Pp16-27.

34. Ozdemir R, Kilinç H, Unlü RE, Uysal AC, Sensöz O, Baran CN.Anatomicohistologic study of the retaining ligaments of the face and use in face lift: retaining ligament correction and SMAS plication. Plast Reconstr Surg. 2002 Sep 15;110(4):1134-47; discussion 1148-9.

35. Hargiss JL. Surgical anatomy of the eyelids. Trans Pac Coast Otolaryngol Ophthalmol Soc 1963: 44: 193-202.

36. Muzaffar AR, Mendelson BC and Adams WP. Surgical anatomy of the ligamentous attachments of the lower lid and lateral canthus. Plast Reconstr Surg. 2002; 110: (3):873-84; discussion 897-911.

37. Ghavami A1, Pessa JE, Janis J, Khosla R, Reece EM, Rohrich RJ. The orbicularis retaining ligament of the medial orbit: closing the circle. Plast Reconstr Surg. 2008 Mar;121(3):994-1001. doi: 10.1097/01.prs.0000299941.62645.4e.

38. Kikkawa DO, Lemke BN, and Dorxbach RK. Relationship of the superficial musculoaponeurotic system to the orbit and characterization of the orbitomalar ligament. Opthal PRS 1996; 12:77-88.

39. Accioli de Vasconcellos JJ, Britto JA, Henin D, Vacher C. The fascial planes of the temple and face: an en-bloc anatomical study and a plea for consistency.Br J Plast Surg. 2003;56(7):623-9.

40. Letuormeau A and Daniel R. The superficial musculoaponeurotic system of the nose. Plast Reconst Surg. 1988; 82-48.

41. Kakizaki H, Seah LL, Asamoto K, Nakano T, Selva D, Leibovit I.

Dissection of the eyelid and orbit with modernised anatomical findings. The Open Anatomy Journal 2010, 2, 5-24.

42. Hirmand H. Anatomy and nonsurgical correction of the tear trough deformity. Plast Reconstr Surg. 2010;125(2):699-708.

43. Spiegel JH and DeRosa J. The anatomical relationship between the orbicularis oculi muscle and the levator labii superioris and zygomaticus muscle complexes. Plast Reconstr Surg. 2005;116(7):1937-1942; discussion 1943-1944.

44. Lei T, Xu DC, Gao JH, Zhong SZ, Chen B, Yang DY, Cui L, Li ZH, Wang XH and Yang SM. Using the frontal branch of the superficial temporal artery as a landmark for locating the course of the temporal branch of the facial nerve during rhytidectomy: An anatomical study. Plast Reconstr Surg. 2005;116(2):623-629; discussion 630.

45. Teimourian B. Blindness following fat injections. Plast Reconstr Surg. 1988;82(2):361.

46. Dreizen NG and Framm L. Sudden unilateral visual loss after autologous fat injection into the glabellar area. Am J Ophthalmol. 1989;15;107(1):85-87.

47. Antonio CR, Antonio JR, Gracia AC, Correia AA. Glabellar region filling: examining the reasons for the high incidence of complications and blindness. Surg Cosmet Dermatol 2012;4(2):111-3.

48. Chen YH, Tsai YJ, Chao AN, Huang YS and Kao LY. Visual field defect after facial rejuvenation with botulinum toxin type A and polyacrylamide hydrogel injection. Plast Reconstr Surg. 2010;126(5):249e-250e.

49. Rechard L Drake, Wayne Vogl and Adam WM Mitchell. Gray's anatomy for student. International edition (Elsevier Inc.) 2005;p823.

50. Wayne F Larrabee Jr, Kathleen H Makielski and Jenifer Henderson: Surgical anatomy of the face, 2nd Edition, Lippincott Williams and Wilkins.p97,2004,

51. Schaverien MV, Pessa JE and Rohrich RJ. Vascularized membranes determine the anatomical boundaries of the subcutaneous fat compartments. Plast Reconstr Surg. 2009;123(2):695-700.

52. Wayne F Larrabee Jr, Kathleen H Makielski and Jenifer L Henderson. Surgical anatomy of the face. 2nd Edition, Lippincott Williams and Wilkins. p87,2004.

53. Bernstein L and Nelson RH. Surgical anatomy of the extraparotid distribution of the facial nerve. Arch Otolaryngol. 1984;110(3):177-183.

54. Wayne F Larrabee Jr, Kathleen H Makielski and Jenifer L Henderson. Surgical anatomy of the face. 2nd Edition, Lippincott

Williams and Wilkins. p80,2004.

55. Gosain AK, Sewall SR, Yousif NJ. The temporal branch of the facial nerve: How reliably can we predict its path? Plast Reconstr Surg. 1997;99(5):1224-1233; discussion 1234-1236.

56. Lee YH. Facial danger zones, avoiding nerve injury in facial plastic surgery. Translation copyright by ShinHeung Medscience Inc., Korea, Pp30, 2003.

57. Ziarah HA and Atkinson ME. The surgical anatomy of the mandibular distribution of the facial nerve. Br J Oral Surg. 1981;19(3):159-170.

58. Dingman RO, Grabb WC. Surgical anatomy of the mandibular ramus of the facial nerve based on the dissection of 100 facial halves. Plast Reconstr Surg Transplant Bull. 1962 Mar;29:266-72.

59. Hazani R, Chowdhry S, Mowlavi A, Wilhelmi BJ. Bony anatomic landmarks to avoid injury to the marginal mandibular nerve. Aesthet Surg J. 2011 Mar;31(3):286-9. doi: 10.1177/1090820X11398352

60. Knize DM. Reassessment of the coronal incision and subgaleal dissection for foreheadplasty. Plast Reconstr Surg. 1998;102(2):478-89; discussion 490-2.

61. Macedo VC, Cabrini RR, Faig-Leite H. Infraorbital foramen location in dry human skulls. Braz. J. Morphol. Sci., 2009;26(1): 35-38.

62. Bartlett SP, Grossman R, Whitaker LA.Age-related changes of the craniofacial skeleton: an anthropometric and histologic analysis. Plast Reconstr Surg. 1992 Oct;90(4):592-600.

63. Pessa JE, Zadoo VP, Mutimer KL, Haffner C, Yuan C, DeWitt AI, Garza JR. Relative maxillary retrusion as a natural consequence of aging: combining skeletal and soft-tissue changes into an integrated model of midfacial aging. Plast Reconstr Surg. 1998 Jul;102(1):205-12.

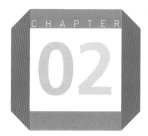

Facial aging

In 1965, Gonzales-Ulloa M and Flores ES first described the external changes of facial aging; the physical symptoms of senility. They explained that the causes of facial aging are the gradual absorption of the adipose tissue, the decrease of the thickness and elasticity of the skin, the decreased adhesion between skin and the subcutaneous tissue, the descent of the soft tissue with attenuation of the facial septa, and progressive craniofacial resorption based on observation[1].

It is not easy to briefly define facial aging because all of the soft tissues of the face interact complexly and diversely and facial aging gradually or simultaneously progresses with the compounding influence of internal and external factors as time passes. Recently, concrete evidence in support of previous hypotheses about the aging process has been found due to advances in molecular biology and the development of cutting-edge diagnostic equipment such as CT and MRI.

Generally, the change in facial contour with age is shown in Figure 1 and 2. Overall facial contours change as aging progresses, as shown in Figure 1. These changes occur not only in bone but also in the soft tissue. However, the change of soft tissue is greater, mainly caused by the redistribution of the subcutaneous fat layer. In general, the facial contour of a young adult is characterized by an inverted triangle or U-shaped outline, whereas that of an old adult is characterized by a trapezoid or rectangle outline due to sagging skin and the downward descent of the soft cheek. This change in geometry is more evident in the female face.

As shown in the following two examples from Figure 2, a notable difference in the regional facial contour can be noted between a young and an old person.

The young face shows full, with an even, ample distribution of fat. It appears homogenized and balanced without demarcation of the aesthetic functional units which abut each other. Three-dimensionally, the young face is a series of important arcs and convexities with smooth transition. In contrast, the

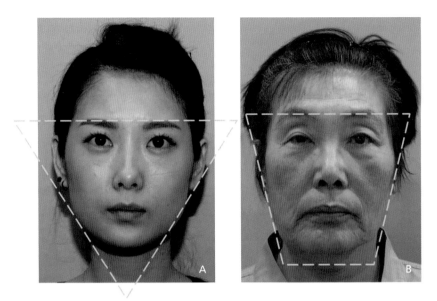

Figure 01 Change of total facial contour with age; 20 years old (A) and 70 years old (B)

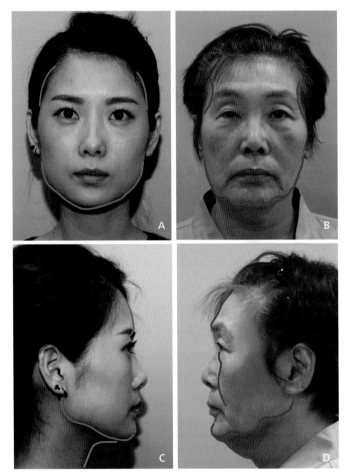

Figure 02 Comparison of the definitive arcs and convexities between a 20 years old women (blue lines of A and C) and a 70 years old women (red lines of B and D).

old face shows a vivid demarcation of the aesthetic units, which leaves the face unbalanced. It is characterized by the disruption of the arcs as broken, wary, or concave shapes. The convexities of temple and suborbital area are decreased. On the contrary, those of jowls and lateral cheeks are increased [19].

A large proportion of the studies have been made about "mid-face" aging process, because not only the mid-face has much more dynamic movement, faster aging processes, and more frequent cosmetic requirements than other facial areas but also the mid-facial aging is hard to be improved by a simple method such as face lifting. Therefore, it is quite important to understand the facial aging process, and to consider characteristics and changing patterns of the structure, for the proper selection of cosmetic procedures in facial rejuvenation. Hence, I would like to introduce several interesting hypotheses and research results regarding factors that cause aging as follows:

1 Causes of aging

In general, these are some of the factors known to cause aging: cell dysfunction by DNA damage, the inhibition of cell division due to disconnection of telomere - a region at the end of a chromosome that has a protective function from chromosomal damage and a combination with other chromosomes, oxidative damage by free radical, an accumulation of toxic substance, and autoimmune response, etc.

The followings are factors that contribute to aging, which can be divided into internal and external factors based on the human body.

Intrinsic factors are physiological and histological changes of all human tissue due to genetically determined biological processes and cellular apoptosis. For reference, the intrinsic factors that cause skin aging are shown in Table 1 [2,3,4]. Extrinsic factors — most long-term damage is caused by environmental factors — including dehydration, improper nutrition, extreme temperature exposure, damage caused by trauma, environmental toxins (ultraviolet radiation, smoking, smoke, drug abuse, food etc.), disease, mental stress and habits, gravity, and so on.

For instance, the result of a follow-up study on identical twins conducted to learn the correlation

Table 01 **Skin aging phenomena by intrinsic factors**

1. Thinning epidermal tissue and decrease in Langerhans cells and melanocytes
2. Variability in the size and shape of the epidermal cells
3. Appearance of atypical nuclei
4. Reduced number of fibroblast, mast cell and blood vessels
5. Shortening of capillary loops
6. Abnormal morphology of nerve endings

between aging and external factors, convinced that there is a statistically significant association in approximately 10 factors as shown in Table 2[5]. To improve the appearance of aging, these external factors need to be carefully considered for the optimal management of patients by the exclusion of all elements that can affect the results after the procedure and for a proper selection of treatment method.

Table 02 Extrinsic factors related to facial aging

1. Sun exposure
2. Duration of cigarette smoking
3. Body mass index
4. Duration of hormonal replacement
5. Marital status
6. Alcoholic consumption
7. History of skin cancer
8. Outdoor activities
9. Lack of sun screen use
10. Radiation therapy and chemotherapy

2 Aging of facial skeleton

1) Craniofacial bony remodeling theory

Following recent trends to prefer a non-invasive treatment, many doctors tend to accept soft-tissue augmentation as a method to recover facial aging. Of course, the atrophy of soft tissue is the main causes of facial volume reduction with aging. However, a claim that facial skeletons have an impor-

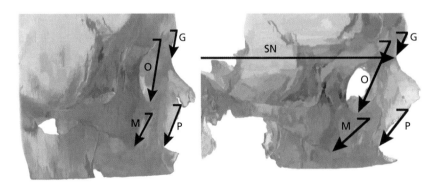

Figure 03 The changes of angles in the mid-facial skeleton with age; a young person (A) and an old person (B). Four angular measurements were recorded in degrees divergent from the sella-nasion (SN) line, which is to say, from the anterior cranial base. These included the glabellar (nasofrontal) angle (G), orbital angle (O), pyriform angle (P), and the angle of the maxillary wall (M).

Table 03 Four angular measurements were obtained relative to the sella-nasion line (SN)

Angles	Definition
Glabellar angle (G)	maximal prominence of glabella to nasofrontal suture
Orbital angle (O)	superior to inferior midorbit
Pyriform angle (P)	nasal bone to lateral inferior pyriform aperture
Maxillary angle (M)	superior to inferior maxilla at the articulation of the inferior maxillary wing and alveolar arch

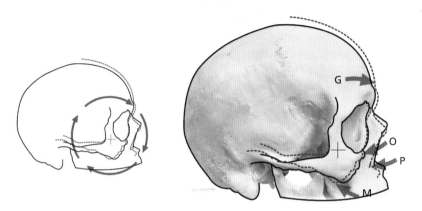

Figure 04 Schematic drawings of Lambro's skeletal remodeling that aging changes in the mid-facial skeleton may be conceptualized as a clockwise rotation of the mid-face relative to the cranial base.

tant and simultaneously core role in the formation of three-dimensional contours of the face is also valid since facial bone supports the soft tissue covering the face. Recently, many studies have shown that changes in the cranial and facial bone play an important role in the aging process. Common discoveries found in these studies are changes in contour of orbital rim, reduction of the height of the central face without teeth, changes in glabella and pyriform aperture, and a reduction of the maxillary angle. Most of the changes occurred in the mid-facial bone.

Pessa JE published the Lambros hypothesis in his article in 2000[6], "When the face is aged, in almost all cases, the mid-facial skeleton changes such as a clockwise rotation against the cranial base."He reported that the glabellar angle, orbital angle, pyriform angle, and maxillary angle are reduced with increasing age, as in Figure 3 and Table 3. He also reported that these results lead to a change in the profile view which consisted of posterior movement of the maxilla and pyriform as shown in Figure 4 and anterior movement of the superior orbit and glabellar. The change shows a characteristic morphological change as a clockwise rotation against the cranial base. In addition, as shown in Figure 5, he has reported that the reduced surface of bone-as a characteristic bone deformity of the infero-lateral orbital rim by aging- serves as a leading cause of soft tissue descent.

Since 2009, Richard MJ et al. reported relatively objective results that support the "Lambros hypothesis" by computed tomography scan[7]. Kahn DM et al. also suggested positive results that are

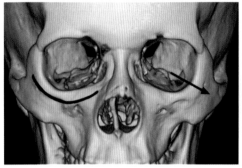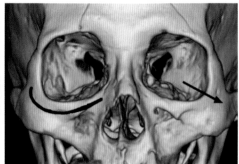

Figure 05 Contour change of the infero-lateral orbital rims with age; a youthful man (A) and a middle-aged man (B). The curve of the orbital rim of a youthful man is relatively shallow and symmetrical and implies that that this patient's face has achieved normal skeletal maturity, whereas that of a middle-aged man is distorted, deep and asymmetrical (shifted to lateral) due to skeletal remodeling. Additionally, the curve type of A is often absent in young patients who show early signs of aging (soft-tissue malposition, early fat show), and it is also frequent in patients with genetic facial deformities.

related to the validity of this hypothesis, by measuring the shape and respective ratio of bone that consists of mid-face and orbit from young and old people's CT scans[8]. Shaw RB Jr et al. recently estimated the changes of facial bone based on age and gender excluding components such as loss of teeth, by increasing the number of the sample. The results are as follows: Orbital aperture size (width, orbital aperture area and height of the superomedial and inferolateral orbital rim), the angle of mandible and the size of pyriform aperture of maxilla increased with increasing age, whereas the angle of glabella, maxilla, mandibular length, and height decreased with increasing age.

2) Skeletal deformity due to selective bony resorption theory

Recently, Mendelson B et al. summarized piecemeal information about the aging process of the facial skeleton that has been studied in various literatures[10]. They also concisely abstracted the research result regarding the features and causes of skeletal deformity, and the impact of the aging process on the soft tissue in each face part. The aging changes in the facial skeletal framework are caused by selective bony resorption in specific areas of the adult facial bone. The areas where bony resorption occurs correspond to more mobile parts of the face during animation, especially the obicularis oculi covering the lateral brow, the lateral orbital crow's feet areas, and the inferolateral orbital rim as shown in Figure 6.

The mobility required for the functioning of these areas is structurally associated with a less ligamentous fixation of soft tissue to the bone. Hence, the attachment of muscles and ligaments to the bone in these areas is attended by little stress[9]. Therefore, the authors suggested that the lack of stress in the long term may be a factor contributing to bone losses in these. The authors' results are also at the base of the bone remodeling theory.

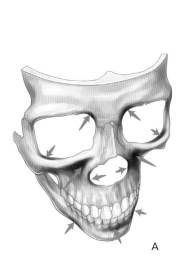
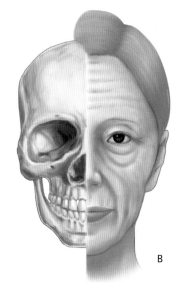

A　　　　　　　　　　B

Figure 06 The close relationship between facial skeletal deformity due to bone resorption and soft tissue changes in the aging process. Arrows indicate the high susceptible areas to bone resorption with aging. The size of the arrow correlates with the amount of resorption (A). The darker areas on the skull are those of the greatest bone loss. The characteristic manifestations of the aging in the facial soft tissues correspond with the areas of weakened skeletal support (B).

3) Impact of the skeletal deformity on aging manifestation of soft tissue.

The shape of the bone is one of the most important components in decision of the entire facial contour.

Firstly, morphology of the facial skeleton has a decisive impact on the aging of soft tissue. following two examples let us know that the congenital shape of the bone shape greatly influence signs of aging. Some people who have an innate strong skeletal structure charicterized as like a prominent supraorbital bar, a strong cheekbone, and a prominent jaw line show a slower sign of aging and maintain a comparatively young appearance. Because the bearing power is strong to support the soft tissue covering bones. Even though bone loss occurs due to aging, the aging signs shown in soft tissue occur considerably late. Conversely, another people with a poor skeletal structure, including a retrusive supraorbital rim, midfacial hypoplasia, poor zygomatic development (extremely seen in Treacher Collins Syndrome), and microgenia are relatively predisposed to manifest aging changes prematurely, even though they are 20s. Regardless of age, the prominent difference in these two examples described above implies that the morphology of the facial skeleton has a decisive impact on the aging of soft tissue. Figure 7 clearly presents the differences of clinical manifestation of aging in these two examples.

Secondly, we need to consider how the facial soft tissue changes by acquired factors such as a facial skeletal deformity. Consider the case of facial bone fracture due to a traffic accident as a simple example. If the zygomatic bone is fractured and pushed posterior, a soft tissue attached to the arch will

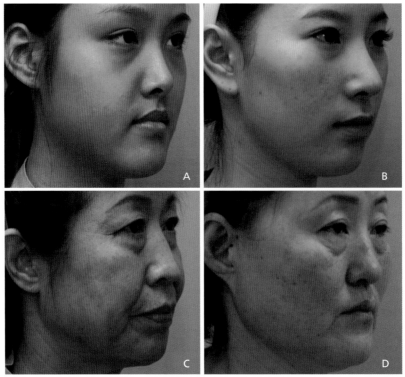

Figure 07 Difference of aging manifestations of soft tissue according to the size of the malar bone; A young girl in her 20's who has small malar bones with poor skeletal support (A) and has strong large malar bones with strong skeletal support (B). An old women in her 50's who has small malar bones with relative poor skeletal support (C) and an old women in her 60's who has large malar bones with strong skeletal support. The stronger skeletal support, the less soft tissue sagging, the later aging signs.

obviously move in the same direction and the surrounding soft tissue will also droop down. As another example, a sagging of mid-face soft tissue can often be seen as a complication after malar bone reduction surgery. The above examples are strong evidences that the location and shape of soft tissues vary with changes in the skeleton.

Thirdly, the skeletal changes of the mid-face in facial aging, effectively decreases the space available to support the overlying soft tissue of the mid-face. In effect, this change creates less available space for the overlying soft tissues to occupy. A "concertina effect" may occur whereby the soft tissues appear to reposition themselves in an accordion-like manner, such as folding in soft tissue over a constricted skeletal platform[11].

These results highlight the importance of skeletal remodeling in determining the soft-tissue contours of the aging face. Even though Rohrich RJ et al. who proposed the pseudo-ptosis theory of soft tissue, recognized the skeletal changes measured by Shaw RB Jr et al. they suggested a question about whether a variety changes of soft tissue occur by direct influence of bone remodeling or not, and emphasized the necessity of verification[12]. The content of Table 4 summarizes the previous reports regarding the possibility of soft tissue changes in facial bone remodeling.

Table 04 Possible soft tissue changes corresponding to facial skeletal remodeling

Facial areas of skeletal remodeling	Possible soft tissue changes
1. Superior orbital rim of frontal bone	
(1) Antero-inferior movement by prominence of supraciliary arch and accentuation of glabella	May lead to the ptosis of medial eyebrow.
(2) Superomedial rim remodeling	May contribute to the unmasking of the medial upper lid fat, a change currently attributed to weakening of the orbital septum.
(3) Acute glabella angle	May also lead to the perceived descent of the medial brow and the formation of glabella skin creases.
(4) Orbital aperture widening (orbital height increase)	May result in the soft tissues rolling into the orbital aperture and thus the appearance of brow descent and lateral orbital hooding,
2. Inferior orbital rim of maxilla	
(1) Orbital aperture widening	The tissues may roll over the recessed bonyledge, leading to a lag of the lower lid, prominence of lower lid fat pockets, and a deepening of the nasojugal groove.
2. Inferolateral orbital rim and maxilla	
(1) A sharp and shallow orbital rim by distortion of the inferolateral orbital rim (lateral suborbital trough deformity)	May lead to the relative increase in the prominence of the zygomatic arch.
(2) A suborbital groove	May result in eyelid malposition such as ectropion, scleral show, lateral bowing, and eyelid bags.
3. Inferomedial orbital rim and maxilla	
(1) Postero-inferior movement	May result in mal-positioned mid-facial soft tissue (malar bag and mid-cheek furrow).
(2) Medial suborbital hypoplasia	May lead to medial tear trough deformity.
4. Zygomatic arch and body	
(1) Deflation of Frankfort line (downward)	May result in the deflation (decreased fullness) and flattened prominent malar.
(2) Postero-inferior movement of cheek bone	May increase the infra-zygomatic concavity (submalar hollow).
5. Pyriform aperture of maxilla	
(1) Large aperture and inferior posterior movement	May result in a deepening of nasolabial fold, nasal ptosis and mal-positioned mid-facial soft tissue (upper lip drooping, perioral wrinkle).
(2) Acute maxillary angle	May lead to decreased skeletal support for the malar fat pad, which may allow the nasolabial crease to become more prominent.
6. Orbital aperture and pyriform aperture	
(1) Increase in size of both apertures	May decrease the bony maxillary surface area available to support the overlying soft-tissue envelope - concertina effect. May affect the formation of the tear trough deformity and tend to display more prominent nasolabial folds.
7. Dimension of the mandible	
(1) Decreased length and height of the mandible body	May lead to having poor skeletal support for the mid-face and perioral soft-tissue repositioning.
(2) Mandibular volume loss	May contribute to the increased laxity of the platysma and soft tissues of the neck.
(3) Increase in mandibular angle	May result in blunting or the loss of definition of the lower border of the face

3 Aging of facial soft tissue

Facial soft tissue consists of skin, fat, muscle, and ligamentous fixation. The basic structures of individual soft tissues are explained in Chapter 1 in detail. Here, I would like to describe the changes of individual soft tissues and facial contour by aging, to the exclusion of the influence of the skeletal aging process.

1) Aging of the skin

The skin also goes through intrinsic aging changes over time due to external and internal factors as previously discussed. Among these, smoking and photo damage leading to characteristic changes as like epidermal thinning, solar elastosis and dermal collagen disorganization, consistent with skin aging. In addition, some have suggested that repetitive and habitual contraction of facial muscles contributes to the appearance of facial rhytids[13]. It is important to understand the changes of skin elasticity by aging, because the skin sagging phenomenon is not only the aging of skin itself but also the secondary factor due to the changes of the underlying bone and soft tissue. I would like to briefly describe the fragmentation mechanism of the dermal collagen matrix that has recently been reported.

A major feature of aged skin is the fragmentation of the dermal collagen matrix. This fragmentation results from the actions of specific enzymes (matrix metaloproteinases) and can be observed in both intrinsic and extrinsic aging. The reduction of extracellular collagen by fragmentation leads to the loss of structural integrity of the skin itself and subsequent impairment of fibroblast functions that produce and organize the collagen matrix. These fibroblasts cannot attach to fragmented collagen and subsequently collapse. Therefore, the aged skin loses its elasticity[14]. Figure 8 shows the models in terms of

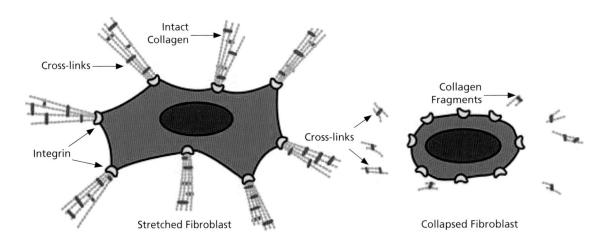

Figure 08 Mechanism of elasticity loss in aged skin.

mechanism of these phenomena in a young and aged person's skin[15].

Elastic filaments of dermis also change during the aging process. Not only does it become thinner, decreased, and fragmented, but it is gradually replaced by collagen of a fibrotic nature; it is one of the major causes of the skin drooping due to the decreasing elasticity of the dermis[16,17]. Additionally, the skin has an ability of the outer skin envelope to adjust to underlying soft tissue volume loss. One should be reminded that both external and internal aging factors affect this ability[18].

For these reasons in particular, once a fat grafting procedure has been performed in aged skin patients to improve facial volume deficiency; the location, level, and amount of the injected fat should be recognized by taking into careful consideration the characteristics of the skin aging.

2) Aging of the muscle

Recently, Le Louran et al. suggested a hypothesis that the shape and action of facial muscles are determined by the position of the underlying fat and that, over time, repetitive contraction of the mimetic muscles contributes to changes in this fat distribution[19]. They speculated this mechanism leads to a loss of the youthful curvilinear contour and an increase in the resting tone of the muscles, resulting in changing the shape, morphology, and three-dimensional topography of the face. Interestingly, this hypothesis is in contrast to the previous traditional concept that facial muscle laxity and weakness causes a downward displacement of the peripheral soft tissue including facial muscle itself.

First of all, we need to take into account changes in the facial contour including wrinkles and depressions depending on the difference of movements between the facial muscles on the right and the left sides of the face. We can observe that the ipsilateral facial wrinkles actually look much softened and the senescent appearance seems to be improved in a patient with unilateral Bell's palsy. In addition, when only one side of the face has been used to chew for a long time, or in the case of vector difference of facial animation between each side of the face being great when people smile or frown, we can also find some differences in wrinkles or depressions between the right and left sides of the face. At this moment, the facial areas with less muscle movement feature a plump appearance with less volume reduction, decreased skin elasticity, and less sagging, whereas the areas with more movement feature a thin appearance with increased skin elasticity, more sagging, and more volume reduction.

This phenomenon convinces that more or less movement of the facial expression muscles considerably affects aging. Especially, one can observe that crow's feet get severe with aging. It is because the resting tone of the muscle increases in order to compensate for the volume and position of the subcutaneous fat changes by the persistence of the orbicularis oculi contraction for a long time. This concept means, in other words, that crow's feet cannot help but become worse, even if the muscle is overused, as long as attenuation of the muscle by the aging process allows a decrease in the resting tone of muscle.

Meanwhile, even though Botulinum toxin significantly improves crow's feet wrinkles, it is not capable of volume restoration. Some patients may often complain that the wrinkles have been reduced, but the soft tissue around the injected area has become more saggy[11,20]. This phenomenon indicates that the redistribution of soft tissue, the resting tone of muscle, and changes to the facial contour, including local aging phenomenon, are intimately related to each other according to the degree of muscle movement. In addition, it reminds the importance of adequate volume restoration under the mimetic muscle in order to improve aging.

3) Aging of the SMAS

SMAS has a function as a distributer and amplifier of the movement of the facial soft tissue through the active animation of the facial expression muscles. So, it is a persuasive argument the facial aging appears much more and faster in the active facial animation area. It is supported by a report[22] concluding that elastic fibers show a degenerative reduction in both dermis and SMAS of the elderly.

In addition, depending on the respective regions of the face, SMAS has different thickness, compositions, and function. It seems likely that the degenerative loss of elastic tissue in the SMAS contributes to the development of the alterations of facial aging, For example, relatively well-developed SMAS of the lateral cheeks is attached to the periosteum of zygoma and it has a function to support the soft tissue of the lower face and neck. In this case, the aging of SMAS here plays a major role in the gravitational descent and sagging of the lateral cheek[23].

4) Aging of the retaining ligaments

The retaining ligaments are tight and thick in youth keeping the mobile superficial face tissues firmly anchored to the underlying skeleton or deep fascia. Years of muscular activity and gravity result in facial laxity and ligamentous attenuation, which in combination with decreased skin elasticity and increased fat in deep compartments, results in the sagging of all elements of the soft tissues. For example, the malar soft tissues are suspended from the zygomatic eminence and maxilla by the zygomatic ligaments laterally and buccal maxillary ligaments medially. With aging, as these ligaments become lax or attenuated, there is inferior migration of malar tissues. This soft tissue ptosis occurs adjacent to the line of fixation along the nasolabial fold. This leads to a prominent nasolabial fold with aging. The attenuation of masseteric ligaments leads to a descent of the cheek soft tissues below the mandibular border and the formation of jowls, because the anterior border of jowls is formed by mandibular ligaments and posterior border by masseteric ligaments.

Also, with aging, the orbital retaining ligament has a laxity which mean a distension, elongation and thinning of ligament due to the decrease of collagen and elastic fiber and loss of intra- and periligamental fat. The laxity of the ligament form a downward displacement of the underlying structures and contributes to the aging phenomenon of the infraorbital and the mid-cheek regions, such as a V-shaped downward angulation (deformity), the appearance of malar mounds, tear trough deformities,

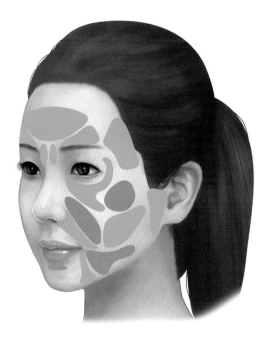

Figure 09 Facial fat redistribution in aging. The areas with loss of soft tissue fullness (green colored areas which are periorbital, forehead, temporal, mandibular, mental, perioral and glabella) and the persistence or hypertrophy (violet colored areas which are submental, nasolabial folds, labiomandibular folds, jowls, infraorbital fat, and malar fat).

and periosteal SMAS ptosis[24].

5) Aging of the fat layer

The superficial and deep fat of the face, along-with the SMAS, forms the basis of facial volume and contour. An obvious example of this can be seen in patients suffering from facial lipodystrophy. With aging, the changes that occur in the two layers of facial fat are different. There is a loss of superficial subcutaneous fat due to decreased vascularity. On the other hand, there is an increased accumulation of fat in the deep fat layer. This is due to the slowing down of metabolism after the 4th decade of life. Particularly, in women, decreasing estrogen levels after the age of 50 further contributes to increased fat in deep depots and paradoxical loss of superficial subcutaneous fat. Figure 9 displays the decreasing or increasing area of subcutaneous fat appearing distinctively in the aging face[25].

The subcutaneous fat layer has attracted attention as a dynamic structure that has been continuously changed, contributing to the formation and maintenance of the facial contour. Furthermore, recently there have been several interesting hypotheses regarding the aging process of the mid-face, which are closely related with the aging of the subcutaneous fat layer. I would like to describe the aging of the fat layer in detail, focusing on these hypotheses.

6) Hypothesis of soft tissue aging in the midface

Generally, when a person of average weight is standing, the aging of the mid-face is characterized by a loss of subcutaneous tissue fullness in the infraorbital area and a prominent nasolabial fold. Of course, there may be variable degrees depending on individual body types. However, generally, facial aging has been understood to appear as sagging by the aging of the soft-tissue itself and the influence of gravity as the environmental factor. Interesting recent studies regarding the reasons for soft tissue aging are largely focused on ptosis hypothesis; in which ageing is caused by a migration of soft tissue, the pseudoptosis hypothesis; in which aging is caused by deflation of soft tissue, and the volume shift hypothesis.

(1) Soft tissue migration

Some interesting research regarding soft tissue migration as a reason for facial aging follows:

① Displacement

Through an analysis of a picture of an elderly mid-face, Yousif NJ et al. argued that the deep naso-labial fold majorly occurring in anterio-inferior displacement is the main cause of the gravitational deflection of the midface[26].

② Redistribution

Gosain AK et al. compared dynamic changes and forms of the nasolabial fold when young and old people smile, by using magnetic resonance imaging (MRI). They concluded that a permanent redistri-bution of the superficial fat of the cheek is the main cause in the formation of a prominent nasolabial fold, accompanying a reduction in the prominence of the infraorbital area located in the superior mar-gin of the malar fat pad at the same time[27].

③ Dynamic displacement

As shown in Figure 10, in the analysis of the dynamic changes of the nasolabial fold using magnetic resonance imaging (MRI), Owsley JQ at el. claimed that when a young person laughs, the levator muscle contract and shorten. And, the lower portion of the cheek fat pad becomes thickened by ex-panding forward due to the increased inner pressure. At this time, the shape of a deep nasolabial fold, that is formed temporarily, is similar with that of an old person[28].

They explained that, in the case of a young person who is doing expression movement frequently, the expansion pressures gradually result in a permanent elongation of the septa. Loss of the intra-fat pad septal support allows the semifluid cheek fat to gradually descend with gravity into the expanded skin envelope at the lower end of the cheek above the nasolabial folds: dynamic displacement. Over years of animation, the skin in the region of the nasolabial fold is expanded to create the permanent nasolabial fold filled with the descended malar fat pad.

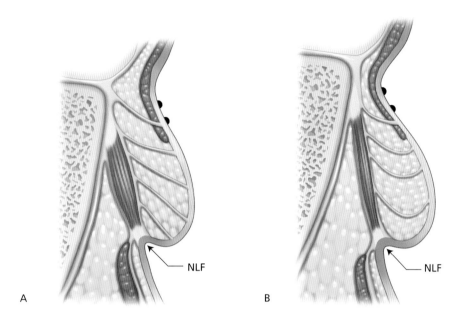

Figure 10 Schematic drawings of the mid-sagittal anatomy of the youthful mid-face in action (A) and the aging face at rest (B). NLF(nasolabial fold).

(2) Soft-tissue volume reduction and deflation

① Deflation hypothesis

Lambros V analyzed a sequence of mid-face aging changes in patients aged between 20 to 40 and announced the result that the nevi - the points located in the infraorbital area - showed minimal descent with the mid-facial aging process. He argued that the cheek skin does not sag significantly in the midface but rather it is atrophy of the cheek fat that produces a deflation of the cheek skin envelope that causes the sagging appearance of mid-face[29].

On the other hand, Owsley JQ, who claimed the dynamic displacement theory has refuted Lambros' deflation theory, explained that fat atrophy is a secondary phenomenon that can be seen in the weight loss of those going through the aging phenomenon. However, he agreed with Lambros V's assertion regarding the phenomenon showing little or no deflection of the skin in the area above the cheek fat pad (or infraorbital area), and explained the reason is the orbital retaining ligament fixes the skin below and above the orbit firmly[28].

② Pseudoptosis hypothesis

After Lambros V's first proposal that deflation hypothesis is a major cause of facial aging, Nicolau PJ. emphasized the importance of volume reduction as an aging factor with released study showing results that injecting artificial fillers into the deep medial fat of the mid-face can cause mid-face projection and improve the aging of the surrounding areas[30].

In addition to this, Rohrich RJ.et al. reported that the V-deformity[31] of the lid-cheek junction and the prominent nasolabial fold has improved by protruding of the mid-face, as the result of an injected saline solution into the deep fat beneath the SMAS in the inner facial area of the zygomatic major of elderly dead bodies. From these results, they claimed that a prominent nasolabial fold is mainly due to the reduction in the protrusion of the mid-face by the deflation of deep medial cheek fat.

Moreover, they emphasized that superficial subcutaneous fat was compartmented by the septum and volume of the fat is reduced only within compartment without movement to another compartment. They explained that nasolabial folds were finally worsened as a form of pseudoptosis because the laxity of skin causes a secondary excess skin due to volume deflation[32]. These views show a significant conceptual difference in the existing theories that have been used for explaining factors of facial aging up until now.

③ Compartmental migration and intra-compartmental shift hypothesis

Gierloff M et al. introduced two concepts of age-dependent changes of the mid-facial fat compartments: an inferior migration of the fat compartments and an intra-compartmental volume shift within the compartments as shown in Figure 11[33].

This inferior migration should not only be attributed to gravity forces. Rather, it should be considered as a consequence of volume loss of the buccal extension of the buccal fat pad. A deflation of this fat compartment will consequently lead to a lack of support for the medial cheek and middle cheek fat, aggravating the descent of these compartments.

The concept of intra-compartmental volume shift suggests a detailed another evidence of pseudoptosis hypothesis that the volume is decreased in the cephalad portion of each of the subcutaneous fat compartments in the mid-face, while it is increased in the inferior portion. For example, the volume

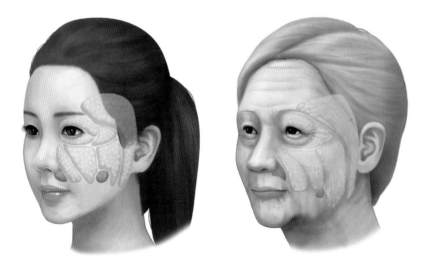

Figure 11 Schematic drawings of aging changes in superficial (yellow-colored) and deep (brown colored) fat compartments: a young women (A) and an old women (B).

loss of the cephalad part of the nasolabial and medial cheek fat will consequently worsen the appearance of the tear trough, the tear trough deformity, and the palpebromalar groove. The volume increase of the inferior part of the nasolabial fats will lead to deep nasolabial folds and pronounced superior jowls.

Based on this concept, they have suggested that to restore a youthful fat distribution for facial rejuvenation, a volume reduction of the inferior portion and a volume augmentation of the cephalic portion would be necessary. It is also evaluated as embodying the fat rebalancing concept of Donofrio LM. in detail[25].

4 Anti-aging approach using lipoplasty

1) Lipoplastic approach for the modification of the facial skeletal framework

Recently, a new controversy has come into focus suggesting that the correction of facial skeletal deformities is important to prevent unnatural and disharmonious outcomes, which have been identified as problems in the traditional treatment of surgical face lift. In addition, based on this hypothesis, there are some results showing that the effect was quietly improved by procedures enhancing skeletal support for the soft tissue using a solid implant or filler in the mid-face.

From these results, Shaw RB Jr et al. further detailed the possibility of soft tissue changes due to skeletal augmentation in each part of the face[9]. Citing Matros E and Flowers RS, they claimed that skeletal implantations can create convex morphology by increasing projection and provide resuspension of sagged soft tissue by a concave bony platform[34, 35]. Synthesizing their claims, the facial aging is occurring due to overall decreasing in bony volume by morphological change of the facial skeleton with increasing age. This results in decreased support and projection of the overlying soft tissue. With accompanying the atrophy of subcutaneous fat, it leads to the appearance of the aged face. This means that skeletal changes are the main influences in the process of facial aging. Additionally, Mendelson B et al. emphasized persuasive opinions, necessity, and enough possibility regarding the fact that restoration of bone volume results in increasing skeletal support for the overlying soft tissues and eventually brings a natural and harmonized outcome[10]. This approach differs with many trials to date which have believed that they one could be effective in improving of the aging process by surgical face lift, with an emphasis on repositioning and redraping of soft tissue, and by soft filler injection for restoration of youthful volume and shape.

The materials used for the purpose of skeletal augmentation such as recovering bone loss or increasing bony projection could be classified under two major groups – implant (autologous or artificial) and filler (artificial filler or autologous fat). Of these, implant (artificial or autologous) is the most effective material in improving facial bone contour, however, it has many constraints in its use due to bone loss and allergic reaction by the artificial implant, the limitation of insertion sites for preserving major nerves and vessels, and increased downtime by invasive surgery. Compared with it, artificial filler is deemed to be inefficient due to the constant injections and allergic reaction even though it is known to be a convenient material.

I would like to propose autologous fat grafting as an alternative to skeletal augmentation on the premise that there is an obvious limitation of improving contour of facial skeleton perfectly using only fat grafting. Nevertheless, there are many advantageous aspects of fat grafting. There is an economic and non-allergic characteristic because fat is autologous tissue with no limitation of the injection (site and depth), no scarring because of it being a non-surgical procedure, and a short recovery time. It also improves bone and soft tissue contour simultaneously. It can be pointed out as a demerit that this technique has an irregular survival rate and longevity dependent upon the patient's condition and the skill level of the doctor. But, recently, many positive results have been reported in relation to the cell

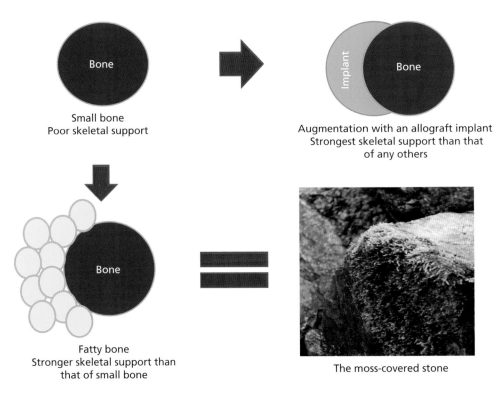

Figure 12 Improvement of skeletal support by the moss-covered stone (Fatty bone) hypothesis.
Even though implanted fat is not as strong as the bone, it is expected to improve bearing capacity of soft tissue if fat grafting is made like moss covered stone, getting larger on the periosteum than moss-uncovered stone is. The no-moss part can be compared to the bone and the moss-covered part can be compared to the shape which looks as if the size of the bone got bigger as the implantation of fat is performed by attaching fat to the bone

assisted lipo-transfer (CAL) method[36,37] and so on.

Is it possible to improve the facial bone contour through fat grafting? I would suggest a look at the hypothesis of "the moss covered stone" as seen in Figure 12. Even though the grafted fat is not as strong as bone, it is expected to improve the skeletal support for soft tissue if the fat grafting is made like a moss covered stone, getting larger on the periosteum than moss-uncovered stone. Modification of bone contour through fat grafting means an improvement of skeletal support to the surrounding soft tissue by attaching fat to the bone like "the moss covered stone". It would be successful if this procedure should bring a final outcome either with a real lifting effect or without any sagging appearance at the minimum.

However, as we know, since aging occurs not only in bone but also in soft tissue, one approach cannot provide a satisfactory and perfect outcome. For instance, it is not a good choice to apply artificial fillers or implants only for recovering youthful morphology of the bone in the old patient whose face has a soft tissue sagging with less elasticity. Therefore, it is strongly suggested that the basic and reasonable approach to facial rejuvenation is the application of combination procedure to improve both bone and soft tissue simultaneously. Also, how and what procedure will be applied must be dependent on each patient's condition.

2) Approach for the improvement of facial aging, according to the type of facial soft tissue contour

On the basis of the change of facial contour with aging, according to the hypothesis of Gonzalez-Ulloa M as shown in Figure 1, to rejuvenate the aged face is to change the facial contour from the rectangular to the reverse triangle outline. Of course, the ideal rejuvenation means the restoration of youthful morphology of bone and soft tissue. But, in reality, it is very rare to do the bone contouring surgery for facial rejuvenation. The Figure 13 shows two types of the typical aging face which are categorized by Fournier F.[38]

The first, true ptosis type, as shown in Figure 13A, can be seen in a fat face, featuring the true ptosis form where the increased amount of tissue makes the flesh of the face outward and sagging under the influence of gravity. This face shows a tension and pressure fold and the totally protruded form of an old face. The second type is a form that can be seen in hollow faces such a Figure 13B. It is a visible form of false ptosis like a laxness due to an influence of relatively reduced gravity with a volume reduction of tissue, from which the flesh of the face entered inwardly. This face makes generally collapsed-shape of an aged face with sag and shrinkage wrinkles[2].

I would like to suggest the possibility of my rejuvenation concept. The characteristics of soft tissue regarding these two types are introduced as following.

Among the hypotheses of soft tissue aging described above, which hypothesis will be correct for ex-

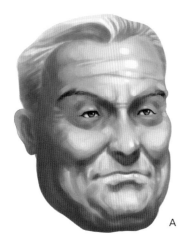
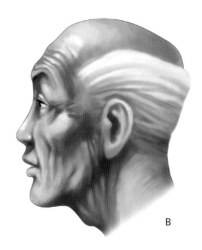

A   B

Figure 13   Two types of the aging face (A: Outward aging, B: Inward aging).

A.True ptosis type face (Outward aging)   B. False ptosis type face (Inward aging)

Example of tissue proliferation   Example of tissue involution, hypotrophy

Gravity acting   Less gravity acting

Ptosis on the outside   Ptosis from the inside

plaining an aged facial type such as Figure 13A? Probably, the true ptosis hypothesis due to the movement of the soft tissue will be a better explanation. Likewise, false ptosis by deflation of the soft tissue shall be deemed to be an explanation for a facial form such as Figure 13B. However, the shape of each is not fully explained because all of the aged facial types of patients cannot be classified into only the two types above and most are a mixture of the two forms with a varied ratio.

In terms of these two cases, what will be the reasonable approaches to rejuvenate facial aging? It is not easy to decide which procedure is best for ideal rejuvenation in detail to each type. However, generally, it can be recommended to perform a liposuction with traditional surgical face lifting for type A and a fat grafting with a complementary surgical face lifting as needed for type B. Then, how to approach to the intermediate type (A and B)? It depends on the demand and cosmetic status of the patient, but the proper combination of above three procedures should be applied. As a matter of course, to achieve better result, it is necessary to perform additional procedures for increasing skeletal support for the soft tissue to each type and it ought to be belonged with the volume rebalancing surgery. In explaining the important sequence of these procedures in details, it is recommended that volume rebalancing surgery should be performed first. For example, in type A, liposuction should be performed first and then face lift be done immediately. However, in type B, surgical face lift after fat grafting should be performed immediately at the same day or can be done at least 3 months after. In intermediate type, I always recommend to do the surface surgery after volume surgery because it is for decreasing of invasiveness and complications by traditional surgical face lift and eventually for achieving more natural and harmonious result.

In addition, in order to gain further improvements, we must analyze the main cause of aging in each patient and then choose the method of approach by determining which type of facial shape it is closer to, between the two types mentioned above, by observing the facial characteristics. After that, select the appropriate procedure considering the type and environment of each individual patient.

3) Lipoplastic rejuvenation focused on the modification of subcutaneous fat layers

To improve facial aging by only modifying subcutaneous fat layers, compartment-specific volume restoration which was proposed by Gierloff M et al. should be recommended[33]. However, it would not be easy to perform fat grafting based on the above hypotheses due to the following reasons: First, it's not easy to precisely draw (= know the locations of) these compartments on the skin. Second, because several compartments abut one another and form layers, the interaction between each compartment has to be considered. The elements related to the interaction of the compartments are the shape and location of each compartment, the presence of ligament fixations, the effect of gravity, and the aging process. Third, the aging is not caused only by deformity of fat layer but caused by dynamic changes of whole facial tissue.

4) The key points of fat grafting which is able to obtain from various aging theories to improve aged face.

Based on the above mentioned several hypothesis, I'd like to describe fundamental factors for ideal fat grafting method.

Fat grafting for correction of congenitally underdeveloped bony skeleton or aging-induced bone resorption can improve skeletal support for the soft tissue. The fat should be injected into deepest layer, on the periosteum. It is summarized from Mendelson B et al.'s bone resorption theory, Lambros' theory, and the moss-covered stone (Fatty bone) hypothesis.

To prevent sagging or pseudoptosis of the superficial fat compartments, it is necessary to inject fat into the deep fat compartments. It is summarized from Rohrich RJ et al.'s pseudoptosis theory and Gierloff M et al.'s inferior migration of compartment theory.

Fat should be grafted into the fat reduced-cephalic portion of the compartment, whereas liposuction should be performed in the fat increased-caudal portion of the compartment. It is summarized from Gierloff M etal.'s intracompartmental volume shift theory and Donofrio LM. rebalancing theory.

Fat can be injected into all atrophic and attenuated soft tissue for volume restoration, because aging occurs with multiple and simultaneous at all tissue. It can be explained from the general concept of facial aging.

In addition it is an extremely common-sense that shape and location of facial soft tissue are influenced by gravitational force,. Especially, it must not be excluded the influence of gravity to facial manifestations of aging, such as sagging appearance which is the most definitive feature of aging, even though it is not a primary but a secondary cause. Eventually, because it is highly likely to increase the risk of sagging appearance by the weight of injected fat after fat grafting. It can be suggested from the concept of gravitation and facial aging process.

Until now, surgical face lifting has been only performed to improve facial sagging with the concept of anti-gravitation. However, recently, significance of the volume restoration surgery is gradually increasing day by day for achieving of natural and harmonious result. From the viewpoint of fat grafting alone for facial rejuvenation, it is necessary to develop another way of fat grafting which is able to overcome the influence of gravity. It also should meet the above mentioned all requirements.

Reference

01. Gonzalez-Ulloa M, Flores ES. Senility of the face - Basic study to understand its causes and effects. Plast Reconstr Surg. 1965;36;239-246.

02. Yaar M, Gilchrest BA. Skin aging: postulated mechanisms and consequent changes in structure and function. Clin Geriatr Med. 2001 Nov;17(4):617-630, v.

03. El-Domyati M, Attia S, Saleh F, Brown D, Birk DE, Gasparro F, Ahmad H, Uitto J. Intrinsic aging vs. photoaging: a comparative histopathological, immunohistochemical, and ultrastructural study of skin. Exp Dermatol. 2002 Oct;11(5):398-405.

04. Rabe JH, Mamelak AJ, McElgunn PJ, Morison WL, Sauder DN. Photoaging: mechanism and repair. J Am Acad Dermatol. 2006;55(1):1-19.

05. Guyuron B, Rowe DJ, Weinfeld AB, Eshraghi Y, Fathi A, Iamphongsai S. Factors contributing to the facial aging of identical twins. Plast Reconstr Surg. 2009;123(4):1321-1331. doi: 10.1097/PRS.0b013e31819c4d42.

06. Pessa JE. An algorithm of facial aging: Verification of Lambros' theory by three-dimensional stereolithography, with reference to the pathogenesis of midfacial aging, scleral show, and the lateral suborbital trough deformity. Plast Reconstr Surg. 2000;106(2):479-88; discussion 489-490.

07. Richard MJ, Morris C, Deen BF, Gray L, Woodward JA. Analysis of the anatomic changes of the aging facial skeleton using computer-assisted tomography. Ophthal Plast Reconstr Surg. 2009;25(5):382-386.

08. Kahn DM, Shaw RB Jr. Aging of the bony orbit: a three dimensional computed tomography study. Aesthet Surg J. 2008 May;28(3):258-264.

09. Shaw RB Jr, Katzel EB, Koltz PF, Yaremchuk MJ, Girotto JA, Kahn DM, Langstein HN. Aging of the facial skeleton: aesthetic implications and rejuvenation strategies. Plast Reconstr Surg. 2011;127(1):374-383. doi: 10.1097/PRS.0b013e3181f95b2d.

10. Mendelson B, Wong CH. Changes in the Facial Skeleton With Aging: Implications and Clinical Applications in Facial Rejuvenation. Aesthetic Plast Surg. 2012 May 12. [DOI 10.1007/s00266-012-9904-3]

11. Pessa JE, Zadoo VP, Yuan C, Ayedelotte JD, Cuellar FJ, Cochran CS, Mutimer KL, Garza JR. Concertina effect and facial aging: Nonlinear aspects of youthfulness and skeletal remodeling, and Why, perhaps, infants have jowls. Plast Reconst Surg. 1999;103(2):635-644.

12. Rohrich RJ, Pessa JE. Discussion: Aging of the facial skeleton: Aesthetic implications and rejuvenation strategies. PlastReconstr Surg. 2011;127(1):384-385.

13. Farkas JP, Pessa JE, Hubbar B, Rohrich RJ. The science and theory behind facial aging, PRS GO 2013;1:e8; doi:10.1097/GOX.0b013e31828ed1da; Published online 5 April 2013.

14. Fisher GJ, Varani J, Voorhees JJ. Looking older; fibroblast collapse and therapeutic implications. Arch Dermatol 2008;144:666-672.4. Fisher GJ, Varani J, Voorhees JJ. Looking older; fibroblast collapse and therapeutic implications. Arch Dermatol 2008;144:666-672.

15. Fitzgerald R, Graivier MH, Kane M, Lorenc ZP, Vleggaar D, Werschler WP, Kenkel JM. Update on facial aging. Aesthet Surg J. 2010;30 Suppl:11S-24S.

16. Kligman AM, Zheng P, Lavker RM. The anatomy and pathogenesis of wrinkles. Br J Dermatol, 1985: 113(1):37-42.

17. Pasquali-ronchetti I, Baccarani-Contri M. Elastic fiber during development and aging. Micros Res Tech. 1997:38(4):428-435.

18. Fitzgerald R, Graivier MH, Kane M, Lorenc ZP, Vleggaar D, Werschler WP, Kenkel JM. Update on facial aging. Aesthet Surg J. 2010 Jul-Aug;30 Suppl:11S-24S. doi: 10.1177/1090820X10378696.

19. Le Louarn CL, Buthiau D, Buis J. Structural aging: the facial recurve concept. Aesthetic Plast Surg. 2007;31:213-218.

20. Guerrissi JO. Intraoperative Injection of Botulinum Toxin A into Orbicularis Oculi Muscle for the Treatment of Crow's Feet.Plast Reconstr Surg. 2000 May;104(6):2219-2225.

21. Baek RM, Park SO, Jeong EC, Oh HS, Kim SW, Minn KW, Lee SY. The effect of botulinum toxin A on fat graft survival. Aesthetic Plast Surg. 2012 Jun;36(3):680-6. Epub 2012 Feb 23.

22. Owsley JQ, Roberts CL. Some anatomical observations on midface aging and long-term results of surgical treatment. Plast Reconstr Surg. 2008 Jan;121(1):258-268. doi: 10.1097/01.prs.0000293872.14916.bb.

23. Owsley, LQ. Aesthetic Facial Surgery. Philadelphia: Saunders, 1994.

24. Kikkawa DO, Lemke BN, Dortzbach RK. Relations of the

superficial musculoaponeurotic system to the orbit and characterization of the orbitomalar ligament. Ophthal Plast Reconstr Surg. 1996 Jun;12(2):77-88.

25. Donofrio LM. Fat distribution: a morphologic study of the aging face. Dermatol Surg. 2000 Dec;26(12):1107-1112.

26. Yousif NJ, Gosain A, Sanger JR, Larson DL, Matloub HS. The nasolabial fold: a photogrammetric analysis. Plast Reconstr Surg. 1994 Jan;93(1):70-77.

27. Gosain AK, Amarante MT, Hyde JS, Yousif NJ. A dynamic analysis of changes in the nasolabial fold using magnetic resonance imaging: Implications for facial rejuvenation and facial animation surgery. Plast Reconstr Surg. 1996;98(4):622-636.

28. Owsley JQ, Roberts CL. Some anatomical observations on mid-face aging and long-term results of surgical treatment. Plast Reconstr Surg. 2008;121(1):258-268.

29. Lambros V. Facial aging: What really happens as we grow old. Presented at the annual meeting of the American society of plastic surgeons, Philadelphia, Pennsylvania, 2004;9-13.

30. Nicolau PJ. Long-lasting and permanent fillers: Biomaterial influence over host tissue response. Plast Reconstr Surg. 2007;119(7):2271-2286.

31. Mendelson BC, Muzaffar AR, Adams WP Jr. Surgical anatomy of the mid-cheek and malar mounds. Plast Reconstr Surg. 2002 1;110(3):885-96; discussion 897-911.

32. Rohrich RJ, Pessa JE, Ristow B. The youthful cheek and the deep medial fat compartment. Plast Reconstr Surg. 2008 Jun;121(6):2107-2112. doi: 10.1097/PRS.0b013e31817123c6.

33. Gierloff M, Stöhring C, Buder T, Gassling V, Açil Y, Wiltfang J. Aging changes of the midfacial fat compartments: a computed tomographic study. Plast Reconstr Surg. 2012 Jan;129(1):263-273. doi: 10.1097/PRS.0b013e3182362b96.

34. Matros E, Momoh A, Yaremchuk MJ. The aging mid-facial skeleton: Implications for rejuvenation and reconstruction using implants. Facial Plast Surg. 2009;25(4):252-259.

35. Flowers RS. Augmentation maxilloplasty. In: Terino EO, Flowers RS, eds. The art of alloplastic facial contouring. St. Louis: Mosby; 2000;129-150.

36. Sterodimas A, de Faria J, Nicaretta B, Papadopoulos O, Papalambros E, Illouz YG. Cell-assisted lipotransfer. Aesthet Surg J. 2010 Jan;30(1):78-81. doi: 10.1177/1090820X10362730.

37. Matsumoto D, Sato K, Gonda K, Takaki Y, Shigeura T, Sato T, Aiba-Kojima E, Iizuka F, Inoue K, Suga H, Yoshimura K. Cell-assisted lipotransfer: supportive use of human adipose-derived cells for soft tissue augmentation with lipoinjection. Tissue Eng. 2006 Dec;12(12):3375-3382.

38. Fournier PF. Fat grafting; My technique. Dermatol Surg. 2000;26(12):1117-1128.

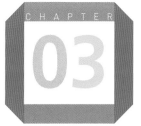

a novel facial fat grafting technique with a concept of volumetric lifting

Various parameters affecting survival of fat grafting

▪1 Adipocyte as endocrine gland

Adipocyte, also known as a lipocyte or a fat cell, is a major component of adipose tissue, specialized in storing energy as fat. And, previously, its function was known as just releasing energy during starved state or cold winter. However, adipocyte is recently known to secrete over 30 types of hormones or cytokine, which are named adipocytokine as in Figure 1. Leptin, one of the hormones made by adipocyte, helps to regulate energy balance by inhibiting hunger. In addition, TNF-∝, IL-6, and PAI-1 were found out to significantly participate in causing diabetes and other endocrine diseases. Now, adipocyte is being regarded as a single independent endocrine organ[1].

▪2 Adipose tissue

Adipose tissue in human body can be classified into 5 types according to anatomy or function.

1) Bone marrow adipose tissue

With aging, the number of osteoblasts decreases while number of adipocytes increases in bone marrow. One example is the increased fat quantity in bone marrow of patients suffering from osteoporosis. This cell not only provides energy to osteoblast, but also promotes osteogenesis and hematopoiesis by

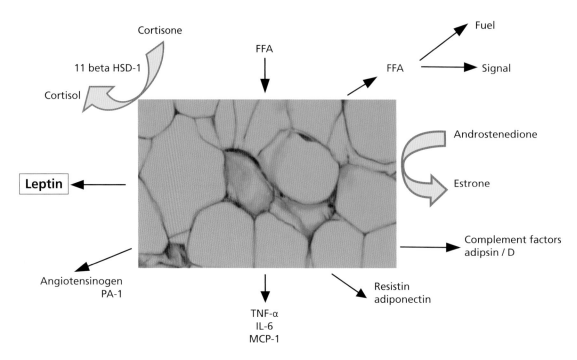

Figure 01   Basic science of adipocyte as an endocrine organ. Over 30 kinds of various hormones and cytokines secreted from adipocytes.

secreting various adipocytokines.

2) Brown adipose tissue (BAT)

Its function is to generate body heat (thermogenesis). Humans do not need it after birth, so it is abundant in newborns and is absent in adults. It is especially abundant in hibernating mammals.

3) Mammary adipose tissue

It is present in breasts, providing nutrients or energy during lactation.

4) Mechanical adipose tissue

Even though it does not provide energy, it supports important structures for retrobulbar area and palm's fat pads.

5) White adipose tissue (WAT)

White adipose tissue is a topic of great interest in fat grafting and other various researches. It plays a role in providing energy and has function of insulation. It also contains the most abundant number of stem cells compared to the other four adipose tissues.

◼3◼ Hypotheses on fat graft survival

Gap filling mechanism which describes what process is used to fill the volume-deficient area during fat grafting can be explained by hypotheses below.

1) Host replacement hypothesis

This hypothesis was announced by Neuhof H and Hirshfeld S in 1929. They claimed that much of the grafted adipocytes barely survive in host tissues and is replaced by fibrotic tissue or newly generated metaplastic fat. Death of adipocytes in the tissue after fat grafting can cause inflammation and diverse fibrosis. It is ultimately same as dead cell debris injection[2].

2) Survival hypothesis

30 years after the announcement of the host replacement hypothesis, Peer LA reported that approximately 50% of grafted adipocytes survived. This hypothesis suggests that grafted connective tissues containing fibroblasts, vascular system, and endothelial cells survive and new blood vessels are formed (angiogenesis) at the beginning. Then, they link to the host's vascular system and lead to the survival of grafted adipocytes[3].

3) Recent concepts

After the announcement of the survival theory, almost every research about grafted fat survival was focused on the survival theory rather than the host replacement theory. Fibroblast and vascular endothelium which play major roles in early angiogenesis are included in adipose derived stem cells (ADSCs). The dominant concept is that survival and roles of preadipocytes and adipose derived stem cells are more significant in survival of grafted adipose tissue rather than survival of mature adipocytes.

This is because mature adipocytes are more vulnerable to impacts and prone to damage by suction, harvest, separation and injection compared to preadipocytes and ADSCs. And, mature adipocytes require more nutrients and oxygen[4, 5] for survival and the chance of their survival is very scarce after grafting. And, hence it is reasonable that only most of the preadipocytes and adipose derived stem cells survive. Recently, many researchers have interests on the roles of ADSCs on self-replication, angiogensis and related clinical application of growth factors.

4) Grafting process of transplanted fat

Bilings and May reported that grafted adipocytes undergo a series of engraftment as shown in Table 1 and Figure 2[6].

Table 01 Histology of fat at various times after grafting

Time (days)	Histology
First 3 days	Cellular infiltrate: polymorphonuclear cells, plasma cells, lymphocytes, eosinophils. With vessels of graft: red blood cells were clumped together, white blood cells were in process of diapedesis (passage of blood cells through intact vessel walls). No degeneration of graft endothelial cells and fibroblasts of the stroma.
Day 4	Engorgement and dilation of smaller stromal vessels with abundant red blood cells and diapedetic white blood cells. (Anastomoses between smaller graft vessels and host red blood supply.) Increased number of eosinophils in cellular infiltrate. Foreign-body type Giant cells often seen.
10 days	Areas of necrotic adipose tissue. Regenerative proliferation of original fat cells mostly at periphery of lobules-includes proliferating adipose cells of the graft and host round "histiocyte-like" cells that took up lipid and enlarged.
14-21 days	Further adipose cell breakdown. Increasing number of large host histiocytes that appear to be picking up lipid with formation of droplets within their cytoplasm.
30-60 days	Increasing numbers of large histiocytes which peak at 2 months. Coalescing of fat globules in the cytoplasm.

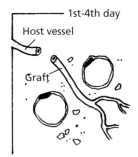

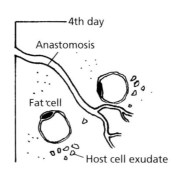

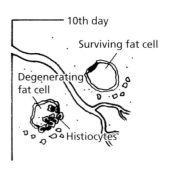

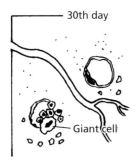

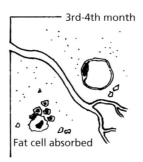

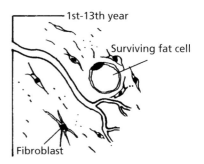

Figure 02 The contrasting face of two adipose cells in free fat autografts. The adipose cell on the left does not survive fatty content and is removed by host histiocytes. The fat cell on the right survives grafting and constitutes the apparently normal adipose tissue seen in the grafted area 1 year or more after grafting.

■4■ Parameters affecting adipocytes survival in fat grafting

Diverse parameters affecting the adipocytes survival in fat grafting are described as follows.

1) Fat harvest

(1) Harvest method

Factors affecting the survival of grafted fat during harvest are instruments, pressure, cannula size, and drugs used for harvest.

It is reported that when fat is harvested for the purpose of fat grafting, approximately 90% of adipocytes is destructed by mechanical liposuction[7]. It is also reported that Coleman's method of maintaining 1-2cc of air in 10cc syringe damages mature adipocytes much lesser compared to using the pressure of general mechanical liposuction[4,8,9]. Moreover, Witort EJ et al. recently reported that Coleman's method is safer than than mechanical liposuction using negative pressure of -680mmHg[10] by measuring the concentration of apoptosis-activating enzymes and cytochrome C which is essentially secreted during apoptosis of ADSCs. Meanwhile, when negative mechanical pressure was used to harvest fat for fat grafting, the lowest negative pressure used for liposuction was 20cm H_2O[11]. According to the results above, the negative pressure used in the harvest method is a crucial factor, and fat should be harvested by the lowest pressure.

There are many researches about cannula size used for liposuction. It has been reported that diameter of 4mm shows double survival rate compared to 2mm, and diameter of 6mm has greater survival rate than 4mm[12]. Their research only focused on giving little damage to fat tissues during suction and grafting.

On the other hand, some surgeons claim that using 2mm-thick cannula provide greater survival rate. They claimed that the smaller cannula they used, the larger mature adipocyte damage they got. And, because these damaged cells are removed as free oil during centrifuge, the possibility of injecting smaller and healthier preadipocytes is considerable. It is also creating expectation of easier injection that results in little damage and better neovascular supply. However, there are yet no obvious objective results of the comparisons in terms of the detailed parts. Currently, diameter between 2.5mm~4mm is the most commonly used size for fat harvesting[13].

Recently, research result by Tonnard P et al. is quite interesting. They classified harvested fats into macrofat, microfat, and nanofat according to the applications of different aspiration cannulas and mechanical emulsification[14]. Macrofat was defined as fat harvested by using standard 3-mm liposuction cannula with large side holes (2 × 7 mm). Microfat was defined as fat harvested by using multiport 3-mm cannula with. However, generally, the harvested fat be air-blocked and stored at 4°C, throughout the whole separation and purification processes, is affirmed to be much safer then room temperature. side holes (1 mm in diameter). Nanofat was made by an application of mechanically-emulsified technique which was achieved by shifting the microfat between two 10cc syringes connected to each other by a transfer and additional filtering process with a sterile nylon cloth with 0.5-mm pore size. They suggested that the nanofat showed remarkable improvements in skin rejuvenation without any complications and other unwanted side effects. This report classified the forms of the injected fats by their sizes, which is a point that is quite interesting in clinical application. If the research results are reported objectively on the grafted survival rates of these three kinds of fats, it can provide important information on the selection of ideal cannular size.

There are many reports that the components of tumescent solution for fat harvest such as lidocaine, epinephrine, and sodium bicarbonate do not influence on the survival rate of adipocytes[15,16].

(2) Donor site

Recent survey on surgeons suggested that the most common harvesting sites for facial fat grafting is abdomen, followed by thigh, flank, gluteal region, and medial knee[17]. In general, since most of the facial fat graftings are operated in the supine position, the abdomen, flank, and medial thigh are the most accessible and easy to be used as fat harvest sites. However, whole body areas from which can be taken be the subject of donor site for fat grafting.

There are more interesting results regarding donor site for fat grafting as below.

Coleman SR reported that, in case of thin male, harvesting fat from lateral thigh and inferior lateral buttock can be recommended since their abdomen and love handles may consist mostly from fibrous tissue with little available fat [18].

Trepsat F reported that the medial knee fat is most suitable for fat grafting to the lower palpebral areas because it is less fibrous in nature, softer, suppler and consisted of smaller individual tissue prarticles[19] than other donor sites. Additionally, Hudson DA et al. reported that size of cells from femoral sites are somehow larger and have greater lipogenic activity than other sites[20]. On the contrary, Rohrich R et al. reported that no statistical differences in adipocyte viability during the first 5 hours after harvest between fats harvested from abdomen, thigh, flank, and knee[21] were demonstrated.

In the latest research, Padoin AV et al. reported that the lower abdomen and the inner thigh may have higher processed lipoaspirate cell concentrations[22], Also, Jurgens W et al. suggested that abdomen seems to be preferable to the hip/thigh region for harvesting adipose tissue, although no differences were detected in differentiation capacity between ADSCs from both harvesting sites[23].

There is another interesting result, Schipper BM et al. reported that the superficial abdomimal region located above Scarpa's fascia is a better harvest site compared to the deep fatty layer due to its stronger resistance against ADSCs apoptosis[24].

Judging from the results in search of the optimal donor site for fat grafting, although we know that all fat is not the same in nature, there is no existing evidence of a superior harvest site for fat viability. From the above results, the superficial fatty layer of the lower abdomen is considered to be the most suitable site, and the thigh comes next. However, additional researches are expected to clarify the controversial issue about the most suitable harvest site.

(3) Age of the patient

Below shows the interesting reports related to the effects of patient's age on the fat survival rate.

According to an experiment, the older the laboratory animal, the lower the lipogenesis-promoting enzyme activitty[25]. It is also reported that young individuals' ADSCs have significantly greater adhesion and proliferation ability but there is no difference in differentiation ability compared to those of older individuals. Particularly, young individuals' ADSCs are reported to have faster proliferation rate[26].

Jurgens W et al.[24], Heunar H et al.[27], and van Harmelen et al[28]. have demonstrated that there is no correlations between BMI, age and numbers of ADSCs per gram of adipose tissue.

On the other hand, Cartwright MJ et al.[29], Kirkland JL et al.[30], and Karagiannides I et al.[31] reported that the replication and differentiation capabilities of preadipocyte, which accounts for 15 to 50 percents of the total adipocytes, decline with aging. The decline in fat depot size with aging is not due to the decrease in adipocyte numbers, but rather caused by decreased adipocyte size[32,33]. Sepe A et al. reported that the proliferation and differentiation also decline with aging, which likely contribute to increased systemic exposure to lipotoxic free fatty acids and to increased inflammation, eventually lead to further reduction in adipogenesis[34].

By inference from the above results, it is suggested that there is still exists the possibility about influence of aging on fat survival rate, but, it may remain debatable because there is no exact evidence yet.

2) Purification and separation

(1) Air exposure and temperature

There is a report that claimed that cytoplasmic lysis occurs in 50% of total adipocytes due to temporary air exposure[35]. On the other hand, Ramon Y et al. have reported that even when the fat, which was dried on towel exposed to air, were grafted, there were no significant decrease of graft survival rate[36]. This report is in contradiction to our general assumption of air exposure effect on graft survival rate.

Besides, there are diverse opinions on the air exposure and storage temperature. However, it is affirmed to be much safer that the harvested fat must be air-blocked and stored at 4°C but not the room temperature. Moreover, it is ideal that harvested adipocytes should be grafted as quickly as possible if it is preserved at room temperature (about 2 hours in maximum). However, it is possible to use aspirated adipocytes which can be stored if it is preserved at 4°C for 12 hours under the sufficient nutrition without any contamination[37].

(2) Separation

Methods for separating harvested fat include sedimentation, centrifugation, and towel-dry technique[38,39]. Recently, the usage of the towel-dry technique has decreased due to concerns such as contaminations or cell damage by air exposure. Whichever method is used, the purpose of separation is to increase the concentration of the adipocytes, to remove lipid, blood cells, water-soluble ingredients such as proteases and lipases, and lidocaine from fat aspirates[40].

For sedimentation method about an hour is required to precipitate fat aspirates. Meanwhile, the centrifugation method requires only approximately 3 minutes at 1,200g and is known as the most appropriate method for fat separation[36,41,42].

It is inappropriate to designate r.p.m.(revolution per minute) for centrifuge speed because the diameter of centrifuge's rotor is dependent on different devices. For example, even if two centrifuges have the same 3000 r.p.m., g value is 1207g for centrifuge with diameter of 12cm while it is 1811g for diameter of 18cm. The relationship between g and r.p.m. is $g=(1.118 \times 10^{-5})RS^2$, where R is the radius of rotor(center of rotor to sample) and S is speed which refers to r.p.m.. Also, most of the centrifuges designate g value and r.p.m.'s correlation for reference.

After centrifugation of the harvested adipose tissue from liposuction, it shows the result as shown in Figure 3. After centrifugation, specimen is divided into 5 portions: The upper most oil layer contains lipid which is generated from destroyed adipocytes. The second upper layer is a floating adipocyte layer which is composed of mature adipocytes filled with lipid droplets. In the lowermost part of the mature adipocytes layer, there is a thin white frothy layer that contains multipotential progenitor cells. The lower denser fluid portion is a sero-sanguinous fluid layer composed of tumescent solution and plasma. At the bottom, cell precipitates contains preadipocytes, endothelial cells, immune cells, and mesenchymal stem cells including preadipocytes[43].

Rose JG et al. reported that the cell viability was higher in samples processed by sedimentation compared with those by centrifuging, because the fat cell is healthy and have well-maintained intercellular distances[38]. However, Rohrich RJ et al. reported that there is no difference in cell viability quantity when compare the two methods[21]. Besides, Kurita M, et al. reported that excessive centrifugation can destroy adipocytes and adipose-derived stem cells, but appropriate centrifugation concentrates them, resulting in enhanced survival rate by concentrating adipocytes, enriching ADSCs and extracellular matrix, and eliminating RBC and fibrin. It is because extracellular matrix contributes to the volume increase even for a short period of time. Macrophage activation by RBC presence causes the decline of adipocytes[48], and modification (tangling or solidification) of adipocytes by fibrin is known

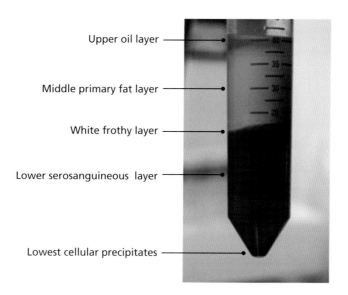

Upper oil layer

Middle primary fat layer

White frothy layer

Lower serosanguineous layer

Lowest cellular precipitates

Figure 03 Separation of the aspirated fat by centrifugation. The upper most layer is supranatant which contains least dense consisting of lipids. The middle portion is primarily consisted of fatty tissue. The white frothy layer between the fat layer and the serosanguinous layer contains multipotent progenitor cells. And the lower layer is infranatant which is composed of blood, tissue fluid, and local anesthetic. The lowest precipitate contains cellular component.

to complicate injection and decrease the survival rate[49].

On the other hand, since adipocytes separated by sedimentation contain relatively more fluid, the number of fat cells per unit volume is lower than that of centrifugation. Therefore, when these adipocytes are grafted, it is not so easy to control the precise volume adequate for the augmentation because of the relatively greater water content. Especially, in the case of mass fat grating, the surgeon should keep in mind the possibility of edema and inflammation due to the accumulation of fluid and free oil. Nevertheless, there are some surgeons who prefer to use precipitated fat for the orbital or peri-orbital fat grafting. This attempt is to inject fat easily and smoothly or to decrease the possibility of overcorrection, irregularity and lumpiness. However, there are no objective comparison results proving that this method is more successful.

Recently, separation by centrifugation is preferred over precipitation method, because it can saves time, concentrates the fat cells and ADSCs more significantly, avoid infections and contaminations, and fully eliminates enzymes that give negative effects on fat survival.

The latest results below suggest very interesting facts.

Ramon Y et al. reported there were no significant differences of fat survival rate between closed centrifugation technique and an operating room cotton towel technique which is used as a platform for concentrating the fat cells and separating them from fluids, oil, and debris. Histologic evaluation of the grafts revealed significantly less fibrosis within the cotton towel technique group[36].

Moreover, Min KW et al.[48] examined fat survival rates of three fat preparation methods- centrifugation, metal sieve, and cotton towel in vivo. Same with Ramon Y et al., they reported that the closed centrifugation method has no advantage over the open cotton towel technique in terms of fat graft viability and the metal sieve concentration technique is deficient as a preparation method because fat prepared by that technique has decreased survival rate and severe inflammation. What should be taken note of is that there is no difference in fat survival rate between closed centrifugation technique and cotton towel technique, and the fat harvested from centrifugation technique contains more fibrous tissues than those of cotton towel technique. To sum up, it may means that the quality of the fat grafts by cotton towel technique was better.

As seen in various research results above, more interesting research results regarding the effect of air exposure and centrifugation are expected to be reported in the future.

(3) Washing solution

The most crucial part in cell washing is that the washing process should not affect the cellular metabolism and should maintain the steady state of the cells. For washing adipocytes, normal saline solution, phosphate-buffered saline, 5% dextrose solution, and lactated Ringer's solution can be used.

Marques A et al. explained that the fat survival rate increased when the harvested fat was washed with lactated Ringer's solution due to removal of inflammation mediators which make inflammation responses of recipient[49]. Furthermore, ADSCs increased glucose consumption and lactate production in a hypoxic environment, and only exhibited osteogenic differentiation in physiologically normal to high glucose and oxygen conditions[50]. Glucose is not only used for the energy source in every cell but also has a special function in certain cells. Based on the research results, lactated Ringer's solution added to glucose can be regarded as a better washing solution for cellular protection and nutrients supply.

(4) Disaggregation

The aspirated fat contains not only single fat cells but also small tissues which are composed of fat cells and connective tissue cells. Theoretically single cells may have higher survival rate because single cells get more chance to contact with new vessels and to absorb nutrients by diffusion from peripheral tissues.

When multi-cell spheroids were cultured in vitro, all spheroids eventually reached a dormant phase with a population of approximately 10^6 cells in a diameter of 3-4mm. In the dormant spheroid, newly generated cells at the periphery balanced those lost by necrosis in the center. This shows an importance of the spheroidal size to eliminate catabolites and absorb nutrients for their survival. For reference, the distance capable of nutrient diffusion after fat grafting is within 100μm[51].

Sometimes, the harvested fat is being observed as tangled together in agglomerates, which is advised to be cut into smaller pieces with scissors. To make the agglomerated adipose tissues into single cells, it is necessary to undergo the treatment process by collagenase for enzymatic digestion.

3) Recipient bed condition

The survival rate of fat grafting can be affected by the conditions of the recipient bed such as levels of vessel distribution, mobility of facial muscle altered osmotic pressure, and presence of scar and fibrous tissue.

Guerrerosantos J et al. monitored fat graft (into cystic space and muscles) over a period of 3, 6, 9, and 12 months. According to their report, most of the fat injected into cystic space disappeared and only some fats survived near fascia, whereas 40% of the fat injected into muscle survived even after 12 months[52]. They presented evidences that there is a close relationship vessel distribution and fat survival rates in the recipient bed. And their report directly influenced the development of FAMI technique.

Carpaneda CA et al. demonstrated that the ability of grafted fat to obtain nutrition through plasmatic imbibition occur approximately 1.5±0.5 mm from the edge of the vascularized tissue and only 40% of grafted fat are viable from the graft edge at 60 days[53]. And the authors demonstrated, in subsequent study, that the percentage of fat graft viability depends on the thickness and geometric shape of the graft in the recipient bed. The grafted fat become to surrounded by a collagen capsule and ischemia occurs nearer to the core, that leads to necrosis and results in scar tissue, which eventually felt hard or lumpiness[7,41,45] as in Figure 4. Eto H et al. also suggested the fate of grafted adipocytes after nonvas-

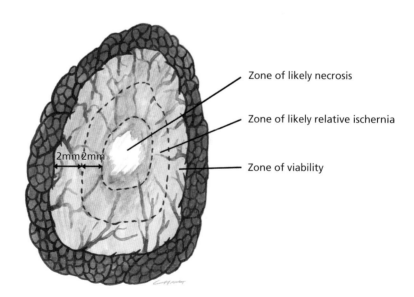

Figure 04   Fat survival depends on available oxygenated blood. Fat within 2mm of an artery will survive; more distant fat becomes necrotic and dies, leaving a cicatrix. Clinically this appears as a "lumpy bumpy" appearance and palpable contour abnormalities.

Table 02 The fate of adipocytes after nonvascularized fat grafting.

	In vitro study	In vivo study
On day – On day 1	Adipocytes are susceptable to death under ischemic conditions, meanwhile, ADSCs can remain viable for 3 days	Most adipocytes in the graft began to die on day 1
For 3 days		The number of proliferating cells increased from day 3
7 days		Increased in viable adipocytes area was detected from day 7

cularized fat grafting as shown in Table 2. They also described three zones from the periphery to the center of the graft: the surviving area, the regenerating area, and the necrotic area as an evidence of dynamic remodeling of adipose tissue after grafting as shown in Figure 5[54]. These above two research confirmed that the arterial distribution (oxygenation) is the most important factor of early engraftment of injected fat.

Recently, as the result of animal research, it has been reported that the gross weight and volume of the fat grafts and cellular integrity were considerably higher compared with control subjects in the regions for which Botulinum toxin was injected[55]. The researchers assumed that, within the first 4 days of revascularization period of grafted fat, Botulinum toxin induce immobilization of mimetic muscles and it leads to a stable contact with new vessels, peripheral vasodilatation based on the inhibition of the norepinephrine secretion and stimulates the proliferation of endothelial cells. This animal study convinces one that a concomitant use of fat grafting with Botulinum toxin produces a more effective treatment outcome for the correction of facial volume deformities. Based on this research finding, it

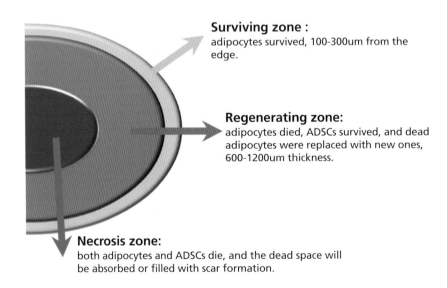

Surviving zone :
adipocytes survived, 100-300um from the edge.

Regenerating zone:
adipocytes died, ADSCs survived, and dead adipocytes were replaced with new ones, 600-1200um thickness.

Necrosis zone:
both adipocytes and ADSCs die, and the dead space will be absorbed or filled with scar formation.

Figure 05 A schematic explanation of the formation of three zones after fat grafting.

is suggested that the areas of active facial expression, such as nasolabial folds, forehead, glabella, and lips may have lower survival rate of grafted fat. The reasons are suggested as follows. First, active facial expressions may apply physical pressure to grafted fat during the process of engraftment. It may damage the fat cells directly and decreases the chance of contact with new blood vessels. Second, just after grafting, active facial movements increase the possibility of migration or agglomeration incidence of grafted fat.

When aspirated fat is injected into face, it itself constitutes to dilutional hypotonic environment in recipient bed even though isotonic Klein's solution was used for harvest. It is because Klein's solution dilutes the concentration of interstitial protein in recipient bed tissue[56]; thus, colloid osmotic pressure declines. It causes gross edema and damages adipocytes, resulting in shrinkage of grafted fat.

4) Grafting method

With the assumption that fat separation and purification is performed perfectly, the most critical step in following procedures is the injection method into recipient bed. The goal of successful injection is to maximize survival rate, by providing better blood vessel contact for the injected fats. This can be achieved by injecting the fats evenly and finely to the recipient bed's tissues.

(1) Usage of needle or cannula

In 1926, Charles Conrad Miller reported that depositing fat through hollow metal cannula resulted in a better long term correction and a more natural-appearing change in facial and body contours than fat grafting through an open incision[57]. Even though he reported good results, the technique he described never became popular since liposuctioned-fat become used for fat grafting. Until 1990, sharply pointed syringe needle (14G or 18G) was commonly used. Blunt cannula has been generally used in the late 1990s after Coleman type cannula released in the late 1990s. The most common type of cannula produced and used for injection today is also based on Coleman type cannula.

(2) Thickness of cannula

Thickness of cannula for injection is an important factor. It is designated in gauge (G) and external width in millimeter (mm), and the correlation between gauge and millimeter is described as in Table 3. Average thickness of cannula for fat grafting ranges from 14G to 19G.

Coleman SR used 17G blunt cannula connect with 1cc syringe[18]. Trepsat F reported that he used 0.33mm and 19G blunt cannula in case of fat grafting which is injected under the orbicularis oculi muscle[19]. Tzikas T reported he used a 16G bullet shaped cannula with a hole in the end to connect with 1cc syringe. He reported that this cannula prevents tissue damage because it slides smoothly when it passes through the tissue[58].

To sum up the reports above, various blunt cannulas are widely used. Nonetheless, there is still an

Table 03 The relationship between gauge (G) and milimeter(mm).

Gauge (G)	mm	Gauge (G)	mm
23G	0.6mm	18G	1.2mm
22G	0.7mm	17G	1.5mm
21G	0.8mm	16G	1.6mm
20G	0.9mm	15G	1.8mm
19G	1.0mm	14G	2.0mm

argument about the correlation between cannula thickness and the survival rate of grafted fat. Referring to Min KH et al.'s recent report, their research team harvested fat with 12G cannula and centrifuged (500g, 2 min) it. Then, they charged the harvested fat to three 1cc Luer-Lok syringes each connected with 17G, 18G, and 19G injecting cannula respectively. They passed the fats through the cannulas by regular speed (1 cc/20sec) and measured the survival rates of mature adipocytes and pre-adipocytes. They reported that there was no significant difference on the survival rate of fat passed through cannula with different sizes[59].

They concluded that, thickness of the injected fat should be within 2mm for survival through blood vessel supply and it is reasonable to use cannulas with external diameter of 1.0mm (19G) in minimum to 2mm (14G) in maximum. But it is important to pay attention that injected fat should not be coalesced and form agglomeration. I usually uses 18G cannula that is connected to 1.0 cc Luer-Slip disposable syringe. However, 19G cannula is used for intraorbital fat graftings which require fine handling.

(3) Size and shape of syringe which is connected with cannula

Internal diameter of syringe which is connected to cannula is important as well because the greater the difference in internal diameter between barrel of the syringe (include needle adaptor) and cannula, the greater the pressure is applied on the passing-through fat. 1.0cc Luer-Lok syringe is used in most cases. However, there are some points which have to be aware of when using this syringe. In case of cannula blockade by large fat agglomerations or fibrous tissues, use of excessive force increase the pressure inside the syringe and cause damages to adipocytes. Also, excessive volume may be injected into a single region abruptly. In this respect, a disposable Luer-Slip syringe instead of Luer-Lok syringe as shown in Figure 6 is more useful in preventing the problem since cannula and disposable syringe are separated when exposed to excessive pressure. Additionally, in comparison to 1.0ml Luer-Lok syringe, 1.0 ml Luer-slip syringe is more comfortable when Asian surgeons or any surgeons who have small hands perform fat injection using Baton grip technique because it is smaller with less slippery outer surface of the syringe.

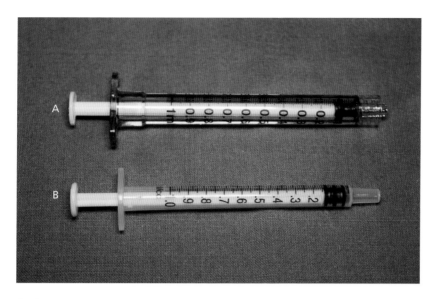

Figure 06 2 Kinds of 1.0 ml syringe for fat injection. Luer-Lok B/D syringe (A), Luer-Slip disposable syringe (B).

(4) Injection volumes per a pass

As yet there are no objective reports about how much volume should be injected when fat is injected into desired region. Merely, Fournier PF injected 0.25~0.5cc per cm by 14G needle[60] while Coleman SR recommended the grafting of 0.1~0.2ml in minimum per pass by 17G cannula, and 0.03~0.02cc for orbital or peri-orbital injection according to his clinical experience[61]. I use 1ml Luer-Slip disposable syringe with 18G blunt cannula. Around 0.06~0.1ml can be injected per pass and 10-15 passes are available with 1ml of fat using Baton grip I developed.

(5) Fine and even injection method

Even though many surgeons say that, in order to acquire the optimal survival rate, the harvested fat should be injected finely with minimal amount by several layers without contact with each other, they do not mention about a particular technique in detail. Then, the most important factor for the fine injection is being able to control while injecting the desired injection volume accurately; and it is depend on the method of holding the syringe which is connected to cannula.

The shapes of injected fat are depending on the injection method. The smaller the injected shape, the better; and discontinuous shape is more favorable compared to continuous shape with the same thickness. But, injecting discontinuous injection takes more time and it would be difficult to inject the fats in regular shapes.

When choosing the best method for injecting fats into hollow areas of a patient's face, the basis criteria is to find a method that can maximizes the surface area of transplanted fat in contact with peripheral vasculature. Injection method which is closest to the criteria above and most commonly used is "fanning-out technique". This technique inserts cannula into tissue, build numerous tunnels, and inject small fat into the built tunnels. The injections and tunnels should be intersected horizontally[62].

(6) Local or systemic approach

Also, in order to recover the facial deficiency area by fat grafting, it is important to determine whether to inject artificial filler into only that area using a simple concept of local augmentation or to inject into the whole face or several areas by considering balance of whole face, level of aging, degree of facial expression and gravity.

(7) Personal differences of surgeons

The one of the critical factors, besides the considerations mentioned above for fat injection, is the surgeon's aesthetic sense and surgical skills. It is because the survival rate and aesthetic result of surgery showed great difference among individuals.

5) Frozen fat storage

Generally, frozen fat refers to the remaining fat stored in freezer for possible future autologous fat grafting after liposuction or first fat grafting.

Tzakas TL et al. and Bertossi D et al. reported that the architecture of fats which are frozen for 12 months are maintained relatively well[41,63]. On the other hand, Lidagoster MI et al. had grafted three different groups of purified fat into laboratory animals. First group was grafted immediately after purification. Second and third group were grafted after storage in refrigerator (1°C) and freezer (-16°C) for 1-2 weeks, respectively. They reported that the fat stored in refrigerator or freezer has decreased in viable adipocytes and increased in signs of inflammation and fat necrosis[64]. Later, Pu LL et al. reported that purified fat stored in freezer with cryoprotective agent (CPA) showed greater survival rate compared to control group[65]. The result above suggested that clinical application is required as the innovative method of using frozen fat. Therefore, it is necessary to look into alteration of adipocytes by freezing and application of CPA as shown below.

Adipocytes are relatively large in size and have very thin cell membranes as if they are balloons fully filled with water. When the adipocytes are stored in freezer, sharp isocrystals will be formed if they are kept in phosphate buffered solution or normal saline solution. This isocrystals cause the death of most adipocytes due to dehydration and mechanical damage. In order to prevent the death of adipocytes, CPA that hinders isocrystal formation must be added when the remaining fat is to be stored in freezer.

Frequently used CPA are 10% dimethyl sulfoxide (DMSO), combination of 7.5% polyvinyl-pyrrolidone (PVP) and 7.5% dimethyl sulfoxide, combination of 0.5M dimethyl sulfoxide and 0.2M trehalose, and 10% glycerol[66,67]. DMSO, most frequently used CPA, has chemical poisoning effect which makes adipose tissues soft and fragile in room temperature after defrost and it is inconvenient to remove it from the defrosted tissue. Recently, trehalose, a non-reducing disaccharide of sugar presents in many organisms naturally, is known as superb CPA without poisoning effect and hence it does not have to be removed[68,69]. Nonetheless, the safety of the practical application of CPA to store frozen fat in clinic should be guaranteed through more systematic researches.

Temperature is also very important in storing frozen fat. There was a report saying that frozen fat stored in -20°C within 3 months is relatively safe and effective, but later on this temperature was reported to be insufficient[70]. A liquid nitrogen tank is more stable than a freezer when it comes to maintaining the temperature between -70~80°C for more effective storage of fat. But, fat is immediately put in the liquid nitrogen tank with addition of CPA, even though it freezes too quickly, and the freezing process itself physically can damages the cells. To minimize the physical damage, decrease 1°C per minute until it drops to -80°C. Generally, in laboratory, it is performed after 1 or 2 hours of freezer storage with CPA treatment to drop the temperature to -20°C and move the fat to freezer of -70°C before finally storing it in the liquid nitrogen tank[71]. However, the whole process is impractical to be performed in private clinics. Recently, Lee JE et al. reported their results of cell viability staining and differentiation of ADSCs after defrosting the fats stored for 1 year with or without CPA and in different temperature of freezers. The cell viability was about 30% at -20°C without CPA while it was 87% at -80°C with CPA. Moreover, ADSCs were not detected when it was frozen directly without CPA whereas the number of ADSCs was maintained at -80°C with CPA for 1 year and also differentiated into adipocytes. However, when stored in -20°C under the same condition, the number of ADSCs rapidly decreased within 1 month of storage[72].

It is necessary to carefully understand the cell viability measurement as the laboratory result and its meaning. The laboratory result of 30% of cell viability in CPA non-treated frozen fat does not mean that 30% was actually alive. This is because even though cell viability is 30%, it is common that when the cells are re-cultured, living adipocytes are hardly being found. Likewise, it is reasonable to regard that those cell are hardly living cells including stromal vascular fraction in this case. Shortly, direct grafting of frozen adipocytes which are thawed 3 or 6 months later is the same as inserting dead cell debris, resulting in various inflammation responses such as macrophage activation to eliminate them. It ultimately leads to gap filling through fibrosis. In other words, it is associated with the replacement of fibrosis instead of fat cell. This phenomenon is the reason for necrosis and inflammation in case of frozen fat grafting and also provides the evidence of scar and touchable solid lumpiness and calcification in the patient's face.

6) Additives

Addition of various substances has been attempted to enhance the survival rate of the grafted fat. There are many addictives culture medium with various growth factors such as insulin growth factors and fibroblast growth factors, hyperbaric oxygen, albumin for maintaining normal osmotic pressure, and Linger's lactate solution, insulin as selective β-1 blocker involved in adipocytes metabolism, and collagen which is a major substance of connective tissues[73-78]. They were all reported to increase survival rate of grafted adipocytes compared to the control group.

In terms of adipocytes activation, platelet rich plasma[79] and growth factors[80] are the most interesting addictives; so, they will be briefly described below.

(1) Platelet rich plasma

Platelet rich plasma (PRP) is blood plasma that has been enriched with highly concentrated platelets. PRP has been used for the purpose to heal wound with assistance of various growth factors secreted to plasma and to decrease infection, pain, and bleeding after surgery. Lately, it is also used as an additive in old skin regeneration and fat graft.

① Platelet and cytokines

Platelet or thrombocyte is one of the substances constituting blood, which contains 140-400 thousands units on average per $1mm^3$. It is present mostly in buffy coat layer after centrifugation and approximately 2-5μm in size. Platelet has no nucleus because it is developed by falling out from megakaryocytes cytosol. Thus, it is incapable of replication, and dies in 10 days[81]. Platelet has known as one of the participant in the coagulation pathway and wound healing in the past, but later found out that they also secrete numerous cytokines. The cytokines are proteins of 25,000 dalton, which were subsided in α-granule. The cytokines are small proteins (5~20 kDa) that are important in cell signaling and are in platelet α-granule. They are secreted externally by cellular activation and degranulation. Following initial extrusion, they become complete through meeting with histones and carbohydrate side chains in a wound site and resulting in "active" cytokine[82,83].

Platelet activation is performed by thrombin and calcium chloride[84], while adenosine diphosphate(ADP) is reported to directly activates platelets[85]. α-granules, which are secreted from activated platelet to cell›s exterior by degranulation, contain seven basic protein growth factors (PDGF-αβ, PDGF-ββ, TGF-1, TGF-β2, VEGF, EGF, and IGF-1)[83,86]; their functions are described in Table 4. Fibrin, fibronectin, and vitronectin – the 3 proteins acting on cell adhesion – are present in PRP along with the growth factors.

② Preparation and stabilization of platelet rich plasma

After the blood treated with anticoagulant is centrifuged, it is separated to 3 layers as shown in Figure 7. Buffy coat layer in the middle is constituting 1% of the total volume. 94% of the total platelets, 6% of the total RBC, and 1% of total WBC exist in this layer. The rest of the 6% of platelets are present in the red blood cell button which is RBC layer located just beneath the buffy coat layer. Large and young platelets mostly reside in this layer.

Table 04 **Function of the platelet-derived growth factors.**

Factor	Name	Principal source	Effects	Reference
PDGF-αβ PDGF-ββ	Platelet Derived Growth Factors	Activated thrombocytes	chemotactic effect on monocytes, neutrophils,fibroblasts, mesenchymal stem cells, and osteoblasts powerful mitogen for fibroblasts and smooth muscle cells and is involved in all three phases of wound healing, including angiogenesis, formation of fibrous tissue, and reepithelization.	86
TGF-1, TGF-β2	Transforming Growth Factors	Activated thrombocytes	mitogen for fibroblasts, smooth muscle cells, and osteoblasts. promotes angiogenesis and extracellular matrix production	87.88
VEGF	Vascular Endothelial Growth Factor	Activated thrombocytes	promotes angiogenesis and can promote healing of chronic wounds and aid in endochondral ossification	88.89
EGF	Epidermal Growth Factor	Activated thrombocytes	mitogen for fibroblasts, endothelial cells, and keratinocytes, and also is useful in healing chronic wounds	88
IGF-1	Insulin-like Growth Factor	Activated thrombocytes	regulates bone maintenance and is also an important modulator of cell apoptosis, and in combination with PDGF, can promote bone regeneration	90

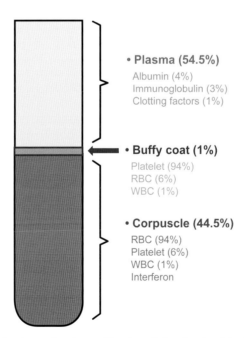

Figure 07 Distribution of separation layers for the purification of the platelet rich plasma from whole blood.

During PRP preparation, what should be taken note of is how to efficiently separate as much platelets as possible and prevent secretion of growth factors from damaged or activated platelets. Platelet damage may appear during blood and mainly due to excessive centrifugation.

General sampling process is described to concentrate platelet from autologous blood.

First, it is recommended to use needle which is thicker than 18G to prevent platelet damage or activation, which may occur by thin needle or strong suction. Blood sample should be collected from relatively large veins such as anterior cubital vein. When separating platelet, the optimal anticoagulant for platelet membrane stabilization is acid citrate dextrose (ACD-A). Separation under low gravity force is recommended[91,92]. Anticoagulant ACD-A is prepared in a syringe beforehand. It is then combined with blood drew from patient in a ratio of 10cc of blood to 1.4cc of the anticoagulant.

Double centrifugation should be performed in 2 steps as below.

First step is separation spin and separate the RBCs from plasma which contains platelet, WBCs, clotting factors. More than 95% of platelets are separated by centrifuge for 4 minutes in 1000g. After centrifugation, move upper layer's plasma, buffy coat layer, and RBC button to other tubes and do second concentration spin (8-9 minutes at 800g). To acquire high concentration of PRP, remove great amount of upper platelet poor plasma (PPP)and, to acquire low concentration of PRP, remove little amount of PPP.

When extracting 1ml of the bottom layer including buffy coat layer after primary and secondary centrifugation of 10ml of adult's blood, the average platelet number should be over 1,000,000units/$\mu\ell$ in minimum and at least 4 times more compared to the peripheral blood.

Clotting of the PRP should be done only at that time of use. Clotting activates platelets and which begin secreting stored cytokines immediately. And then they synthesize additional amount of cytokines about 8 days until they are depleted and die. So, clinicians should only clot PRP when they are ready to use.

Since developed PRP kit contains anticoagulant, the condition can be maintained until coagulation begins. It can be used in the operation or even when the operation is delayed because it can be stored at room temperature for more than 8 hours. However, it is advised not to use PRP which is stored for more than 8 hours[93].

Although the number of separated platelet is important, the viability degree is equally important. Platelet viability can be examined by P-selection test[94]. P-selectin is protein present in platelet's α particle membrane. It is detected on the surface of platelet when α particle membrane fuses with that of activated platelets[95]. Stable platelet rich plasma prepared normally has P-selectin value of 10-20% while it increases to 40-60% when reacted with ADP (Adenosine diphosphate), the platelet activator. If P-selectin value does not change even after ADP reaction, it means that the platelets are already activated or damaged.

There is another way of designating coagulation degree to % after reacting 200mg/m of collagen fibers to platelets. If the value is lower than 60%, it is evaluated to have no platelet activity[93].

③ **Platelet rich plasma use for fat grafting**

Still there are debates over the effect of injecting PRP combination to increase fat survival rate. In vitro researches report, injecting PRP combination is effective, whereas in vivo researches report yet question the effect.

For example, Nakamura S et al.[96] and Peres Fraga MF et al.[97] reported that they have better outcomes in laboratory animal research while Por YC et al.[98] reported that there were no effect after 10 days of grafting, but survival rate increased due to fine vessel development promotion 120 days after fat grafting.

On the other hand, Cervelli V et al.[99,100] reported that when PRP-combined fat was injected into facial concavity, there were enhanced survaval rate and volume maintenance compared to fat-only injection. Nevertheless, Salgarello M et al.[101] reported that there were no effects in breast augmentation.

From the reports above, it was also reported that surgery result differs depending on the ratio of injected fat and PRP. Mostly, the combination ratios of fat and PRP in various researches were 9:1 (10%)[98,101], 4:1 (20%)[96,98] and 2:1 (33%)[99,100]. Cases with ratios of 9:1 and 4:1 were reported to have no effect, whereas cases with 2:1 ratio were reported to be effective, suggesting that this concentration is appropriated[101].

It is possible that using PRP greatly affects survival in fat. But, yet there are no clear results or proofs to confirm the effects of the survival rate increase in human body researches. However, there are possibilities that PRP positively affects fat grafting as summarized below.

First of all, PRP contains albumin, globulin, fibrinogen and etc. to prevent osmotic pressure decline in recipient bed and, as a result, can provide appropriate environment for fat engraft[75,102].

Second, prior to vessel supply, transplanted adipocytes acquire nutrients by diffusion from plasma in about 48 hours after grafting.

Third, through the effects of various activators including growth factors secreted from activated platelets, healing process and angiogenesis in recipient bed will be promoted.

Fourth, some reports from practical laboratory researches[103,104] suggest that PRP positively affect angiogenesis or ADSCs proliferation. Of course, researches of PRP effects on vascular endothelium[105], bone marrow stromal cell[106], and umbilical vein endothelium[107,108]. Some also reported that there is a positive effect in 5% PRP concentration, while the proliferation decreased in 20% PRP concentration due to thrombospondin-1's oversecretion[106].

According to the results above, the potentiality of PRP for fat engraft is not skeptical. But, adipose tissue undergoes more complicated processes such as basement membrane breakdown during angiogenesis, vasculogenesis, angiogenesis, angiogenic remodeling, vessel stabilization, vascular permeability and etc. Therefore, there is a huge possibility that the effect may be restricted.

Fifth, even though the tissue-engineering application of PRP in fat grafting are not satisfactory yet, the recent research result shows that PRP improve maintenance and function of fat graft in patients who underwent plastic reconstructive surgery, possibly by stimulating adipose-tissue-derived stem cell proliferation[99,100].

④ **Contraindication in using PRP**

Platelet rich plasma is prohibited to be used to patients with platelet disorders, thrombocytopenia, anti-aggregating therapy, bone marrow aplasia, uncompensated diabetes, sepsis, cancer, osteomyelitis, and chronic or post-traumatic scar of over 50% of tissue damage in arms or legs after treatment[114].

⑤ **Platelet rich plasma separation kit**

There are various kinds of PRP separation Kits available in the market now as shown in Table 5. The table content shows the results from independent test of each company.

(2) Growth factors involved in angiogenesis

The most effective way to increase the survival rate after fat grafting is to supply new vessels to transplanted adipocytes by promoting neovascularization in recipient bed. The most definite method would be using growth factors that can promote angiogenesis[110].

There is no pure single ingredient in growth factors yet to be injected into patients for promoting angiogenesis clinically. It is currently in development and is expected to be practically applied soon. In this chapter, basic mechanism involved in angiogenesis and characteristics of the most interesting

Table 05 Various kinds of PRP kit.

	Yes PRP® Kit	Mycells® Kit	SmartPrep® 2 system	Arteriocyte Magellan®
Picture				
Company	Zizion Group, LLC	Estar Technologies Inc	Harvest Technologies Corp	Arteriocyte Medical Systems, Inc.
Type of automation	Manual	Manual	Automatic	Full automatic
Separation method	Centrifuge (1300gX9 min)	Centrifuge (1500g x10min) and Z-gel separator	Centrifuge and 2 spaces in one plasma chamber	Centrifuge
Blood Draw Volume	20ml	10-12ml	30 – 240 ml	60ml
Website	http://yesprpkit.com/	http://www.estar-medical.com/history	http://www.terumo-cvs.com/products/Product-Families.aspx?groupId=72&country=1	http://www.arteriocyte.com/

growth factors will be explained briefly.

① Development mechanism of angiogenesis

Figure 8 shows the process of vessel formation. Vasculogenesis refers to developing primary vasculature which is immature vessel, while angiogenesis refers to developing mature vessels by angiogenic remodeling. Vascular endothelial growth factor (VEGF), angiopoietin-1 (Ang-1) and ephrin-β2 (Ephβ) play pivotal roles in angiogenesis[111,112].

Among them, vascular endothelial growth factor (VEGF) is crucial for the formation and maintenance of blood vessels. It forms primary vasculature that is consisted of poorly organized immature hemorrhagic "leaky" vessel and is required to initiate the further development of immature vessels by

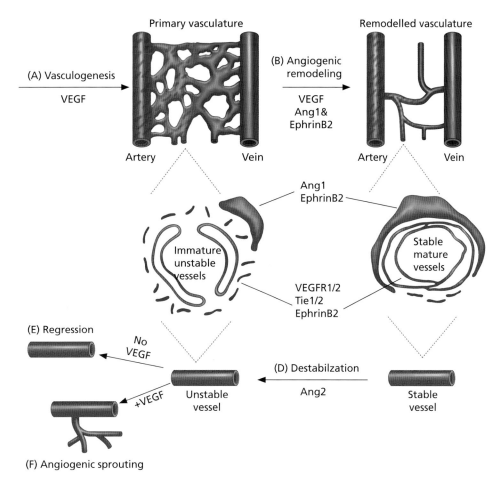

Figure 08 Schematic representation of the roles of VEGF, Ang1, Ang2 and ephrin-B2 during vessel formation. The processes include vasculogenesis (stage A), angiogenic remodelling (B), stabilization and maturation (C), destabilization (D), regression (E) and sprouting (F). An attempt is made to assign the indicated vascular growth factors to the various processes, and to indicate their expression patterns. Although not noted in the figure, expression of ephrin-B2 marks arterial vessels from the earliest developmental times.

angiogenic sprouting as new branching from premature vessels.

The angiopoietins-1 (Ang-1) seems to be one of the VEGF's most important partners. Vascular leakage is caused by either VEGF or inflammation, Ang-1 induces production of stable mature vessels that are resistant to leak. This resistance seems to be related to the ability of Ang-1 to maximize interactions between endothelial cells and their surrounding cells and matrix.

The ephrin-B2 is a necessary growth factor which apparently not only required during the earliest stages of arterial/venous determination, but also may continue to be important during the development of arteries, perhaps by regulating interactions between endothelial and smooth muscle cells involved in the formation of arterial muscular walls[117].

② **Growth factors involved in angiogenesis**

Growth factors involved in angiogenesis known are described in Table 6. The most crucial and strong growth factors are vascular Endothelial Growth factor (VEGF) and Angiopoietin-1.

Effects of growth factors involved in angiogenesis are described in Table 4. The most crucial and strong growth factors are Vascular Endothelial Growth factor (VEGF) and Angiopoietin-1 (Ang-1).

7) Causes of volume loss after fat grafting.

Possible mechanisms and theories explaining the fat graft volume loss are as follows[123].

First, in a short period of time after grafting, grafting volume is decreased due to reabsorption of tumescent solution and blood, and disappearance of edema induced by tissue damage and hyposmolarity.

Second, inflammation caused by apoptosis or extracellular lipid results in tissue fibrosis and contraction of the transplanted fat[6,124]

Third, as partially confirmed in animal studies, it was reported that the relative deficiency of ADSc may induce postoperative long-term atrophy of transplanted fat [125-128].

Fourthly, as a predictable hypothesis based on many laboratory researches [4,128-131,] the concept of cellular volume loss, or "adipocyte atrophy," by dedifferentation may play an important role in fat graft volume change after fat grafting.

Fat graft volume can be decreased according to several causes mentioned above. Are there any possible approaches to prevent the fat graft volume decrease?

Firstly, 120-130% of overcorrection has been commonly performed to compensate for volume decrease based on clinical experiences, yet there are no objective research reports to the effectiveness of overcorrection. Nevertheless, the quantity of tissues in recipient bed is the crucial factor to keep in mind in overcorrection. If the fat grafting is performed with overcorrection when recipient bed holds absolutely small volume of tissues, grafted fat will easily agglomerate together and become a large lump-like mass. Consequently, it will decrease the possibilities of the grafted fats to be in contact with neo-vasculature. So, when there is absolutely little volume in recipient bed, it is recommended to graft

Table 06 Growth factors affecting angiogenesis in adipose tissue.

Name	Effects	Reference
Vascular Endothelial Growth factor (VEGF)	The only true endothelial cell growth factor. Initiate the formation of immature vessels. Hypoxia-inducible factor (HIF). Highest in omental fat. Insulin induce VEGF induction during rebound weight gain after diet restriction.	113, 114
Angiopoietin (Ang)-1, 2	acting via the Tie-2 receptor, increases association of endothelial cells with pericytes/ vascular smooth muscle cells (VSMC) to remodel, stabilize, and mature newly formed blood vessels, whereas the angioinhibitory factors, Ang-2 and thrombospondin-1 (TSP-1), act to disassemble blood vessels.	115
Ephrin-β2/Ephβ4	Cell-to-cell interaction because it should be membrane bound form to activate.	116
Matrix metalloproteinase (MMP) MMP-2, MMP-9, TIMP	Degradation of extracellular matrix and remodeling during adipose tissue expansion.	117
Plasminogen activator inhibitor-1 (PAI-1)	Inhibit t-PA and u-PA. Influence migration of endothelial, smooth muscle cells and preadipocytes. Induced by hypoxia.	118, 119
Integrin αvβ3	participates in the activation of vascular endothelial growth factor receptor-2 (VEGFR-2), providing a survival signal to the proliferating vascular cells during new vessel growth.	120
Growth factors/Cytokines	Platelet derived growth factor(PDGF); recruits pericytes to preformed capillaries. Transforming growth factors(TGF-β1); formation of vessel tubes by modulating the synthesis of ECM(extracellular matrix). Tumor necrosis factor-α(TNF-α); endothelial cell tube formation. Fibroblast growth factor (FGF).	121, 122

small volume repeatedly.

Secondly, the best way to prevent tissue damage and bleeding during fat grafting is to monitor the surgeon's handling skill to be smooth with little force. In this respect, it is not recommended to carry out pre-tunneling before grafting. For quick recover of the damaged tissue, PRP application is a good method to be considered.

Thirdly, to prevent grafted adipocyte's death caused by ischemia, the accessibility of neighboring vessels should be enhanced by injecting small volume finely and evenly into the recipient beds. It is not exaggerated that this stage is absolutely depending on the handling skills of the surgeon. From the view of angiogenesis in recipient bed, applying angiogenetic growth factors, which are currently under development, to fat grafting is expected to have great assistance in increasing/ to greatly increase the survival rate of grafted fat.

Fourthly, it is considered that the post-operative long term atrophy induced by relative deficiency of ADSCs in transplanted lipoaspirates is sufficiently prevented by Cell-Assisted Lipotransfer (CAL) because it not only enhance survival rate but also maintain relative ratio of ADSCs and adipocyte during the replacement process of the adipose tissue.

Fifthly, if the grafted mature adipocyte has dedifferentiated in recipient bed, its cellular volume m ay be decreased and eventually the total grafted fat volume also may decrease. Fortunately, the volume of grafted fat may be maintained by dynamic equilibrium of adipocyte de-differentiation and re-differentiation in the body. At this moment the recovery of fat volume can be carried out by re-differentiation, but it depends on adipogenic condition which induces re-differentiation.

Reference

01. Kershaw EE, Flier JS. Adipose tissue as an endocrine organ. J Clin Endocrinol Metab. 2004;89: 2548-2556.

02. Neuhof H, Hirshfeld S. The transplantation of tissues. New York: D. Appleton, 1923. Pp. 1-297.

03. Peer LA. Cell survival theory versus replacement theory. Plast Reconstr Surg. (1946). 1955;16(3):161-168.

04. Von Heimburg D, Hemmrich K, Haydarlioglu S, Staiger H, Pallua N. Comparison of viable cell yield from excised versus aspirated adipose tissue. Cells Tissues Organs. 2004;178(2):87-92.

05. Wolter TP, von Heimburg D, Stoffels I, Groeger A, Pallua N. Cryopreservation of mature human adipocytes: In vitro measurement of viability. Ann Plast Surg. 2005;55(4):408-413.

06. Billings E Jr, May JW Jr. Historical review and present status of free fat graft autotransplantation in plastic and reconstructive Surgery. Plast Reconstr Surg. 1989;83(2):368-381.

07. Nguyen A, Pasyk KA, Bouvier TN, Hassett CA, Argenta LC. Comparative study of survival of autologous adipose tissue taken and transplanted by different techniques. Plast Reconstr Surg. 1990;85(3):378-86; discussion 387-389.

08. Ersek RA. Transplantation of purified autologous fat: A 3-year follow-up is disappointing. Plast Reconstr Surg. 1991;87(2):219-27; discussion 228.

09. Torio-Padron N, Huotari AM, Eisenhardt SU, Borges J, Stark GB.Comparison of pre-adipocyte yield, growth and differentiation characteristics from excised versus aspirated adipose tissue. Cells Tissues Organs. 2010;191(5):365-71. Epub 2010 Jan 14.

10. Witort EJ, Pattarino J, Papucci L, Schiavone N, Donnini M, Lapucci A, Lulli M, Lo Russo G, Mori A, Dini M, Capaccioli S. Autologous lipofilling: Coenzyme Q10 can rescue adipocytes from stress-induced apoptotic death. Plast Reconstr Surg. 2007 1;119(4):1191-1199.

11. Kuhbier JW, Weyand B, Radtke C, Vogt PM, Kasper C, Reimers K. Isolation, characterization, differentiation, and application of adipose-derived stem cells. Adv Biochem Eng Biotechnol. 2010;123:55-105.

12. Ozsoy Z, Kul Z, Bilir A. The role of cannula diameter in improved adipocyte viability: a quantitative analysis. Aesthet Surg J. 2006;26(3):287-289.

13. Carpaneda CA, Ribeiro MT. Percentage of graft viability versus injected volume in adipose autotransplants. Aesthetic Plast Surg. 1994;18(1):17-9.

14. Tonnard P, Verpaele A, Peeters G, Hamdi M, Cornelissen M, Declercq H. Nanofat grafting: basic research and clinical applications. Plast Reconstr Surg. 2013 Oct;132(4):1017-26. doi: 10.1097/PRS.0b013e31829fe1b0.

15. Moore JH Jr, Kolaczynski JW, Morales LM, Considine RV, Pietrzkowski Z, Noto PF, Caro JF. Viability of fat obtained by syringe suction lipectomy: effects of local anesthesia with lidocaine. Aesthetic Plast Surg. 1995;19(4):335-339.

16. Shoshani O, Berger J, Fodor L, Ramon Y, Shupak A, Kehat I, Gilhar A, Ullmann Y. The effect of lidocaine and adrenaline on the viability of injected adipose tissue--an experimental study in nude mice. J Drugs Dermatol. 2005;4(3):311-316.

17. Kaufman MR, Bradley JP, Dickinson B, Heller JB, Wasson K, O'Hara C, Huang C, Gabbay J, Ghadjar K and Miller TA. Autologous fat transfer consensus survey: Trends in techniques for harvest, preparation, and application, and perception of short- and long-term results. Plast Reconstr Surg. 2007;119(1):323-331.

18. Coleman SR. Structural fat grafting. Quality Medical Publishing, Inc. 2004.

19. Trepsat F. Periorbital rejuvenation combining fat grafting and blepharoplasties. Aesthetic Plast Surg. 2003;27(4):243-253.

20. Hudson DA, Lambert EV, Bloch CE. Site selection for fat autotransplantation: some observations. Aesthetic Plast Surg. 1990 14(3):195-197.

21. Rohrich RJ, Sorokin ES, Brown SA. In search of improved fat transfer viability: a quantitative analysis of the role of centrifugation and harvest site. Plast Reconstr Surg. 2004;113(1):391-395; discussion 396-397.

22. Padoin AV, Braga-Silva J, Martins P, Rezende K, Rezende AR, Grechi B, Gehlen D, Machado DC. Sources of processed lipoaspirate cells: influence of donor site on cell concentration. Plast Reconstr Surg. 2008;122(2):614-618.

23. Jurgens WJ, Oedayrajsingh-Varma MJ, Helder MN, Zandiehdoulabi B, Schouten TE, Kuik DJ, Ritt MJ, van Milligen FJ. Effect of tissue harvesting site on yield of stem cells derived from adipose tissue: implications for cell-based therapies. Cell Tissue Res. 2008;332(3):415-426.

24. Schipper BM, Marra KG, Zhang W, Donnenberg AD, Rubin JP. Regional anatomic and age effects on cell function of adipose-derived stem cells. Ann Plast Surg. 2008;60(5):538-544.

25. Nogalska A, Pankiewicz A, Goyke E, Swierczynski J. The age-related inverse relationship between ob and lipogenic enzymes genes expression in rat white adipose tissue. Exp Gerontol. 2003;38(4):415-422.

26. Zhu M, Kohan E, Bradley J, Hedrick M, Benhaim P, Zuk P. The effect of age on osteogenic, adipogenic and proliferative potential of female adipose-derived stem cells. J Tissue Eng Regen Med. 2009;3(4):290-301.

27. Hauner H, Entenmann G. Regional variation of adipose differentiation in cultured stromal-vascular cells from the abdominal and femoral adipose tissue of obese women. Int J Obes. 1991 Feb;15(2):121-6.

28. van Harmelen V, Skurk T, Röhrig K, Lee YM, Halbleib M, Aprath-Husmann I, Hauner H. Effect of BMI and age on adipose tissue cellularity and differentiation capacity in women. Int J Obes Relat Metab Disord. 2003 Aug;27(8):889-95.Aging and Regional Differences in Fat Cell Progenitors – A mini-Review

29 Cartwright MJ, Tchkonia T, Kirkland JL. Aging in adipocytes: potential impact of inherent,depot-specific mechanisms. Exp Gerontol 2007; 42: 463–471.

30 Kirkland JL, Hollenberg CH, Gillon WS. Age, anatomic site, and the replication and differentiation of adipocyte precursors. Am J Physiol 1990; 258:C206–C210.

31 Karagiannides I, Tchkonia T, Dobson DE,Steppan CM, Cummins P, Chan G, Salvatori K, Hadzopoulou-Cladaras M, Kirkland JL. Altered expression of C/EBP family members results in decreased adipogenesis with aging. Am J Physiol Regul Integr Comp Physiol 2001; 280:R1772–R1780.

32 Bertrand HA, Lynd FT, Masoro EJ, Yu BP. Changes in adipose mass and cellularity through the adult life of rats fed ad libitum or a life-prolonging restricted diet. J Gerontol 1980; 35: 827–835.

33 Spalding KL, Arner E, Westermark PO, Bernard S, Buchholz BA, Bergmann O, Blomqvist L, Hoffstedt J, Naslund E, Britton T, Concha H, Hassan M, Ryden M, Frisen J, Arner P. Dynamics of fat cell turnover in humans. Nature 2008; 453: 783–787.

34. Sepe A, Tchkonia T, Thomou T, Zamboni M, Kirkland JL. Aging and regional differences in fat cell progenitors - a mini-review. Gerontology. 2011;57(1):66-75. Epub 2010 Jan 29.

35. Aboudib Junior JH, de Castro CC, Gradel J. Hand rejuvenescence by fat filling. Ann Plast Surg. 1992;28(6):559-564.

36. Ramon Y, Shoshani O, Peled IJ, Gilhar A, Carmi N, Fodor L, Risin Y and Ullmann Y. Enhancing the take of injected adipose tissue by a simple method for concentrating fat cells. Plast Reconstr Surg. 2005;115(1):197-201; discussion 20220-3.

37. Matsumoto D, Shigeura T, Sato K, Inoue K, Suga H, Kato H, Aoi N, Murase S, Gonda K, Yoshimura K. Influences of preservation at various temperatures on liposuction aspirates. Plast Reconstr Surg. 2007;120(6):1510-1517.

38. Rose JG Jr, Lucarelli MJ, Lemke BN, Dortzbach RK, Boxrud CA, Obagi S, Patel S. Histologic comparison of autologous fat processing methods. Ophthal Plast Reconstr Surg. 2006 May-Jun;22(3):195-200.

39. Jackson IT, Simman R, Tholen R and DiNick VD. A successful long-term method of fat grafting: Recontouring of a large subcutaneous postradiation thigh defect with autologous fat transplantation. Aesthetic Plast Surg. 2001;25(3):165-169.

40. Kurita M, Matsumoto D, Shigeura T, Sato K, Gonda K, Harii K, Yoshimura K. Influences of centrifugation on cells and tissues in liposuction Aspirates: Optimized centrifugation for lipotransfer and cell isolation. Plast Reconstr Surg. 2008;121(3):1033-41; discussion 1042-1043.

41. Cook T, Nakra T, Shorr N, Douglas RS. Facial recontouring with autogenous fat. Facial Plast Surg. 2004;20(2):145-147.

42. Gutowski KA. ASPS Fat Graft Task Force. Current applications and safety of autologous fat grafts: A report of the ASPS Fat Graft Task Force. Plast Reconstr Surg. 2009;124(1):272-280.

43. Kaufman MR, Miller TA, Huang C, Roostaeian J, Wasson KL, Ashley RK, Bradley JP. Autologous fat transfer for facial recontouring: is there science behind the art? Plast Reconstr Surg 2007;119(7):2287-2296.

44. Matsudo PK, Toledo LS. Experience of injected fat grafting. Aesthetic Plast Surg 1988;12(1):35-38.

45. Niechajev I, Sevćuk O. Long term results of fat transplantation: Clinical and histologic studies. Plast Reconstr Surg. 1994 Sep;94(3):496-506.

46. Shiffman MA, Mirrafati S. Fat transfer techniques: the effect of harvest and transfer methods on adipocyte viability and review of the literature. Dermatol Surg 2001;27(9):819-826.

47. Nguyen A, Pasyk KA, Bouvier TN, Hassett CA, Argenta LC. Comparative Study of Survival of Autologous Adipose Tissue Taken and Transplanted by Different techniques. Plast Reconstr Surg. 1990 Mar;85(3):378-386; discussion 387-389.

48. Minn KW, Min KH, Chang H, Kim S, Heo EJ. Effects of fat

preparation methods on the viabilities of autologous fat grafts. Aesthetic Plast Surg. 2010 Oct;34(5):626-31. doi: 10.1007/s00266-010-9525-7. Epub 2010 May 5.

49. Marques A, Brenda E, Saldiva PH, Amarante MT, Ferreira MC. Autologous fat grafts: A quantitative and morphometric study in rabbits. Scand J Plast Reconstr Surg Hand Surg. 1994;28(4):241-247.

50. Wilson A, Butler PE, Seifalian AM. Adipose-derived stem cells for clinical applications: a review. Cell Prolif 2011;44(1):86-98. doi: 10.1111/j.1365-2184.2010.00736.x.

51. Folkman J, Hochberg M. Self-regulation of growth in three dimensions. J Exp Med. 1973;138(4):745-753.

52. Guerrerosantos J, Gonzalez-Mendoza A, Masmela Y, Gonzalez MA, Deos M, Diaz P. Long-term survival of free fat grafts in muscle: an experimental study in rats. Aesthetic Plast Surg 1996;20(5):403-408.

53. Carpaneda CA, Ribeiro MT. Study of the histological alterations and viability of the adipose graft in humans. Aesthetic Plast Surg 1993;17(1):43-47.

54. Eto H, Kato H, Suga H, Aoi N, Doi K, Kuno S, Yoshimura K. The fate of adipocytes after nonvascularized fat grafting: evidence of early death and replacement of adipocytes. Plast Reconstr Surg. 2012 May;129(5):1081-1092. doi: 10.1097/PRS.0b013e31824a2b19.

55. Baek RM, Park SO, Jeong EC, Oh HS, Kim SW, Minn KW, Lee SY. The effect of botulinum toxin A on fat graft survival. Aesthetic Plast Surg. 2012 Jun;36(3):680-6. Epub 2012 Feb 23.

56. Kaminski MV, Wolosewick JJ, Smith J. Preservation of interstitial colloid: A critical factor in fat transfer. In J. Niamtu (Ed.), Oral and MaxillofacialS urgery Clinics of North America, Vol.12, 4th Ed. Philadelphia :Saunders, 2000;Pp.631-639.

57. Miller JJ, Popp JC. Fat hypertrophy after autologous fat transfer. Ophthal Plast Resconstr Surg. 2002;18(3)228-231.

58. Tzikas TL. Lipografting: Autologous fat grafting for total facial rejuvenation. Facial Plast Surg. 2004 ;20(2):135-143.

59. Min KH, Heo CY, Lee EH, Eun SC, Chang H, Kim S, Minn KW, Park SS. Correlation analysis of injection cannula's diameter and fat cell viability in autologous fat graft. J Korean Soc Aesthetic Plast Surg. 15(1);31-34,2009.

60. Fournier PF. Fat grafting : my technique. Dermatol Surg. 2000;26(12):1117-1128.

61. Coleman SR. Structural Fat Grafting: More Than a Permanent Filler. Plast Reconstr Surg. 2006;118(3 Suppl):108S-120S.

62. Linder RM. Permanent lip augmentation employing polytetrafluoroethylene grafts. Plast Reconstr Surg. 1992;90(6):1083-90; discussion 1091-1092.

63. Bertossi D, Zancanaro C, Trevisiol L, Albanese M, Ferrari F, Nocini PF. Ultrastructural evaluation by transmission electron microscopy of injected adipose tissue. Arch Facial Plast Surg. 2003;5(5):392-398.

64. Lidagoster MI, Cinelli PB, LeveéEM, Sian CS. Comparison of autologous fat transfer in fresh, refrigerated, and frozen specimens. An animal model. Ann Plast Surg. 2000 May;44(5):512-515.

65. Pu LL, Cui X, Fink BF, Cibull ML, Gao D. Long-term preservation of adipose aspirates after conventional lipoplasty. Aesthet Surg J. 2004 Nov-Dec;24(6):536-541. doi: 10.1016/j.asj.2004.09.002.

66. Moscatello DK, Dougherty M, Narins RS, Lawrence N. Cryopreservation of human fat for soft tissue augmentation: viability requires use of cryoprotectant and controlled freezing and storage. Dermatol Surg. 2005;31:1506-1510.

67. Pu LL, Cui X, Fink BF, Gao D, Vasconez HC. Adipose aspirates as a source for human processed lipoaspirate cells after optimal cryopreservation. Plast Reconstr Surg. 2006;117:1845-1850.

68. Karlsson JO, Toner M. Long-term storage of tissues by cryopreservation: Critical issues. Biomaterials 1996;17(3):243-256.

69. Gao D, Critse JK. Mechanisms of cryoinjury in living cells. ILAR J. 2000;41(4):187-196. Review.

70. Kim YK, Park HS, Lee HJ. Studies on the proper storage period and change of -20°C cyropreserved adipocyte, J. Korean Soc Aesth Plast Surg. 2006;12(1):33-42.

71. Wolter TP, von Heimburg D, Stoffels I, Groeger A, Pallua N. Cryopreservation of mature human adipocytes: in vitro measurement of viability. Ann Plast Surg. 2005 Oct;55(4):408-13.

72. Lee JU, Kim IO, Kim MH. Adipose differentiation of human adipose tissue-drived stem cells obtained from cryopreserved adipose aspirates. Dermatol Surg 2010;36;1078-1083.

73. Huss FR, and Kratz G. Adipose tissue processed for lipoinjection shows increased cellular survival in vitro when tissue engineering principles are applied. Scand J Plast Reconstr Surg Hand Surg. 2002;36(3):166-171.

74. Shoshani O, Ullmann Y, Shupak A, Ramon Y, Gilhar A, Kehat I, Peled IJ. The role of frozen storage in preserving adipose tissue obtained by suction-assisted lipectomy for repeated fat injection procedures. Dermatol Surg. 2001 Jul;27(7):645-647.

75. Smith J, Kaminski MV Jr, Wolosewick J. Use of human serum albumin to improve retention of autologous fat transplant.

Plast Reconstr Surg. 2002 Feb;109(2):814-816.

76. Har-Shai Y, Lindenbaum ES, Gamliel-Lazarovich A, Beach D, Hirshowitz B. An integrated approach for increasing the survival of autologous fat grafts in the treatment of contour defects. Plast Reconstr Surg. 1999 Sep;104(4):945-954.

77. Yuksel E, Weinfeld AB, Cleek R, Wamsley S, Jensen J, Boutros S, Waugh JM, Shenaq SM, Spira M. Increased free fat-graft survival with the long-term, local delivery of insulin, insulin-like growth factor-I, and basic fibroblast growth factor by PLGA/PEG microspheres. Plast Reconst Surg. 2000;105(5):1712-1720.

78. Palma PC, Vidal B, Riccetto CL, Herrmann V, Dambros M, Thiel M, Netto NR Jr. Effect of purified collagen on lipograft survival: experimental basis for periurethral lipoinjections. J Endourol. 2003 May;17(4):255-259.

79. Eppley BL, Pietrzak WS, Blanton M. Platelet-rich plasma: a review of biology and applications in plastic surgery. Plast Reconstr Surg. 2006 Nov;118(6):147e-159e.

80. Yoshimura K, Sato K, Aoi N, Kurita M, Hirohi T, Harii K. Cell-assisted lipotransfer for cosmetic breast augmentation: Supportive use of adipose-derived stem/stromal cells. Aesth Plast Surg 2008;32:48-55

81. Welsh WJ. Autologous platelet gel: Clinical function and usage in plastic surgery. Cosmetic Derm. 11: 13, 2000

82. Harrison P, Cramer EM. Platelet alpha-granules. Blood Rev. 1993;7(1):52-62.

83. Eppley BL, Woodel JE, Higgins J. Platelet quantification and growth factor analysis from platelet-rich plasma: Implications for wound healing. Plast Reconstr Surg. 2004;114(6):1502-1508.

84. Tischler M. Platelet rich plasma: The use of autologous growth factors to enhance bone and soft tissue grafts. NY State Dent J 2002;68(3):22-24.

85. Kevy SV, Jacobson MS, Blasetti L, et al. Preparation of growth factor enriched autologous platelet gel. Plast Reconstr Surg. November 2006; 158e; 262. Transactions of the Society for Biomaterials 27th Annual Meeting, St. Paul, Minn. 2001; April: 24-29.

86. Weibrich G, Kleis WK, Hafner G, et al. Growth factor levels in platelet-rich plasma and correlations with donor age, sex, and platelet count. J Craniomaxillofac Surg. 2002;30(2):97-102.

87. Hosgood G. Wound healing : The role of platelet-derived growth factor and transforming growth factor-beta. Vet Surg 1993;22(6):490-495.

88. Bennett SP, Griffiths GD, Schor AM, Leese GP, Schor SL.Growth factors in the treatment of diabetic foot ulcers. Br J Surg. 2003 Feb;90(2):133-46.

89. Maes C, Carmeliet P, Moermans K, Stockmans I, Smets N, Collen D, Bouillon R, Carmeliet G. Impaired angiogenesis and endochondral bone formation in mice lacking the vascular endothelial growth factor isoforms VEGF164 and VEGF188. Mech Dev. 2002 Feb;111(1-2):61-73.

90. Spencer EM, Tokunaga A, Hunt KT. Insulin like growth factor binding protein-3 is present in the granules of platelets. Endocrinology 1993;132(3):996-1001.

91. Marx RE. Platelet-rich plasma (PRP): What is PRP and what is not PRP? Implant Dent 2001;10(4):225-228.

92 Gonshor A. Technique for producing platelet-rich plasma and platelet concentrate: Background and process. Int J Periodontics Restorative Dent 2002 ;22: 547-557.

93. Robert E Marx and Arun K Garg. Dental and craniofacial applications of platelet-rich plasma. Bae C, Park JE, Yoon GI. koonja, 2006;Pp35.

94. Blann AD, Nadar SK, Lip GY: The adhesion molecule P-selectin and cardiovascular disease. Eur Heart J 2003;24(24):2166-2179.

95. Mayadas TN, Johnson RC, Rayburn H, Hynes RO, Wagner DD. Leukocyte rolling and extravasation are severely compromised in P selectin-deficient mice. Cell 1993;74(3):541-554.

96. Nakamura S, Ishihara M, Takikawa M, Murakami K, Kishimoto S, Nakamura S, Yanagibayashi S, Kubo S, Yamamoto N, Kiyosawa T. Platelet-rich plasma (PRP) promotes survival of fat-grafts in rats. Ann Plast Surg 2010;65(1):101-106.

97. Pires Fraga MF, Nishio RT, Ishikawa RS, Perin LF, Helene A Jr, Malheiros CA. Increased survival of free fat grafts with platelet-rich plasma in rabbits. J Plast Reconstr Aesthet Surg 2010;63(12):e818-822. Epub 2010 Aug 13.

98. Por YC, Yeow VK, Louri N, Lim TK, Kee I, Song IC. Platelet-rich plasma has no effect on increasing free fat graft survival in the nude mouse. J Plast Reconstr Aesthet Surg. 2009;62(8):1030-1034. Epub 2008 Jun 11.

99. Cervelli V, Palla L, Pascali M, De Angelis B, Curcio BC, Gentile P. Autologous platelet-rich plasma mixed with purified fat graft in aesthetic plastic surgery. Aesthetic Plast Surg. 2009 Sep;33(5):716-721. Epub 2009 Jul 9.

100. Cervelli V, Gentile P, Scioli MG, Grimaldi M, Casciani CU, Spagnoli LG, Orlandi A. Application of platelet-rich plasma in plastic surgery: clinical and in vitro evaluation. . Tissue Eng Part C Methods. 2009 Dec;15(4):625-34. doi: 10.1089/ten.

TEC.2008.0518.

101. Salgarello M, Visconti G, Rusciani A. Breast fat grafting with platelet-rich plasma: a comparative clinical study and current state of the art. Plast Reconstr Surg. 2011 Jun;127(6):2176-2185.

102. Smith J, Kaminski MV Jr, Wolosewick J. Use of human serum albumin to improve retention of autologous fat transplant. Plast Reconstr Surg. 2002 Feb;109(2):814-816.

103. Kakudo N, Minakata T, Mitsui T, Kushida S, Notodihardjo FZ, Kusumoto K. Proliferation-promoting effect of platelet-rich plasma on human adipose-derived stem cells and human dermal fibroblasts. Plast. Reconstr Surg. 2008;122:1352-1360.

104. Abuzeni PZ, Alexander RW. Enhancement of autologous fat transplantation with platelet rich plasma. Am J Cosm Surg 2001;18:59-70.

105, Eppley BL, Pietrzak WS, Blanton M. Platelet-rich plasma: A review of biology and applications in plastic surgery. Plast Reconstr Surg. 2006;118:147e-159e.

106 Hu Z, Peel SA, Ho SK, Sa´ndor GK, Clokie CM. Platelet-rich plasma induces mRNA expression of VEGF and PDGF in rat bone marrow stromal cell differentiation. Oral Surg Oral Med Oral Pathol Oral Radiol Endod. 2009;107:43-48.

107. Rughetti A, Giusti I, D'Ascenzo S, Leocata P, Carta G, Pavan A, Dell'Orso L, Dolo V. Platelet gel-released supernatant modulates the angiogenic capability of human endothelial cells. Blood Transfusion. 2008 Jan;6(1):12-17.

108. Giusti I, Rughetti A, D'Ascenzo S, Millimaggi D, Pavan A, Dell'Orso L, Dolo V.Identification of an optimal concentration of platelet gel for promoting angiogenesis in human endothelial cells. Transfusion. 2009 Apr;49(4):771-8. doi: 10.1111/j.1537-2995.2008.02033.x. Epub 2008 Dec 23

109. Pietro Gentile and Valerio Cervelli. Autologous platelet-rich plasma: Guidelines in plastic surgery. Plast Reconstr Surg. 2010;126(5)269e.

110. Hausman GJ, Richardson RL. Adipose tissue angiogenesis, J Anim Sci 2004. 82(3):925-934. http://jas.fass.org/cgi/content/full/82/3/925.

111. Yancopoulos GD, Davis S, Gale NW, Rudge JS, Wiegand SJ, Holash J. Vascular-specific growth factors and blood vessel formation. Nature. 2000 Sep 14;407(6801):242-248.

112. Karamysheva AF. Mechanisms of Angiogenesis, ISSN 0006-2979, Biochemistry (Moscow), 2008, Vol. 73, No. 7, pp. 751-762. © Pleiades Publishing, Ltd., 2008.

113. Ferrara N. Vascular endothelial growth factor: Basic science and clinical progress. Endocri Rev. 2004;25:581-611.

114. Shibuya M. Vascular endothelial growth factor-dependent and-independent regulation of angiogenesis (mini review). BMB reports 2008; 41(4): 278-286.

115. Bonagura TW, Aberdeen GW, Babischkin JS, Koos RD, Pepe GJ, Albrecht ED. Divergent Regulation of Angiopoietin-1 and -2, Tie-2, and Thrombospondin-1 Expression by Estrogen in the Baboon Endometrium. Mol Reprod Dev. 2010 ; 77(5): 430--438. doi:10.1002/mrd.21163.

116. Wang HU, Chen ZF, Anderson DJ. Molecular distinction and angiogenic interaction between embryonic arteries and veins revealed by ephrin-B2 and its receptor Eph-B4. Cell 1998;93(5):741-753.

117. Chavey C, Mari B, Monthouel MN, Bonnafous S, Anglard P, Van Obberghen E, Tartare-Deckert S. Matrix metalloproteinases are differentially expressed in adipose tissue during obesity and modulate adipocyte differentiation. J Biol Chem 2003 ;278(14):11888-11896. Epub 2003 Jan 15.

118. Hoover-Plow J, Ellis J, Yuen L. In vivo plasminogen deficiency reduces fat accumulation. Thromb Haemost. 2002 Jun;87(6):1011-1019.

119. Morange PE, Bastelica D, Bonzi MF, Van Hoef B, Collen D, Juhan-Vague I, Lijnen HR. Influence of t-pA and u-PA on adipose tissue development in a murine model of diet-induced obesity. Thromb Haemost 2002 ;87(2):306-310.

120. Soldi R, Mitola S, Strasly M, Defilippi P, Tarone G, Bussolino F: Role of alphavbeta3 integrin in the activation of vascular endothelial growth factor receptor-2. EMBO J 1999;18(4):882-92.

121. Pandya NM, Dhalla NS, Santani DD. Angiogenesis--a new target for future therapy. Vascul Pharmacol 2006 ;44(5):265-274. Epub 2006 Mar 20.

122. Bhadada SV, Goyal BR, Patel MM. Angiogenic targets for potential disorders. Fundam Clin Pharmacol. 2011 Feb;25(1):29-47. doi: 10.1111/j.1472-8206.2010.00814.x.

123. Tholpady SS, Aojanepong C, Llull R, Jeong JH, Mason AC, Futrell JW, Ogle RC, Katz AJ. The cellular plasticity of human adipocytes. Ann Plast Surg. 2005 ;54(6):651-656.

124. Hausberger FX. Quantitative studies on the development of autotrans plants of immature adipose tissue of rats. Anat Rec 1955;122(4):507-515.

125. Mastumoto D, Sato K, Gonda K, Takaki Y, Shigeura R, Sato T et al. Cell-assisted lipotransfer: supportive use of human adiposederived cells for soft tissue augmentation with lipoinjection. Tissue Eng. 2006;12:3375–3382.

126. Masuda T, Furue M, Matsuda T. Novel strategy for soft tis-

sue augmentation based on transplantation of fragmented omentum and preadipocytes. Tissue Eng. 2004;10:1672-1683.

127. Moseley TA, Zhu M, Hedrick MH. Adipose-derived stem and progenitor cells as fillers in plastic and reconstructive surgery. Plast Reconstr Surg. 2006;118(3 Suppl):121S-128S.

128. Sugihara H, Yonemitsu N, Miyabara S, Yun K: Primary cultures of unilocular fat cells: characteristics of growth in vitro and changes in differentiation properties. Differentiation. 1986;31(1):42-49.

129. Sugihara H, Yonemitsu N, Miyabara S, Toda S. Proliferation of unilocular fat cells in the primary culture. J Lipid Res, 1987;28(9):1038-1045.

130. Tavassoli M. In vivo development of adipose tissue following implantation of lipid-depleted cultured adipocyte. Exp Cell Res. 1982;137(1):55-62.

131. Green H, Kehinde O. An established preadipose cell line and its differentiation in culture. II. Factors affecting the adipose conversion. Cell 1975;5(1):19-27.

132. Mastumoto D, Sato K, Gonda K, Takaki Y, Shigeura R, Sato T et al. Cell-assisted lipotransfer: supportive use of human adipose derived cells for soft tissue augmentation with lipoinjection. Tissue Eng. 2006;12:3375–3382.

Concept of stem cell and adipose-derived stem cells

Recently, medical application of stem cell is rapidly growing. The use of adipose-derived stem cells (ADSCs) in autologous fat grafting has become more popular to increases survival rate and longevity of grafted fat and some positive results have been reported on the use of ADSCs. Therefore, I would like to briefly introduce basic concepts of stem cell and ADSCs which need to know as a cosmetic surgeon

1 Stem cell

1) Definition

Stem cell is a type of nucleated cell which has self-renewal ability with multipotency to proliferate and possess division and differentiation ability turned into a cell has another function. It can continue normal self-regeneration in particular part of the body where be threatened for survival of organ or damage by senescence.

2) Differentiation

The primitive totipotential stem cells that differentiated into monopotential stem cells which maintain certain tissues[1]. Zygote fertilized by sperm and ovum is the first totipotential stem cell and it cleavages to blastomeres to form morula and then blastocyst. Morula forms blastocyst which contains inner cell mass which will become embryo, and outer cell mass which will become placenta. The two

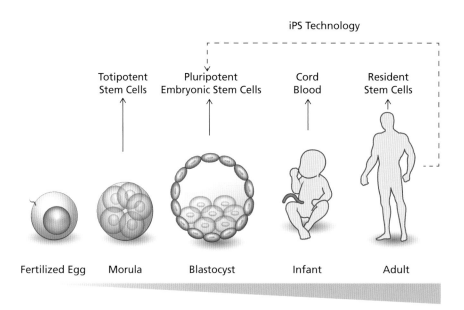

iPS Technology

Totipotent Stem Cells · Pluripotent Embryonic Stem Cells · Cord Blood · Resident Stem Cells

Fertilized Egg · Morula · Blastocyst · Infant · Adult

Figure 01 Stem cells and the different developmental stages of life.

cell masses have irreversible fate and become pluripotent stem cells since then as shown in Figure 1.

The pluripotent stem cells differentiate into ectoderm, mesoderm and endoderm and develop into cells that constitute tissues and organs originating from each germ layer to become multipotent stem cells. Each germ cell is made in each of the germ layers and become monopotent stem cells which differentiate into particular organs developed from each germ layer as shown in Table 1.

Recently, iPS technology was innovatively developed by Takahashi and Yamanaka in 2006[2]. They produced embryonic stem cell like "induced pluripotent stem" (iPS) cell. Adult somatic cells can be reprogrammed into iPS cells by activation of four transcription factors. And then those cell can be de-differentiated into all the embryonic lineages: ectoderm, mesoderm, and endoderm as shown in Figure 2. Although the iPS cells stood out as new stem cells, which would overcome ethical controversy of

Table 01 Stem cells in differentiation cascade

Stem cell	Description	Example
Totipotent	Give rise to both embryo and placenta	Zygote, first blastomere, somatic nuclear transferred enucleated oocytes.
Pleuripotent	Give rise to all three germ later	Inner cell mass of blastocyte, epiblast, blastocyst derived from embryonic stem cells
Multipotent	Differentiate into one of ectoderm, mesoderm or endoderm	Mesenchymal stem cells, hematopoietic stem cells, neural stem cells
Monopotent	Give rise to cells of one lineage	Epidermal stem cells, liver stem cells

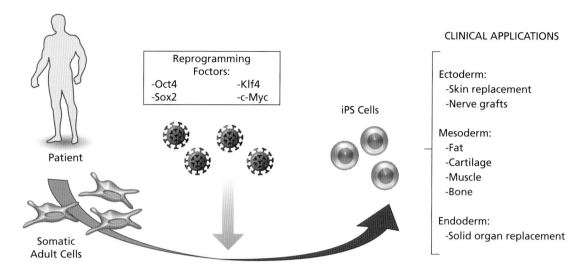

Figure 02 A schematic illustration of iPS technology.

embryonic stem cell and biological limit of the adult stem cell's division and differentiation, there remains a problem of causing cancer by host DNA alteration due to retrotranscriptional virus vector and some genes.

For reference, in stem cell research, somatic nuclear cell transfer was used before multipotent stem cell inducing method. Blastocyte (embryonic stem cell: ES cell) can be produced by transferring nuclei from postnatal somatic cells into an enucleated ovum. It would then allow the design of novel therapies as shown in **Figure 3**. Dolly the cloned sheep was born in this principle[3]. This stem cell has advantage of high proliferation rate and differentiation ability, yet is greatly restricted due to ethical

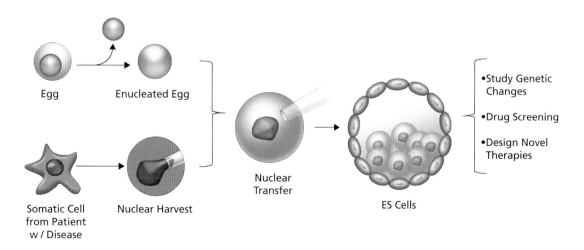

Figure 03 A schematic illustration of somatic nuclear cell transfer.

controversy that extracting cells by destroying embryo which is regarded as a living organism, immunological problems between different organisms, and possibility of becoming teratoma during transplantation.

Many experts today prefer iPS technology over somatic nuclear cell transfer method, and are looking forward to iPS technology which will possibly satisfy present standards and many restrictions of using human embryonic stem cell in regenerative medical field[4].

3) Types

Stem cells are classified to embryonic stem cells and adult stem cells by the acquired time.

• Embryonic stem cells

Embryonic stem cells are derived from the inner cell mass of blastocyte during embryonic period, and refer to stem cells which are capable of differentiating into any tissue constituting body. But the most fatal problem is that the embryo must be killed to obtain ES cell. This brings up the major key issue in bioethical controversy.

• Adult stem cells

Adult stem cells are multipotent stem cells which are considerably differentiated. They are derived from umbilical cord blood after birth, placenta, infant and adult. They have the advantage of avoiding bioethical controversy involved with fetal tissue harvest, but limited division and differentiation are pointed out as drawbacks yet. This stem cell group can be categorized into bone marrow stem cells and mesenchymal stem cells.

International society for cellular therapy defined mesenchymal stem cells by three requirements in minimum as in Table 2[5,6]. Mesenchymal stem cells are derived from bone marrow[7,8], umbilical cord[9], adipose tissue[10,11] and etc.

From them, adipose tissue is the most convenient area for mesenchymal stem cell harvest. Requirements fulfilling ADSCs as successful clinical material in using mesenchymal stem cells in regenerative application is as in Table 3[1,12].

Table 02 Definition of mesenchymal stem cell by the mesenchymal and tissue stem cell committee of the international society for cellular therapy.

1) They are plastic-adherent when maintained in standard culture condition.
2) They express the surface markers CD73, CD90/CD105, and lack expression of CD14/CD34/CD45, CD11b/CD79, and CD19/HLA-DR.
3) They are capable of differentiation into osteoblast, chondrocyte, and adipocytes in vitro.

Table 03 The adipose tissue–derived stem cells in particular fulfill several requirements proposed for successful clinical use in regenerative applications.

1. They should be found in abundant quantities (up to billions of cells).
2. They should be harvested with a minimally invasive procedure.
3. They should be able to differentiate along multiple cell lineage pathways in a controllable and reproducible manner.
4. They should be safely and effectively transplanted into an autologous or allogeneic host.
5. They can be manufactured in accordance with good manufacturing practice guidelines.

According to the conditions above, among mesenchymal stem cells, adipose-derived stem cells (ADSCs) have more advantages than bone marrow stem cells. Thus application of ADSCs with related field is expected to grow continuously.

2 Adipose-derived stem cells(ADSCs)

1) Definition and characteristics

Adipose-derived stem cells (ADSCs) are one kind of adult stem cells, which are mononuclear cell population derived from processing adipose tissues. ADSCs grow in plastic adherent manner in culture disc during cell culture, and have diverse differentiation ability into not only adipocytes but also myocytes, chondrocytes, nerve cells, vascular endothelial cells and osteocytes, thus are actively ap-

Table 04 Clinical implications of tissue engineering in relation to cell-specific differentiation programs of adipose-derived stem cells.

Type of differentiation	Clinical implications
Adipogenic	Breast soft tissue reconstruction after tumor surgery for breast cancer, breast asymmetry, and soft tissue and subdermal defects after trauma, surgery, or burn injury
Chondrogenic	Cartilage repair in joint and disc defects, plastic reconstruction of ear and nose defects
Osteogenic	Skeletal regeneration of inherited and tumor- or trauma-induced bone defects
Myogenic	Tissue reconstruction after trauma and surgery, dystrophic muscle disorders
Cardiomyogenic	Heart muscle regeneration, functional improvement after myocardial infarction, heart failure
Vascular/endothelial	Neovascularization, ischemic diseases
Neurogenic	Brain injury, stroke, peripheral nerve injury
Pancreatic/endocrine	Insulin-secreting cells, type 1 diabetes mellitus
Hepatic	Chronic liver failure, hepatic regeneration, hepatocyte transplantation
Hematopoietic	GVHD(graft-versus-host disease), bone marrow support

plied in tissue engineering as shown in Table 4[13]. In the beginning, ADSCs were classified as fibroblasts but later were classified as preadipocytes, vascular endothelium, pericytes and etc., and subsequently they were all reported to have functions as stem cells.

ADSCs have characteristics of surface markers as in Table 5[13]. They increase angiogenesis, capillary density, and blood supply in the early stages of fat grafting. They are also reported to act as preadipocytes themselves and differentiate into adipocytes to increase survival rate protractedly[14-16]. These cells reside plentifully in both floating fatty portion and infranatant fluid portion of liposuction aspirates. When stromal vascular fraction (SVF) is separated from them by collagenase and centrifugation, ADSCs will be included in the fraction.

Table 05 Minimal prerequisite expression of surface markers and genes for adipose-derived stem cells (ADSCs).

ADSC-positive cellular markers and genes	ADSC-negative cellular markers and genes
CD73	CD11b
CD90	CD14
CD105	CD19
-	CD34
-	CD45
-	CD79α
-	HLA-DR
-	c-kit

Note that all of the gene and surface marker expression profiles apply to in vitro-expanded cells, not primary cells. Abbreviations: ASMA, smooth muscle cell-specific alpha actin; ATMSC, adipose tissue-derived mesenchymal stem cells; HLA, human leukocyte antigen.

2) Nomenclature

Stem cells acquired from adipose tissue were designated as various names as below.

- Adipose derived stem/stromal cells (ASCs)
- Adipose-derived adult stem (ADAS) cells
- Adipose-derived adult stromal cells
- Adipose-derived stromal cells (ADSCs)
- Adipose stromal cells (ASCs)
- Adipose mesenchymal stem cells (AdMSCs)
- Lipoblast, Pericyte, Preadipocyte, Processed lipoaspirate (PLA) cells

The term "adipose derived stem cell (ADSC)" which is being used today was designated in annual academy (2nd annual meeting) of International fat applied technology society (IFATS) held in Pittsburgh in 2004[17]. Those cells were first named processed lipoaspirate cells but are now more commonly called ADSCs (or ASCs, which can be confused with ASCs for adult stem cells)

3) Body distribution and amount

Of the various adipose tissues distributed in human body, the most abundant of stem cells are in white adipose tissues. In particular, the stem cell ratio is diverse depending on the areas of body where the white adipose tissues are located. Arm is reported to have higher stem cell ratio compared to thigh, abdomen and etc[16,18].

4) Principle of applying ADSCs to fat grafting

Yoshimura K et al. reported that Cell-Assisted Lipotransfer(CAL) method which adds ADSCs in fat grafting as shown in Figure 4[19,20], showed significantly increased survival rate(approximately 70%) and longevity compared to previous methods which did not add ADSCs[21]. The CAL method was based on the backgrounds of the following research results.

As partially confirmed in animal studies, the results explained that relative deficiency of ADSCs (approximately half in number) in aspirated fat compared to excised whole fatmay induce postoperative long-term atrophy after fat grafting.

There are three main reasons for this relative deficiency. First, a major portion of the ADSCs is located around large vessels and left in the donor site after liposuction. Second, a part of the ADSCs is

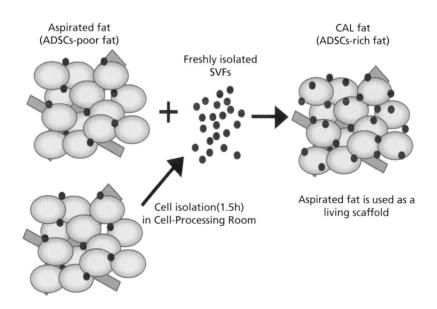

Figure 04　Schematic explanation of cell-assisted lipotransfer (CAL).

released into the fluid portion of liposuction aspirates. Third is mechanical injury during liposuction procedure and digestion by endogenous proteases during the surgery or subsequent storage periods [15,20,22,23].

As summarized in Figure 4, ADSCs-poor aspirated fat was converted to ADSCs-rich aspirated fat by supplementing ADSCs isolated from the other half of the aspirated fat. As a result, the ratio of adipocyte and ADSCs in adipose tissue be grafted was nearly same as that of the patient's body [15,19].

Then what actions ADSCs do after grafting? From recent research results, some confirmed the roles of ADSCs are confirmed explained as below.

First, ADSCs are involved in tissue regeneration by self-produced differentiation into adipocytes [20].

Second, ADSCs are reported to have possibility of differentiating into vascular endothelium or pericytes [22,24,25].

Third, hypoxia condition in the acute phase after fat grafting may accelerate releasing of angiogenic soluble factors such as VEGF and HGF [26].

Fourth, surgical injury accompanying the grafting, subsequent hypoxia condition and wound healing process appear to trigger ADSCs differentiation into adipocytes, vascular endothelial cells, and mural cells [27].

Fifth, ADSCs are reported to increase fat survival rate by preventing fibrosis and fat necrosis through differentiating into endothelium when grafted together with adipocytes [28].

Sixth, according to recent and more detailed result, ADSCs are reported to differentiate into adipocytes and also maintain the adipocytes survival by preventing apoptosis by expressing VEFG and IGF-1 which are angiogenic growth factors [29].

On the other hand, along with the results above, ADSCs role of maintaining the numeral ratio of ADSCs and adipocytes is emphasized. After fat grafting, most of the mature adipocytes which were grafted into body die and the dead adipocytes signal nearby ADSCs to induce new adipocyte production. The presence of adequate number of ADSCs to respond to the signal is very important matte rbecause if the number of stem cells is relatively few, the dead adipocytes' signals cannot be delivered [30]. This also may affect the coming turnover of the fat tissue.

According to the research above, CAL is expected to have great possibility of developing the fat grafting procedure through improvement of survival rate, longevity and complexity of predicting results which were pointed out as the biggest problems.

5) Concept and hypotheses about ADSCs

(1) Differentiation concept

Differentiation concept is based on the survival theory and refers to adipocyte production by differentiation of ADSCs and tissue-specific resident stem cells. ADSCs present in grafted tissue, act as preadipocytes and produce new adipocytes through differentiation[31]. Also, besides embryonic stem cells and mesenchymal stem cells, tissue-specific resident stem cells are found in every tissue and organ[32]. These stem cells reside in the most optimal characteristic location and maintain multipotency by the complex environmental stimuli[33]. They are reported to have function of regenerating damaged tissue and maintaining stable state by self-renewal and differentiation along the organism's whole lifespan[32,34]. The tissue-specific stem cells are studied well in skin. In the case of epidermal stem cells, they undergo cell division in two ways as shown in **Figure 5**[35]. Based on the concepts above, grafted adipose tissue or tissue-specific stem cells in host also produce new adipocytes and ADSCs by the process explained above.

(2) De-differentiation theory

De-differentiation theory is also based on the survival theory. Recently, there is a concept which suggests that some grafted mature adipocytes may undergo de-differentiation again. In other words, the concept proposed that differentiated mature cells might undergo proliferation again, where proliferation means the increase of cell number and de-differentiation means adipocytes differentiate into stem cells[36]. In easier words, the stem cells differentiated into mature cells normally lose proliferation capability but, caused by some unknown reasons, they turn into the stem cells have proliferation capability in increased number.

The de-differentiation process of mature adipocytes is simply explained in **Figure 6**[37]. SVF and mature adipocytes can be acquired from adipose tissue by enzyme digestion respectively. When they are put in the culture disc, SVF precipitate and adhere to the bottom of the tissue culture flask due to their heavy weight and adherence property of stem cell to plastic surface of the flask, whereas mature adipocytes float on the upper surface. During ceiling culture, the mature adipocytes attached to the upper surface of the flask followed by conversion to flattened fibroblast-like dedifferentiated fat (DFAF)

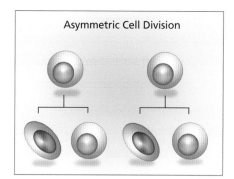 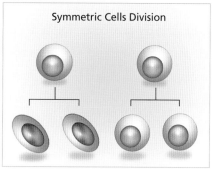 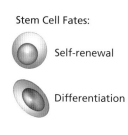

Figure 05 Two possible ways of epidermal cell division in differentiation.

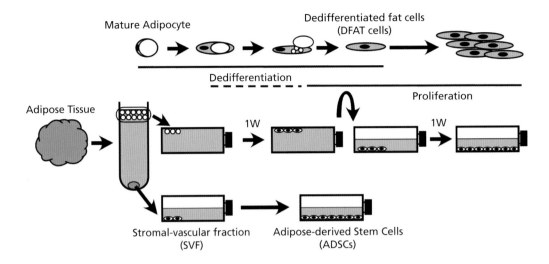

Figure 06 Dedifferentiation of mature adipocytes by conventional ceiling culture methods. 1 W : 1 week.

cells without intracellular lipid. The DFAT cells were cultured at inverted flasks under conventional methods. According to the series of research results, there is possibility that even after grafting, mature adipocytes may become stem cells by de-differentiation in the presence of appropriate culture conditions[37]. Nevertheless, there are not many people who completely approve this hypothesis.

(3) Re-differentiation hypothesis

When DFAT cell is exposed to certain adipogenic growth condition, it is able to re-accumulate intracytoplasmic lipid droplets and eventually become the mature adipocyte again. It is called re-differentiation. Von Heimburg D et al[38]. supported the possibility of this concept through the below interesting animal study. When tissue expanders were placed within the inguinal fat pad of rats, the tissue expanded fat pads had lost over half of their original volume, and the adipocytes had become DFAT cells (become atrophied fat pad). The atrophied expanded fat pads were then auto-grafted to a distant location in the same animal. Interestingly, after the grafting, they regained their previous volume.

(4) Possibility of allogenic ADSCs grafting

Comparing autologous and allogenic ADSCs, the autologous ADSCs are certainly more reasonable because there are more advantages from the view of better regulatory, histocompatibility and infection prevention. However, it lacks of human lymphocyte antigen (HLA-DR) and does not induce alloactivity of incompatible lymphocytes in vitro. It also has immune suppression function which suppresses mitogen-induced mixed lymphocyte reaction and lymphocyte proliferative response ex vivo[39]. Also when compared to freshly isolated ADSCs, passaged isolated ADSCs are known to have characteristics of decreased expression of surface histocompatibility and no longer stimulate mixed lymphocyte reaction[13]. This immunosuppression of ADSCs decreases tissue rejection during allogenic ADSCs grafting, hence strongly implies the strong possibility of allogenic ADSCs grafting bu tsafety cannot be completely excluded.

6) Future solutions in order to use ADSCs

1. Quality controlled stem cell extraction method should be established, furthermore, there should be made to find away to acquire larger amount of stem cells.

2. Qualified and safe culture medium should be developed. Since various growth factors are needed for cell growth, human serum is the principle cell culture medium. However, fetal bovine serum is being used currently instead of it. It will be valuable to develop a serum protein free culture medium to avoid issues related to bovine spongiform encephalopathy or other xenogeneic infections.

3. Controlled ADSCs storage condition should be established. There are still problems of how to store ADSCs, what kind of containers should be used, how to designate them, how to move them to the needed place, how long the storage lifespan should be determined and etc.

4. How long should ADSCs be cultured in vitro is also a problem because it can develop into cancer in prolonged period. It is also confirmed that malignant transformation occurs in ADSCs cultured for more than 4 months ex vivo[40].

5. Although there is no distinct relation yet, it is necessary to have definite research for possibility and further risk of cancer recurrence in recipient bed area when ADSCs is grafted to patients who have malignant cancer history in the past or have certain areas treated with radiotherapy[41]. In other words, there is yet no information of over 5 to 10 years that could consider safety when ADSCs are applied in clinic. It should at least be proved first by appropriate animal experiments.

7) Basic equipment necessary for stem cell and its related research

Table 6 shows the types and usages of basic equipments for culturing stem cell and its researches at laboratory level. Besides, there are additional equipments as requirements: culture roomequipped with facilities to maintain constant temperature, moisture, and antibacterial condition and with inverted microscope; micropipette; culture box, and centrifuge tube etc.

8) Extraction method of ADSCs

Extracting ADSCs means the separation of stromal vascular fraction (SVF) from fat aspirates, because SVF includes mesenchymal stem cells such as endothelial cells, immune cells, preadipocytes and etc.

While harvesting adipose tissue by liposuction, adipocytes are not extracted as a single cell but a mixture of small tissue particles and adipocytes, where ADSCs are located in the stroma of adipose tissue. Therefore, to obtain ADSCs from fat aspirates, it is required to separate stromal ADSCs from

Table 06 Basic and essential instruments for the stem cell culture[42].

Instrument	Picture	Function and Performance
(a) Clean bench		It has a filter (HEPA filter, etc.) which can purify extremely small particles by generating vertical laminar flow of air in physically-isolated box structure. It satisfies temperature, moisture, CO_2 concentration, cleanness condition in particle or bacteria-free environment, Thus; it is devised to control without dispersing particle, microorganisms, gene, DNA etc. It is an essential for living cell culture in hospital's operation room and genetic engineering laboratory.
(b) CO_2 incubator		It is a box-like incubator to culture organisms or their part (e.g. cells) in regular temperature. It is installed with a controlling device to maintain fixed internal temperature, moisture, and CO_2 concentration. It is generally used for bacterial culture in microbiological field. It is also called CO_2 pyrostat because it is designed to keep fixed CO_2 concentration for animal cell culture.
(c) Shaker		It is an instrument which shakes the contents in container in regular speed in order to regularly mix or extract certain reagent in room or certain temperature.
(d) Constant temperature water bath		This is installed with temperature controlling device to maintain a certain degree of temperature. It keeps precise constant-temperature; thus, is used for enzymatic reaction, lipid assay, and solvent extraction, culture in medicine, clinical pathology, pharmacology and microbiology. Some products are installed with shaker inside the bath.
(e) Autoclave		This refers to a sterilizer which uses pressure of 1.0~1.1kg/cm^2 (approximately 15 pounds/$inch^2$, 2 atmC), and heats for 120~121°C for 15~20minutes, utilizing high-pressure vapor. It is composed of iron structure to bare high pressure, vapor generator, and electrical heater.
(f) Drying oven		It is an instrument which dries the object by heating, vacuum and circulating heat wave. It can be used to remove moisture of instrument, reagents, drugs, or volatile substance. It is also used to quantitate moisture, and for sterilization as in the case of heating. It is called constant-temperature drying oven if it maintains the fixed temperature.
(g) Vortex mixer		By using the rapid vortex-like vibration, it mixes solution in a small container. It is composed of electrical motor main body and rubber part which is concave as a cup shape.

(h) Liquid nitrogen storage tank		Liquid nitrogen is generated by compressing clean air in 200kg/cm², and liquefying after cooling by adiabatic expansion, and finally being separated from oxygen in rectifying tower. 1kg of liquid nitrogen evaporates in -196C° and takes 48kcal (47.65kcal) of latent heat from surroundings. Using this latent heat, moisture in handling material turns into delicate ice crystals. This does not harm cytoplasm and also suppress oxygen reactivity, maintaining genetic moiety of cell. It also enables the prolonged storage period and recovery by sudden defrosting.
(i) Centrifuge		It is used to separate, concentrate, wash, and purify substances, cellular, or tissue matter that vary in components or weight by using centrifugal force.
(j) Particle meter		It measures concentration of particles in laboratory or inside of clean bench to measure the contamination degree of the space.

small adipose tissue particles. There are two methods, enzymatic and non-enzymatic, commonly used for ADSCs isolation. For enzymatic isolation method, proteolytic enzyme such as collagenase or trypsin are used to digest adipose tissue. And for non-enzymatic isolation method, physical forces such as shear force, centrifugal force, radiation force, and pressure etc. are used to separate the cells or cell aggregates from adipose tissue.

Aronowitz JA et al. reported an overview of differences between enzymatic and non-enzymatic SVF

Table 07 Mechanical vs enzymatic methods for isolation of ADSCs.

	Enzymatic	Non-enzymatic	Reference
Principle of method	Collagenase digestion	Washing, shaking, filtration, vibrating, centrifugation, ultrasonic stimulation	41
Processing time	30-120 min	15-30 min	42
Total nucleated cells/cc lipoaspirate	350,000	10,000	43
	240,000	12,000	44
	480,000	25,000	45
	368,000	140,000	46
SVF content(%)*	15	5	42
CD34⁺ progenitor deficiency	-	+	47
Viability (%)	57-90	65-90	41
Cost (equipment or disposables)	High	Low	41

*=Number of SVF/Number of total nucleated cellX100

isolation systems (Table 7) as follows[41].

First, mechanical techniques, such as simple washing or centrifugation are simple, quick and generally not associated with expensive equipment or disposables.

Second. while more expensive and slower processing time, enzymatic methods yield more nucleated cells with a higher number of progenitor cells per volume of lipoaspirate processed, but overall viability tends to be unaffected by processing method.

Third, while mechanical methods may be cost-effective in the laboratory setting, enzymatic methods provide a superior SVF output for use in the clinical setting.

Fourth, the method that a certain lab or facility uses ultimately, depends upon their needs and financial capabilities.

Fifth, there are differences in the number of adipose stem cells present in the various adipose tissue deposits of an individual and significant variation between individuals but adipose tissue in general.

They concluded that, non-enzymatic, mechanical methods is equally safe, less costly and less time consuming but the product contains fewer ADSCs compared to enzymatic method, so it is attractive

Table 08 Comparison of two products of collagenase.

Maker	SIGMA	SERVA	
Country of origin	U.S.A	Germany	
Grade	R&D[48] (Research and Development)	Sterile	GMP[49](Good Manufacturing Practice)
Composition	Crude collagenases area mixtures of enzyme (mostly proteases) secreted by Clostridium histolyticum. This preparation contains collagenase, non-specific proteases and Clostripain.	Collagenase 1 (class I and class II) as well as a balanced ratio of proteolytic activities such as Clostripain(EC3.4.22.8), Trypsin-like activity and neutral protease	
Specification	Research Laboratory	1. International GMP-guidelines 2. Sterility according to Pharm. Eur 3. Medicinal Products (Pharm. Eur)	
Microbiological Examination	X	1. Sterility Test (Pharm. Eur) 2. Absence of Clostridia Test 3. Abnormal Toxicity Test : General-Safety-Test (Pharm. Eur.)	
Activities	Irregular	Regular	
Viral Safety	X	X	O
Lot. Certificate	X	O	
Storage Conditions	0°C~4°C	2°C~8°C	
Price	Sterile Grade ≒ 2 high	Low	High (Reasonable)

Table 09 Two kinds of SERVA collagenases for tissue dissociation.

Collagenase	Properties	Application	Package
Collagenase NB 5 Sterile Grade From C. Histolyticum	Contains class I and class II. Collagenases and a balanced ratio of proteolytic actives. Aseptic production according to European Requirements for medicinal products.	Isolation of various cell types including hepatocytes, cardiomyocytes, pancreatic islets, adipocytes, and others. Sterile and thus ready to use	1g/vial (conc. : 1g/1L)
Collagenase NB 6 GMP Grade From C. Histolyticum	Contains class I and class II. Collagenases and a balanced ratio of proteolytic actives. Aseptic production according to European Requirements for medicinal products. Manufactured according to international cGMP guideline.	Isolation of various cell types including hepatocytes, cardiomyocytes, pancreatic islets, adipocytes, and others. Production of cells or tissue engineering for transplantation into humans.	1g/vial

when smaller quantities of ADSCs are sufficient. When consider practical aspects, proteolytic enzymes affords significantly greater efficiency to the separation process. Therefore, although the use of enzymes is accompanied with high costs, the most common isolation technique is still based on enzymatic digestion of adipose tissue to obtain the SVF.

(1) Enzymatic isolation method
Zuk PA et al[11]. first separated SVF and their method has been the most commonly used.

① Choosing the enzyme for SVF extraction.
Collagenase, the most frequently used in laboratory or clinic[43], will be briefly described below. Two types of collagenase currently sold in the market are shown in Table 8. From these two, the author uses NB 5 sterile Grade and 6 GMP grade as in Table 9 and Figure 7, which are collagenases for hu-

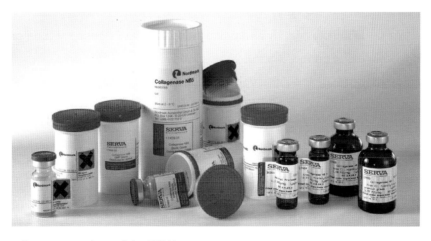

Figure 07 Various collagenase products of the SERVA company.

man, produced by SERVA[46] and sold by Vivagen, Inc. in Korea[47].

② Extraction method

Generally, clean bench, centrifuge, and shaking incubator have been used for cell culture in laboratory. I would like to explain the basic procedure for extraction of SVF from fat aspirates.

Method of SVF extraction by using clean bench is explained as shown in Figure 8.

The first step is to centrifuge suctioned fat (Figure 8: 1~7).

• Centrifuge (100g, 3 minutes) harvested adipocytes and tissue in 50ml conical tube.

• Eliminate the supernatant free oil and its lower layer which includes blood and tumescent by using micropipette

The second step is to mix centrifuged fat and collagenase solution (Figure 8: 8~10).

• 0.1% collagenase solution is prepared as follows. Add and dissolve 100mg of collagenase to 100ml of physiological saline. Put 10 ml of the mixture into 10 conical tubes each. Close the lids and keep them in freezer of -20°C. Defrosting in room temperature or sudden defrost is recommended. SERVA products are convenient to use since they are packaged frozen by the unit of 20mg/20ml.

• Mix the processed fat after the first step and 0.1% collagenase solution in 1:1 ratio. Just before treating enzyme, agglomerated adipose tissues are recommended to be cut finely with scissors; however, should be careful of contamination.

• Activate in shaking incubator(37°C, 200 r.p.m.) for 30 minutes.

The third step is to centrifuge fat reacted with collagenase solution. (Figure 8: 11~13)

• Centrifuge processed fat after the second step. (800~1000g, 3~5 minutes)

• Gradually eliminate oil layer, dissolved fat residue layer, and collagenase solution layer with micropipette. It is recommended to eliminate the collagenase solution layer as whole as possible. However, stem cell layer may be suctioned as well if suction is excessive. Thus, remain 5ml of lower layer to continue to the next step.

The fourth step is to neutralize and wash collagenase (Figure 8: 14~21)

• Centrifuge (1000g, 3 minutes) 10ml of the patient's blood and acquire 5ml of serum. Take double amount of plasma of the desired volume.

• Centrifuge(300g, 3minutes) the mixture of 5ml of the third step, 5ml of the patient's plasma and 20ml of physiological saline of 4°C.

• Leave 5ml of mixed layer of oil layer and plasma by micropipette after centrifuge. Repeat Step 4-) for 3-5 times. This is to lower the collagenase solution concentration to 1/1,000 ~ 1/100,000 times.

The fifth step is to eliminate the final impurities by using cell strainer. (Figure 8: 22~24)

• Install the cell filter(100μm) on the top of the new conical tube and let the purified sample of the fourth step to finally eliminate impurities. It is recommended to let the sample pass through by pipette even though Figure 8:23 illustrates to pour the tube.

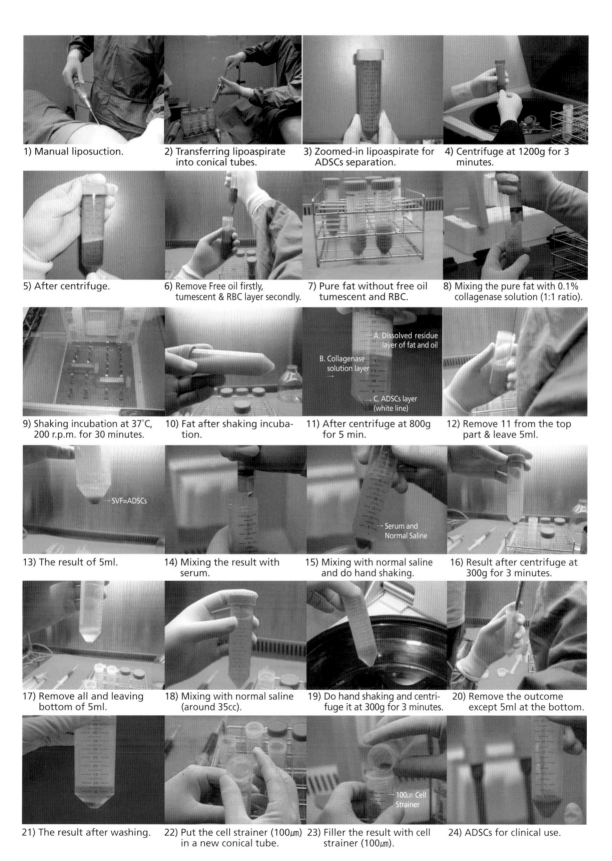

1) Manual liposuction.

2) Transferring lipoaspirate into conical tubes.

3) Zoomed-in lipoaspirate for ADSCs separation.

4) Centrifuge at 1200g for 3 minutes.

5) After centrifuge.

6) Remove Free oil firstly, tumescent & RBC layer secondly.

7) Pure fat without free oil tumescent and RBC.

8) Mixing the pure fat with 0.1% collagenase solution (1:1 ratio).

9) Shaking incubation at 37°C, 200 r.p.m. for 30 minutes.

10) Fat after shaking incubation.

11) After centrifuge at 800g for 5 min.

A. Dissolved residue layer of fat and oil
B. Collagenase solution layer
C. ADSCs layer (white line)

12) Remove 11 from the top part & leave 5ml.

13) The result of 5ml.

SVF=ADSCs

14) Mixing the result with serum.

15) Mixing with normal saline and do hand shaking.

Serum and Normal Saline

16) Result after centrifuge at 300g for 3 minutes.

17) Remove all and leaving bottom of 5ml.

18) Mixing with normal saline (around 35cc).

19) Do hand shaking and centrifuge it at 300g for 3 minutes.

20) Remove the outcome except 5ml at the bottom.

21) The result after washing.

22) Put the cell strainer (100μm) in a new conical tube.

23) Filler the result with cell strainer (100μm).

100μm Cell Strainer

24) ADSCs for clinical use.

Figure 08 Extraction of SVF(ADSCs) from fat aspirates using clean bench, centrifuge, and shaking incubator.

Table 10 Various enzymatic adipose tissue-derived cell isolation systems

Device	Multistation	Medi-Kan Lipokit with MaxStem	Cha-station	Unistation	CDI300	Stempeutron™
Picture						
Company	PNC – International, Inc	Medikan Inc	PNC – International, Inc	Neogenesis Co., Ltd	ICELL. Inc	Stempeutics Rese arch Pvt. Ltd.
Homepage	http://www.pncint.com/	http://www.edikan.com/?r=en	http://www.pncint.com/	http://www.neogenesis.co.kr/eng/main/	underconstruction	http://www.stempeutics.com/index.html
Method & Enzyme	Collagenase digestion	Collagenase digestion	Collagenase digestion	Collagenase digestion	Collagenase digestion	Collagenase digestion
Type of automation	Manual	Manual	Semi-automatic	Semi-automatic	Automatic + Manual/Final Concentration	Full automatic
Reference	50	50	50	-	-	51

Device	TGI	Celution® 800/CRS	HuriCell	Sepax2	Stem-X1s	Robo-Station
Picture						
Company	Tissuegenesis, Inc.	Cytori Therapeutics, Inc	Hurimbiocell, Inc	Biosafe Group SA	Medikan Inc	PNC–International, Inc
Homepage	http://tissuegenesis.com	www.cytoritx.com	http://www.hurimbiocell.com/eng/main.php	http://www.biosafe.ch/	http://www.medikan.com/?r=en	http://www.pncint.com/
Method & Enzyme	Collagenase digestion	Collagenase digestion	Collagenase digestion	Collagenase digestion	Collagenase digestion	Collagenase digestion
Type of automation	Full automatic	Full automatic	Full automatic	Full automatic	Full automatic	Full automatic
Reference	52	50	50, 53	54	55	-

Device	AdiStem™ Kit/AdiLight	Smart Kit® system	Stempro® Human ADSCs Kit	A-Stromal™ Kit	Apparatus and Methods for Cell Isolation
Picture					
Company	AdiStem Pty Ltd.	Donggu Bio & Pharma Co., Ltd	ThermoFisher Scientific Co.Ltd	Cellular Biomedicine Group, Inc./Cellular Biomedicine Group Hk, Ltd.	Ingeneron, Inc.
Homepage	http://www.adis-tem.com/technolo-gy/adipose-derived-adult-stem-cells/	http://dongkoo.co.kr	www.thermofisher.com	http://cellbiomed-group.com/news-room/new-product-new-license.	http://www.ingen-ero.com/
Method & Enzyme	Collagenase digestion	Collagenase digestion	Collagenase digestion	Collagenase digestion	Collagenase digestion
Type of automation	Manual	Manual	Manual	Manual	Manual
Reference	56	57	58	-	59

- RBC is present in the final harvest. It can be used after eliminating RBC by red blood cell lysis buffer depending on the purpose of use. If the purpose is not a research but extracting fat, elimination of RBC is not essential in this step when blood contamination is sufficiently prevented.
- After mixing the final harvest (about 5ml of SVF purified from 50ml of fat) of the fifth step and extracted fat of the patient in the ratio of 1:1, use this for the next grafting.

③ **Various kinds of enzymatic isolation machines**

Please refer to Table 10 which shows the types of enzymatic SVF extraction machines available in current market.

(2) Non-enzymatic isolation method

Recently, several groups have focused on non-enzymatic isolation methods, but similar to the enzymatic cell isolation methods, the range of protocols and methods shows also high variations. Table 11 summarizes a survey of currently patented, published, or commercially available non-enzymatic AD-SCs isolation systems.

Table 11 Various non-enzymatic adipose tissue-derived cell isolation systems.

Device	Puregraft™	Fastkit (Fastem)	LipiVage™	Lipogems®
Picture				
Company	Bimini Technologies LLC	CORIOS Soc. Coop.	Genesis Biosystems Inc.	Lipogems International S.p.A
Homepage	www.cytori.com http://www.puregraft.com/	http://www.fastkit.it/	http://genesisbiosystems.com/products/lipivage/	http://www.lipogems.eu/
Method	Washing & Filtration		Irrigation	Microfragmentation
Type of automation	Manual	Manual	Manual	Manual
Reference	60	61	62	63

Device	IntelliCell®	Filler Geller	ULTRA Stem Cell®
Picture			
Company	BioSciences Inc.	Medikan Co,. Ltd.	Medi futures.Co., Ltd.
Homepage	http://www.intellicellbiosciences.com	http://www.medikan.com/	www.medifutures.net
Method	Ultrasonic cavitation	Fat Condens & fat microfragmentation	Ultrasonic separation and Filtering
Type of automation	Semi-automatic	Semi-automatic	Semi-automatic
Reference	64	65	–

01. Behr B, HeeKo S, Wong VW, Gurtner GC, Longaker MT. Stem Cells. Plast Reconstr Surg. 2010;126(4):1163-1171.

02. Takahashi K, Yamanaka S. Induction of pluripotent stem cells from mouse embryonic and adult fibroblast cultures by defined factors. Cell 2006;126:663-676.

03. Wilmut I, Schnieke AE, McWhir J, et al. Viable offspring derived from fetal and adult mammalian cells. Nature 1997;385:810–813.

04. Pera MF. Stem cells. A new year and a new era. Nature 2008;451:13-136.

05. Dominici M, Le Blanc K, and Mueller I, et al. Minimal criteria for defining multipotentmesenchymal stromal cells: The International Society for Cellular Therapy position statement. Cytotherapy 2006;8:315-317.

06. Horwitz EM, Le Blanc K, Dominici M, et al. Clarification of the nomenclature for MSC: The international society for cellular therapy position statement. Cytotherapy 2005;7:393-395.

07. Sekiya I, Larson BL, Smith JR, Pochampally R, Cui JG, Prockop DJ. Expansion of human adult stem cells from bone marrow stroma: conditions that maximize the yields of early progenitors and evaluate their quality. Stem Cells. 2002;20(6):530-541.

08. Gronthos S, Zannettino AC, Hay SJ, Shi S, Graves SE, Kortesidis A, Simmons PJ. Molecular and cellular characterisation of highly purified stromal stem cells derived from human bone marrow. J Cell Sci. 2003 May 1;116(Pt 9):1827-35.

09. Lee OK, Kuo TK, Chen WM, Lee KD, Hsieh SL, Chen TH. Isolation of multipotent mesenchymal stem cells from umbilical cord blood. Blood. 2004 Mar 1;103(5):1669-1675. Epub 2003 Oct 23.

10. Zuk PA, Zhu M, Ashjian P, De Ugarte DA, Huang JI, et al. Human adipose tissue is a source of multipotent stem cells. Mol Biol Cell. 2002;13:4279-4295.

11. Zuk PA, Zhu M, Mizuno H, Huang J, et al. Multilineage cells from human adipose tissue: implications for cell-based therapies. Tissue Eng. 2001 Apr;7(2):211-228.

12. Gimble JM. Adipose tissue-derived therapeutics. Expert Opin Biol Ther. 2003;3(5):705-713.

13. Schäffler A, Büchler C. Concise review: adipose tissue-derived stromal cells-basic and clinical implications for novel cell-based therapies. Stem Cells. 2007;25(4):818-827.

14. Lin K, Matsubara Y, Masuda Y, Togashi K, Ohno T, Tamura T, Toyoshima Y, Sugimachi K, Toyoda M, Marc H, Douglas A. Characterization of adipose tissue-derived cells isolated with the Celution system. Cytotherapy. 2008;10(4):417-426.

15. Yoshimura K, Shigeura T, Matsumoto D, Sato T, Takaki Y, Aiba-Kojima E, Sato K, Inoue K, Nagase T, Koshima I, Gonda K. Characterization of freshly isolated and cultured cells derived from the fatty and fluid portions of liposuction aspirates. J Cell Physiol2006 ;208(1):64-76.

16. Gimble JM, Katz AJ, Bunnell BA. Adipose-derived stem cells for regenerative medicine. Circ Res. 2007 May 11;100(9):1249-1260.

17. Kuhbier JW, Weyand B, Radtke C, Vogt PM, Kasper C, Reimers K. Isolation, characterization, differentiation, and application of adipose-derived stem cells. Adv Biochem Eng Biotechnol. 2010;123:55-105. doi: 10.1007/10_2009_24.

18. Schipper B, Marra KG, Rubin JP. Regional anatomic and age effects on cell function of human adipose-derived stem cells. Fourth Annual International Fat Applied Technology Society. October 21–24, 2006, Baton Rouge, La. Abstract.

19. Sterodimas A, De Faria J, Nicaretta B, Papadopoulos O, Papalambros E, Illouz YG. Cell-assisted lipotransfer. Aesthet-Surg J. 2010;30:78-81.

20. Mastumoto D, Sato K, Gonda K, Takaki Y, Shigeura R, Sato T et al. Cell-assisted lipotransfer: supportive use of human adipose derived cells for soft tissue augmentation with lipoinjection. Tissue Eng. 2006;12:3375–3382.

21. Yoshimura K, Sato K, Aoi N, Kurita M, Hirohi T, Harii K. Cell-assisted lipotransfer for cosmetic breast augmentation: Supportive use of adipose-derived stem/stromal cells. Aesth Plast Surg. 2008;32:48-55.

22. Masuda T, Furue M, and Matsuda T. Novel strategy for soft tissue augmentation based on transplantation of fragmented omentum and preadipocytes. Tissue Eng. 2004;10:1672-1683.

23. Moseley TA, Zhu M, Hedrick MH. Adipose-derived stem and progenitor cells as fillers in plastic and reconstructive surgery. Plast Reconstr Surg. 2006;118(3 Suppl):121S-128S.

24. Miranville A, Heeschen C, Sengenes C, Curat CA, Busse R,

Bouloumie A. Improvement of postnatal neovascularization by human adipose tissue-derived stem cells. Circulation. 2004;110:349-355.

25. Planat-Benard V, Silvestre JS, Cousin B, Andre M, et al. Plasticity of human adipose lineage cells toward endothelial cells: physiological and therapeutic perspectives. Circulation. 2004;109:656-663.

26. Rehman J, Traktuev D, Li J, Merfeld-Clauss S, Temm-Grove CJ, et al. Secretion of angiogenic and antiapoptotic factors by human adipose stromal cells. Circulation. 2004;109:1292-1298.

27. Considine RV, Nyce MR, Morales LM, Magosin SA, Sinha MK, Bauer TL, Rosato EL, Colberg J, Caro JF. Paracrine stimulation of preadipocyte-enriched cell cultures by mature adipocytes. Am J Physiol. 1996 May;270(5 Pt 1):E895-9.

28. Li J, Gao JH, Lu F, Li HM, Fu BC. Experimental study of the effect of adipose tissue derived stem cells on the survival rate of free fat transplantation. Zhonghua ZhengXing WaiKe Za-Zhi. 2009 Mar;25(2):129-133.

29. Zhu M, Zhou Z, Chen Y, Schreiber R, Ransom JT, Fraser JK et al. Supplementation of fat grafts with adipose-derived regenerative cells improves long-term graft retention. Ann. Plast Surg. 2010; 64:222–228.

30. Yoshimura K. Breast augmentation with autologus fat grafting: optimized adipose remodeling by adipose stem cells. The 8th congress of Oriental cosmetic surgery.Seoul Korea 2010 October 30-31 Abstract Pp72.

31. Kurita M, Matsumoto D, Shigeura T, Sato K, Gonda K, Harii K, Yoshimura K. Influences of centrifugation on cells and tissues in liposuction aspirates: Optimized centrifugation for lipotransfer and cell isolation. Plast Reconstr Surg. 2008 ;121: 1033-41,discussion 1042-1043.

32. Mimeault M, Hauke R, Batra SK. Stem cells: A revolution in therapeutics-recent advances in stem cell biology and their therapeutic applications in regenerative medicine and cancer therapies. Clin Pharmacol Ther. 2007;82:252-264.

33. Moore KA, Lemischka IR. Stem cells and their niches. Science 2006;311:1880-1885.

34. Mimeault M, Batra SK. Recent progress on tissue-resident adult stem cell biology and their therapeutic implications. Stem Cell Rev. 2008;4:27-49.

35. Morrison SJ, and Kimble J. Asymmetric and symmetric stem-cell divisions in development and cancer. Nature 2006;441:1068-1074.

36. Justesen J, Pedersen SB, Stenderup K, Kassem M. Subcutane-ous adipocytes can differentiate into bone-forming cells in vitro and in vivo. Tissue Eng 2004;10(3-4):381-391.

37. Matsumoto T, Kano K, Kondo D, Fukuda N, Iribe Y, Tanaka N, Matsubara Y, Sakuma T, Satomi A, Otaki M, Ryu J, Mugishima H. Mature adipocyte-derived dedifferentiated fat cells exhibit multilineage potential. J Cell Physiol. 2008 Apr;215(1): 210-222.

38. von Heimburg D, Lemperle G, Dippe B, et al. Free transplantation of fat autografts expanded by tissue expanders in rats. Br J Plast Surg.1994;47:470.

39. Rubio D, Garcia-Castro J, Martin MC, de la Fuente R, Cigudosa JC, Lloyd AC, Bernad A. Spontaneous human adult stem cell transformation. Cancer Res 2005;65:3035–3039.

40. Wilson A, Butler PE, Seifalian AM. Adipose-derived stem cells for clinical applications: a review. Cell Prolif. 2011;44:86–98. 2011;44:86–98.

41. Aronowitz JA, Lockhart RA, Hakakian CS. Mechanical versus enzymatic isolation of stromal vascular fraction cells from adipose tissue. Springerplus. 2015 Nov 23;4:713. doi: 10.1186/s40064-015-1509-2. eCollection 2015.

42. Raposio E, Caruana G, Bronomini S, Libondi G.A novel strategy for theisolation of adipose-derived stem cells: minimally manipulated adipose-derivedstem cells for more rapid and safe stem cell therapy. Plast Reconstr Surg. 2014 ;133(6):1406–1409.

43. Markarian FM, Frey GZ, Silveira MD et al. Isolation of adipose-derivedstem cells: a comparison among different methods. Biotechnol Lett. 2014: 36:693–702.

44. Baptista LS, do Amaral RJ, Carias RB, Aniceto M, Claudio-da-Silva C, Borojevic R. An alternative method for the isolation of mesenchymal stromalcells derived from lipoaspirate samples. Cytotherapy (2009) 11(6):706–715.

45. Shah FS, Wu X, Dietrich M, Rood J, Gimble J. A non-enzymatic methodfor isolating human adipose-derived stromal stem cells.Cytotherapy 2013:15:979–985.

46. Millan A, Landerholm T, Chapman JR. Comparison between collagenase adipose digestion and stroma cell mechanical dissociation for mesenchymal stem cell separation. McNair Scholars J CSUS 2014: 15:86–101.

47. Zimmerlin L, Donnenberg VS, Pfeifer ME, Meyer EM, Péault B, Rubin JP, Donnenberg AD. Stromal vascular progenitors in adult human adipose tissue. Cytometry A. 2010 Jan;77(1):22-30. doi: 10.1002/cyto.a.20813.

48. http://en.wikipedia.org/wiki/Research_and_development.

49. http://en.wikipedia.org/wiki/Good_Manufacturing_Practice.

50. Engfeldt P, Arner P, Ostman : Influence of adipocyte isolation by collagenase on phosphodiesterase activity and lipolysis in man. J Lipid Res. 1980 May;21(4):443-448.

51. ttp://www.serva.de/enDE/index.html.

52. http://www.vivagen.co.kr/v2/main/(Tel : 031-737-2080, FAX: 031-737-2083, E-mail: HYPERLINK "mailto:vivagen@vivagen. co.kr"vivagen@vivagen.co.kr).

53. Aronowitz JA, Ellenhorn JD. Adipose stromal vascular fraction isolation: a head-to-head comparison of four commercial cell separation systems. Plast Reconstr Surg. 2013 Dec;132(6):932e-9e. doi: 10.1097/PRS.0b013e3182a80652

54. Do BR, Lee JK, Kim JH, Pak SH, Shin BS. Peristaltic pump, and regenerative cell extraction system using same. 2013. WO 2013089481 A1

55. Doi K, Tanaka S, Iida H, Eto H, Kato H, Aoi N, Kuno S, Hirohi T, Yoshimura K. Stromal vascular fraction isolated from lipoaspirates using an automated processing system: bench and bed analysis. J Tissue Eng Regen Med. 2013 Nov;7(11):864-870. doi: 10.1002/term.1478. Epub 2012 Mar 22.

56. Kaengkan P, Baek SE, Kim JY, Kam KY, Do BR, Lee ES, Kang SG. Administration of mesenchymal stem cells and ziprasidone enhanced amelioration of ischemic brain damage in rats. Mol Cells. 2013 Dec;36(6):534-541. doi: 10.1007/s10059-013-0235-2. Epub 2013 Nov 28.

57. Güven S, Karagianni M, Schwalbe M, Schreiner S, Farhadi J, Bula S, Bieback K, Martin I, Scherberich A.Validation of an automated procedure to isolate human adipose tissue-derived cells by using the Sepax® technology. Tissue Eng Part C Methods. 2012 Aug;18(8):575-582. doi: 10.1089/ten. TEC.2011.0617. Epub 2012 Apr 2.

58. Oberbauer E, Steffenhagen C, Wurzer C, Gabriel C, Redl H, Wolbank S. Enzymatic and non-enzymatic isolation systems for adipose tissue-derived cells: current state of the art. Cell Regen (Lond). 2015 Sep 30;4:7. doi: 10.1186/s13619-015-0020-0. eCollection 2015.

59. Van Pham P, Hong-Thien Bui K, Quoc Ngo D, Tan Khuat L, Kim Phan N.Transplantation of Nonexpanded Adipose Stromal Vascular Fraction and Platelet-Rich Plasma for Articular Cartilage Injury Treatment in Mice Model. J Med Eng. 2013;2013:832396. doi: 10.1155/2013/832396. Epub 2013 Jan 16.

60. Lim JH. ASCs customized to clinical doctors, focusing on SVF-basic. The 104th congress of Japan society of aesthetic surgery, Abstract for presentation. 17th May 2016, p102.

61. Michalek J, Moster R, Lukac L, Proefrock K, Petrasovic M, Rybar J, et al. Autologous adipose tissue-derived stromal vascular fraction cells application in patients with osteoarthritis. Cell Transplant. 2015. doi:10.3727/

62. Stubbers R, Coleman ME. Apparatus and methods for cell isolation. 2015. US 20150056691 A1.

63. Zhu M, Cohen SR, Hicok KC, Shanahan RK, Strem BM, Yu JC, Arm DM, Fraser JK. Comparison of three different fat graft preparation methods: gravity separation, centrifugation, and simultaneous washing with filtration in a closed system. Plast Reconstr Surg. 2013 Apr;131(4):873-880. doi: 10.1097/PRS.0b013e31828276e9.

64. Domenis R, Lazzaro L, Calabrese S, Mangoni D, Gallelli A, Bourkoula E, Manini I, Bergamin N, Toffoletto B, Beltrami CA, Beltrami AP, Cesselli D, Parodi PC. Adipose tissue derived stem cells: in vitro and in vivo analysis of a standard and three commercially available cell-assisted lipotransfer techniques. Stem Cell Res Ther. 2015 Jan 5;6:2. doi: 10.1186/scrt536.

65. Ferguson RE, Cui X, Fink BF, Vasconez HC, Pu LL The viability of autologous fat grafts harvested with the LipiVage system: a comparative study. Ann Plast Surg. 2008 May;60(5):594-7. doi: 10.1097/SAP.0b013e31817433c5.

66. Bianchi F, Maioli M, Leonardi E, Olivi E, Pasquinelli G, Valente S, et al. A new nonenzymatic method and device to obtain a fat tissue derivative highly enriched in pericyte-like elements by mild mechanical forces from human lipoaspirates. Cell Transplant. 2013;22(11):2063–77. doi:10.3727/096368912X657855.

67. Victor S. Ultrasonic cavitation derived stromal or mesenchymal vascular extracts and cells derived therefrom obtained from adipose tissue and use thereof. 2013. US 20130189234 A1. Guasti L1, Prasongchean W, Kleftouris G, Mukherjee S, Thrasher AJ, Bulstrode NW, Ferretti P. High plasticity of pediatric adipose tissue-derived stem cells: too much for selective skeletogenic differentiation? Stem Cells Transl Med. 2012 May;1(5):384-395. doi: 10.5966/sctm.2012-0009. Epub 2012 May 3.

68. Yang H, Lee H. Successful use of squeezed-fat grafts to correct a breast affected by Poland syndrome. Aesthetic Plast Surg. 2011 Jun;35(3):418-25. doi: 10.1007/s00266-010-9601-z. Epub 2010 Oct 17.

Counseling, informed consentand photographing

1 Consideration in counseling, and filling out the informed consent form

Like other surgical procedures, fat grafting also needs to be decided after sufficient counseling and the consent form should be taken. Those are important steps to enhance the patient's comprehension about the fat grafting and built a firm doctor-patient relationship. Eventually, it can minimize complaint and dissatisfaction of the patient after the procedure.

(1) Considerations before consultation

In my case, the followings are important considerations in counseling the patient who needs a fat grafting.

First, before a full-scale consultation, it is good to figure out actual aesthetic characteristics of the patient. When the patient talks about his or her aesthetic problem, you should figure out it through collecting the comprehensive information about contour, ratio, symmetry, degree of aging, and habitual usage of the facial mimic muscleand etc.

Second, notify the patient to be aware of his or her state according to the information gathered in first clause. Most of the patients do not recognize their faces are asymmetry. When counseling, it is important to make the patient to recognize their present state of asymmetry caused by presence of dental problem such as dental extraction and habits when speaking, laughing, frowning, opening and closing the eyes, moving the eyebrows, chewing, or sleeping. All of the above can also cause the asymmetry of the contour and wrinkleof the face. In addition, it is significant to make the patients understand that these characteristic movements and habits may affect the survival rate of engrafted fat significantly after the procedure.

Third, counsel patient's past history of cosmetic and medical treatment thoroughly.

Fourth,you should fully explain about the actual effect and outcome of the fat graftingand also be reduce the excessive expectation of the patient. Sufficient counseling with patients who have too much expectation about fat grafting can reduce postoperative arguments by reducing the initial excessive expectation. On the other hand, it is very important to educate pessimistic patients to understand the reality of fat grafting and to think positively by telling them about the faults and effects of fat grafting. The photographs of patients' younger days can be very helpful in setting the goals and predicting the results of the surgery.

(2) Considerations during consultation

The followings principles should be considered during counseling.

First, investigate the cosmetic treatment history of the patient. Some patients are reluctant to reveal, and do not tell about their past history. Thus, the physicians must precisely check about the patient's past history of facelift surgeries including various threads lift, previous fat grafting, allograft implantation, injection of artificial fillers, and foreign body implantation (silicone or paraffin). Especially, you must notify the possible complications and side effects-such as long lasting edema, high incidence rate of inflammation, low survival rate, and movement of previously existing foreign body. Also, it is important to get as many informationas possible by repeating inquiries while counseling and filling out the consent form because there are many patients who tend to forget their experiences after too much time passed from their procedures.

Second, inspect the basic medical history of the patient. Check the historical records of patients about previous surgery, anticancer treatment, presence of edema, presence of systemic disease — such as hemorrhagic diseases, hypertension, diabetes, and thyroid diseases, presence of food or drug allergy, and neurologic disease like Bell's palsy, etc. Especially, checking the present and past history of mental illness including sleep disorder, depression, and body dysmorphic disorder is an important procedure, and it is good to consider advice from psychiatrists if any consultation or remediation is needed. Especially, body dysmorphic disorder is detected in 1-2% of the total population, with high rate in 15~20 year-old adolescents and unmarried female. Among them, 6-15% visit to cosmetic surgery or dermatologic clinic. However, the results of the treatment often have poor prognosis, accompanying with other mental disorders. Thus, the cooperation of cosmetic surgery and psychiatry is important for early detection of the patient's problems[1]. Those who think that they have their body dysmorphism or defects tend to constantly engross in the thoughts. Eventually, they avoid social situations or jobs due to the anxiety from exaggerating or distorting the minor problems of their appearance.

Third, check the precise information about medications, health foods, and nutritional supplements that are currently taken by patients. For example, since non-steroidal anti-inflammatory drugs, NSAIDs–like aspirins and ibuprofens–and anticoaglutant drugs can cause platelet dysfunction, make sure to discontinue taking the pills 2 weeks prior to the operation and at least 3 days to at most 1 week after the procedure. For pain relievers, lead the patients to take acetaminophen (Pacacetamol[R]) instead of an anodyne like NSAIDs. Check the patients if they are taking any of the oriental medicinal herbs; deer antlers, red ginseng, licorice, ephedra,oleoresin turmeric extract, the health foods and nutritional supplements; garlic, onion liquid, vitamin E (α-tocoperol), and omega(ω)-3 fatty acids and make sure that the patients discontinue taking these supplements at least 1-2 weeks prior to the procedure. When fat grafting and body contouring liposuction are combined simultaneously, oral contraceptive pill (Estrogens) or low dose of estrogen(HRT) for menopausal woman increases the incidence of postoperative thromboembolism. Thus, patients must discontinue taking these drugs 3-4weeks before the procedure and 2 weeks after the procedure. Also, must beware of lidocaine metabolism and related drug interaction. Lidocaine toxicity can occur as a result of adverse drug interactions between lidocaine and drugs that inhibit the hepatic enzymes cytochrome P450 (CYP450) which metabolize lidocaine. Drugs that inhibit CYP450 (CYP3A4), such as sertraline (Zoloft[R]), fluoxetine(Prozac[R]), and diazepam (Valium[R])etc., have the potential for lidocaine toxicity. Antiepileptic drugs, carbamazepine(Tegretol[R]) also appear to compete with lidocaine for CYP3A4 and slow lidocaine metabolism.

Therefore, drugs that interfere with lidocaine metabolism should be discontinued at least 1 or 2 weeks before using the tumescent technique when high doses of lidocaine are anticipated. However, if a drug that might interfere with lidocaine metabolism cannot be discontinued, the surgery should be limited and smaller total doses of lidocaine used.

Fourth, check the weight change of the patient. It is good to record patient's weight change in 3 months right before the procedure and maximally 12 months after the procedure. Generally, the turnover rate for the normal body fat is so slow that it takes about 2 years or more[3]. But grafted fat is reported to be replaced within 2-3 months after the procedure due to transient ischemia resulting from reperfusion[4]. Long-term withdrawal of grafted fat continues commonly up to 6 months[5]. From these results, weight change after the procedure can highly influence the results. But there is no objective evidence yet about the impact of weight change in 3-4 months or within 12 months after the procedure on the survival rate of grafted fat[5]. However, as a rule of the author's thumb, postoperative weight change has a high possibility of bringing unintended outcome, which are different from what the patient and doctor has expected. Considering this fact, it is desirable for the patients to maintain weight at least 6 to 12 months maximally after the procedure. Anyway, according to my experience related with the weight change, more patients were unhappy with weight loss compared to weight gain.

Fifth, notify a patient of the environmental factors that can negatively affect survival rate after fat grafting and how to prevent them.

Surgeon should ask for the pretreatment of botulinum toxin (2 weeks or at least 2-3 days before) to those who habitually use facial mimic muscle and also recommend additional botulinum toxin 3 or 6 months after. It requires explaining the patients what muscle they mostly use when chewing and which side they lie down when sleeping. Particularly, people with jobs that require a lot of talking have more deficiencies such as nasolabial folds, perioral wrinkles, and cheek depressions than other people. So, it is better to notify them in advance about the possibility of low fat survival in these areas after the procedure.

Also, bad impacts of smoking and drinking alcohol on fat grafting and sedation anesthesia must be explained clearly.

Especially, smoking can negatively affect sedation anesthesia by reducing vital capacity and increasing secretion. It also leads to increase wound inflammation and delay recovery due to decreased tissue oxygen tension. Heretofore, abstaining smoking for 4-8 weeks before the procedure was known to reduce the occurrence of postoperative complications. However, recently, Clara K. Chow et al. insisted that stop smoking during the period is meaningless. However, they argued that at least 8 weeks of abstaining is needed to show same complication occurrence rate with that of non-smokers[6]. Over 8 weeks of abstaining smoking is realistically difficult for patients who will be doing fat grafting. However, abstaining smoking has numerous advantages from 1-2 days after it, and at least 12 hours before the fat grafting; and it increases the amount of hemoglobin for oxygen transport by reducing carbon monoxide hemoglobin concentration and shifting the oxygen-hemoglobin dissociation curve to right, which has a significant advantage in sedation and oxygen supply to tissues[7]. Post-operatively abstaining of smoking is also important. Smoking causes vasoconstriction and lowering of tissue oxygen tension, interrupting angiogenesis and increasing inflammation. Generally, safe engraftment of the grafted fat needs 3-4 months after the procedure. Therefore, even though abstaining during this period is ideal, at least 2 weeks to 1 month is highly recommended. It seems to be realistic to recommend patients to quit smoking at least up to 3 months.

Absorbed alcohol in bodyis degraded by alcoholic dehydrogenase(ADH) and microsomal ethanol oxidizing system (MEOS)[9]. It takes about 2-3 days to completely biodegrade alcohol on average with high individual variation. For habitual drunkard, the MEOS is always activated and the anesthetic drugs can be bio-degraded quickly. So, the anesthesia is not only well induced but also wake patient up quickly and consequently need more induction dose. Also, alcohol attenuates liver function and decreases immunity – leading to increase occurrence of hemorrhage, edema, and inflammation and slow down wound healing. Therefore, habitual drunkard must stop drinking at least 1 to 2 weeks before fat grafting, and unhabitual patient should stop at least 3 days to 1 week. It is also recommended to stop drinking at least 2 weeks after the procedure when the postoperative edema almost subsides.

Sixth, surgeon should precisely explain and make the patient understand the process of progressive change and additional procedures after fat grafting. Hemorrhage and edema are common complains that patients feel inconvenient. Normally edema will be subsided within 2 weeks after the procedure. But, the volume of grafted fat will change greatly until 3-4 months after the procedure which is the period of engraftment. So, these points need to be explained to the patient clearly. Also, it is good to inform the patient in advance that if there is a need for additional fat grafting, it should be done 3 months after the first procedure as it is safer and have better effects. Furthermore, surgeon should explain in advance about the reality of using frozen fat and notify the patient of possible side effects such as inflammation, fibrosis, necrosis and calcification.

2 SAFI-specific charts of consultation, operation and anesthesia, and informed consent form

The examples of consultation chart, operation and anesthesia, and informed consent form for SAFI are seen in Table 1, 2 and 3.

3 Photographing

1) Importance of photographing

It is essential to get the patient's consent before taking photographs because protecting patient's portrait right is also the doctor's responsibility. As fat grafting brings dramatic changes in external appearance as time passes, the importance of pre and postoperative photographing cannot hardly be emphasized enough. Especially, keeping the preoperative photographs is more important, because most patients tend to forget their preoperative features easily and there are many cases of dramatic changes of facial contour after the procedure. Doctors or clinic staffs must make a copy of the photographs taken and keep them in separate files for safe custody. I had experienced a ridiculous claim from a patient because of loss of her preoperative photographs.

Close attention should be paid to fix constant condition such as brightness, focus, patient-camera distance, patient-camera height and posture of patient during photographing. Besides, it should be completely obvious to set the same condition in the follow-up photographing since the conditions can

Table 01 An example of consultation chart for the SAFI.

SAFI Consultation Chart

Chart No.		Date	
Name		Sex/Age	
Address		Phone No.	
E-mail		Others	
Chief complaint			

Medical history	DM( ) HTN( ) Hepatitis( ) TBc( ) Allergy( )
	Heart Problem ( ), Psychogenic Problem ( ), Facial trauma Hx ( ), Medication ( ), Nutritional supplements ( )

Aesthetic history	Date	Kinds	Name or area of the procedure
Any fillers			
Foreign body			
Botulinum Toxin			
Operations			

Physical examinations	Vital Sign : BP(/)mmHg PR(/min) RR(/min) BT( ) Body weight : (kg), Recent TBW change ( )

Facial aesthetic examinations

Skin type : Oily / Dry / Mixed( )/( )/( )	Wrinkle : mild / moderate / severe( )/( )/( )
Contour: : Triangular( ) / Inverted Triangle( ) / Pentagonal( ) / Elliptical( ) / Square ( )	Skin drooping : mild / moderate / severe ( )/( )/( )

Facial animations : Severity(+ ~ +++) and Symmetry (Lt>Rt: L, Lt<Rt: R)

Brow or forehead elevation(/) Brow frown (/) Smiling(/)

Lip angle elevation(/) Teeth clamping(/) Oral Puckering (/)

Analysis for the application of SAFI technique

Face	Right Face	Left Face
Patient demand area		
Atrophic area		
Increase area		
others		
Forehead	Right frontal	Left frontal
Patient demand area		
Atrophic area		
Increase area		
others		

Kinds of Anesthesia	Regional A ( ) / IV Sedation( ) / General Anesthesia ( )
Possible combination surgeries	Blepharoplasty ( ),Rhinoplasty( ), Implantation ( ), Face lift( ), Face liposuction( ),Body liposuction( ), Botulinum toxin( ), Filler injection( ), Others( )

Table 02 Example of operation/anesthesia chart for the SAFI.

Name			Age/Male, Female		/M( ),F( )	OP day	
Preop.Lab. test* abnormality					Preoperative medication		
Vital signs	BP(/ mmHg), RR(/min), PR(/min), BT(°C), SpO₂ ( )						
Anesthesia	Regional A.( ), IV sedation( ), General A. ( )						
Time	Operation	: ~ :		Anesthesia	: ~ :		

X-Anesthesia
⊙-Operation
▲-B.T
●-P.R
∨/∧-B.P
Respi.
○-Self
◌-Assist
⊗-Contro

Temp °C: 40, 38, 36, 34, 32, 30, 28, 26
240, 220, 200, 180, 160, 140, 120, 100, 80, 60, 40, 20

Donor site		Site : ( ) ( )	
Tumescent amount (mℓ)	Spin (G for min.)	Amount of aspirates (mℓ)	Refined fat amount (mℓ)

Addictives and mix ratio

ADSCs (mℓ)		PRP (mℓ)	
Mix Ratio	Fat : ADSCs = ( ) : ( )	Fat : PRP = ( ) : ( )	ADSCs-rich Fat : PRP = ( ) :( )

Total Grafted amount for face (ml) and for forehead (ml) / Remaining fat (ml)

Forehead		Face								
Rt Zone	Lt Zone	Rt Area				Lt Area				
1( )	1( )	1( )	6( )	11( )	16( )	1( )	6( )	11( )	16( )	
2( )	2( )	2( )	7( )	12( )	17( )	2( )	7( )	12( )	17( )	
3( )	3( )	3( )	8( )	13( )	18( )	3( )	8( )	13( )	18( )	
4( )	4( )	4( )	9( )	14( )	19( )	4( )	9( )	14( )	19( )	
5( )	5( )	5( )	10( )	15( )	20( )	5( )	10( )	15( )	20( )	

Liposuction or liposysis (amount)

Jowl	Malar	Nasolabial fold	Submental/mandibular
Rt. (mℓ) Lt. (mℓ)	Rt. (mℓ) Lt. (mℓ)	Rt. (mℓ) Lt. (mℓ)	Rt. (mℓ) Lt. (mℓ)
Postoperative medication		Date of bandage removal or stich out	
Operator			(Signature)
Anesthesiologist			(Signature)
Nurses			(Signature)

*Basic list of preoperative laboratory test needed for general anesthesia.
1) Chest PA / 2) ECG
3) Urine analysis
　(1) Chemistry: Color urine, S.G urine, pH urine, Leucocyte Urine, Nitrite Urine, Protein Urine, Glucose Urine, Ketone Urine, Urobilinogen Urine, Bilirubin Urine, and Blood Urine
　(2) Microscopy: WBC/RBC
4) CBC with D/C / 5) Coagulation: PT/aPTT/BT
6) Blood Chemistry(serum) AST/ALT/ALP,T-protein/Albumin, BUN/Cr, Uric Acid, Glucose, Electrolytes(Na/K/Cl), and Total Ca²⁺
7) Infection HBs Ag/Ab, HCV Ab, and HIV Ab

Table 03 An example of informed consent form

1. I understand that unforeseen conditions/accidents may happen during the course of the operation andanesthesia.
2. I thereforeunderstand and I agree to let doctor to perform the other surgery or procedure that is in the exercise of his or her professional judgementnecessary and desirable.
3. I agree to getting required anesthesia injection or anesthesia injections recommended by doctor and understand that complications, injuries or even death may happen during the process of anesthesia.
4. I understand that no one can promise the outcome of the surgery.
5. I promise that if complications happen after surgery, I will go to the clinic that I have undergone surgery to receive treatments and follow the instructions by the doctors who carried out the surgery. If clinic ask me to do extra surgery, I am willing to pay for the cost of the surgery.
6. I allow the clinic to take photographs of certain parts of my body without exposing them to other people. I also allow the clinic to take video of me from a distance.
7. In order to help in promote medical development, I allow the usage of my medical records, photographs and videos for medical, scientific andeducational purposes (conferences, books and papers) and for reference of other doctors. Therefore, I also allow the surgeon to show or send my medical records, photographs, and videos to other doctors via email for further medical consultation.
8. I consent to the disposal of any tissue, medical devices or body parts that may be removed.
9. When required, I allow the use of my name and identity card number partially by related department for registration of medical equipment and medical reports.
10. I agree to send or show my photo and medical record to the other doctors if it needed further medical consultation.
11. Doctor has informed me of the below statements:
    A. Methods and precautions of liposuction and fat grafting
    B. Possibility of extra surgery and treatments
    C. Complications and sequela caused by surgery and treatment
12. I agree to carry out surgery and treatment and the statements stated above (1~10)
13. I am very satisfied with all the explanations above (   ) and I promise to follow the statements stated above (   ) and sign and seal as below.

Year/   Month/   Day

Surgery and clarification doctor: (   ) (Signature)
Patient's name: (   ) (Signature)

significantly affect the comparison of pre and postoperative views. The photographer should keep in mind the effects and be careful in photographing.

2) Preparations for photographing

Black or sky-blue is generally used for background. Especially, sky-blue-colored background is preferred because skin color is expressed better and can have shadow thinning effects.

Flash of camera or strobo in the studio can be used as light source. Strobo flash is a good light source since it is close to natural light. Surrounding light sources have big effects on pre and postoperative photographs so it is good to take photographs under fixed light sources. Thus, it is better to take photograph in darkroom where every surrounding light source is blocked.

Choosing the correct lens is also one of the important factors and how to choose proper lens is explained below.

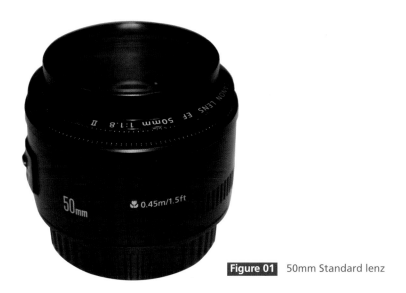

Figure 01 50mm Standard lenz

Standard lens is 50mm and this number represents the distance between the camera and the lens as shown in Figure 1. The smaller the number, the wider the angle of the view is. Why is 50mm a standard lens? This is because camera that has 50mm lens has similar view with human's visual field.Lens that is smaller than 50mm is wide-angle lens and lens that is bigger than 50mm is telephoto lens.

First, wide-angle lens can take wider angle photographs compared to standard lens. Using this lens, subject that is nearer to the lens appears bigger and subject that is further away from the lens looks further away than he or she is in reality. Besides, even if the photographs are taken with a big value of depth, the photograph, near or far places, will come out clear.

Second, telephoto lens is used to make a subject who is far from the camera to look bigger and it is called out focusing photograph. When zoom in, the depth becomes shallow relatively, and the subject who is in the correct focus will appear clear but the background will be blurred.

Third, because the standard lens has similar field of vision with humans, it can express the natural feeling of near and far and real sense of everyday life. Hence, it is widely used in taking pre and post-operative photographs.

Forth, there is a special zoom lens but it cannot be changed and only one lens can be used. The lens is also called trans-focal lens as it can continuously change the focus distance from a fixed point. It is convenient that the lens can change the width and size of the screen by changing the focus distance, but perspective appeared differently. If zoom lens can be used for both wide angle and telescopic view, the zoom can be adjusted to 50mm and can be used as standard lens. However, the author recommends only using standard lens alone.

It is very crucial to take pre and postoperative photographs under the same condition; remove patient's makeup, and put on a hair band to make sure that hair does not cover the patient's face. It is

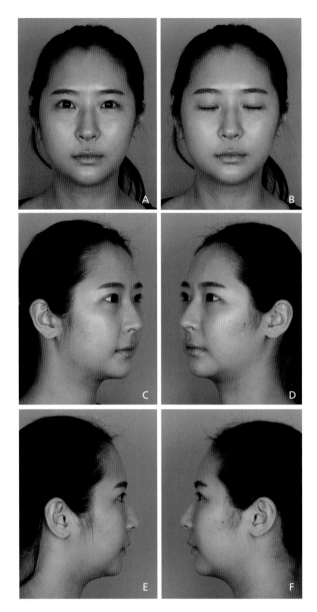

Figure 02 Preoperative photographs for the fat grafting. Frontal view(open eye) (A), Frontal view(closed eye) (B), Right oblique view (C), Left oblique view (D), Right lateral view, and (E), Left lateral view (F).

because the presence of makeup and the change in hair style affect dramatically in comparing pre and postoperative condition. But, it is not easy to ask the patient to be in the exact same conditions during pre and postoperative photographing like making them to remove their makeup.

3) Reality of photographing

Since the distance between patient and camera needs to always be the same while photographing, make sure that the patient stands up or sit at a marked position, and the position of camera must be fixed. Also, patient's face need to be positioned in the center of the monitor using Frankfort line which connects upper rim of external auditory canal and inferior orbital rim as baseline.

Basically, photographs of patients for fat grafting should be taken from frontal view, lateral view, and oblique view as in Figure 2.

For the frontal view, make sure that the patient's eyes look in front, horizontal line to the Frankfort line, and vertical line to the center of nasal bridge. Generally, hair is slightly cropped out, and neck is slightly taken in the picture. Make sure not to lower or raise the head and the shape and position of both ears should be the same in the photograph.

For the lateral view, make sure that the patient's eyes look at the same position as frontal view and horizontal line to the Frankfort line. Whole ear should be appeared in the picture, and opposite eyebrow should not be seen.

For the orbital view, make horizontal line to the Frankfort line, and set the nasal tip to coincide with opposite facial outline.

Reference

01. Pollice R, Bianchini V, Giuliani M, Zoccali G : Early diagnosis of dismorphophobia and others dismorphic disorders: a possible operative model. Clin Ter 2009;160(1):5-10.

02. Bill TJ, Clayman MA, Morgan RF, Gampper TJ : Lidocaine metabolism pathophysiology, drug interactions, and surgical implications Aesthet Surg J. 2004 Jul-Aug;24(4):307-311.

03. Strawford A, Antelo F, Christiansen M, Hellerstein MK : Adipose tissue triglyceride turnover, de novo lipogenesis, and cell proliferation in humans measured with 2H2O. Am J Physiol Endocrinol Metab 2004;286:E577-E588

04. Kotaro Yoshimura, Katsujiro Sato, Noriyuki Aoi, Masakazu Kurit, Toshitsugu Hirohi, Kiyonori Harii : Cell-assisted lipotransfer for cosmetic breast augmentation: Supportive use of adipose-derived stem/stromal cells. Aesthetic Plast Surg 2008;32:48-55.

05. Masuda T, Furue M and Matsuda T : Novel strategy for soft tissue augmentation based on transplantation of fragmented omentum and preadipocytes. Tissue Eng 2004;10:1672-1683.

06. Clara K Chow and PJ Devereaux : The optimal timing of smoking cessation before surgery. Comment on "smoking cessation shortly before surgery and postoperative complications" Arch Intern Med Published online March 14, 2011. doi:10.1001/arch intern med.2011.88. Available at (http://www.physorg.com/news/ 2011-03-shortly -surgery-postoperative-complications.html)

07. The Korean society of anesthesiologist: Anesthesia and pain management, 2nd edition, Elsvier Korea L.L.C, 2009; Pp1316.

08. Jörnvall H, and Harris JI : "Horse liver alcohol dehydrogenase. On the primary structure of the ethanol-active isoenzyme". Eur J Biochem 1970;13(3):565–576.

09. Chales S Lieber : The discovery of the microsomal ethanol oxidizing system and its physiologic and pathologic role. Drug Metabolism Reviews 2004;36:511-529.

06 Practical preparations for fat grafting-Instrument, liposuction and purification

1 Instruments

1) Selecting the type of instrument

Instruments used for fat grafting can be classified by depending on the purposes i.e., tumescent anesthesia, liposuction, centrifugation, fat injection and cleansing. I commonly use the products of Medizone Inc[1]. Especially, almost all cannula are made of stainless steel. But, various products are also introduced in the market, which are coated with gold or titanium inside or outside.

(1) Tumescent anesthesia

When harvesting, infiltration cannula is used for injection of anesthetic tumescent solution into donor areas. The 15G infiltration cannula of 25 cm long with multiple side holes (1.0 mm in diameter) is commonly used. Some facial volume deficiency areas need regional anesthesia with tumescent solution (Figure 1A), 7-10 cm long infiltration cannula of 18G with multiple side holes (0.6 mm diameter) is commonly used (Figure 1B).

(2) Liposuction

For fat harvesting, standard 3 mm liposuction cannula with the length of 25 cm with both side holes (0.8 x 0.3 mm) is mostly used (Figure 1C). The length of the suction cannula is recommended as the same or a little shorter than that of the infiltration cannula. When performing a manual liposuction by syringe, it may be difficult and uncomfortable to maintain appropriate pressure constantly. Wound protector is made of rubber or plastic, which is inserted into the entry site for preventing skin damage

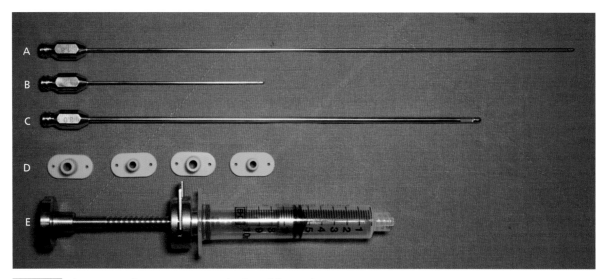

Figure 01 Instruments for tumescent anesthesia and liposuction.
An infiltration cannula for body (15G, 25 cm length) (A), an infiltration cannula for face (18G, 10cm length) (B), a body liposuction cannula (3mm diameter, 25 cm length) (C), wound protectors (D), and a manual vacuum device with 10 cc syringe (E).

during suction (Figure 1D). For convenience, a manual vacuum device, which is attached to a Luer-Lok syringe to maintain a constant intra-barrel pressure, is developed (Figure 1E).

(3) Centrifugation

The rotor type laboratory centrifuge installed with a digital display of timer and RPM (or RCP) and a break system is highly recommended (Figure 2).

The holes of needle adaptor and barrel end should be blocked up with needle adaptor cap and barrel

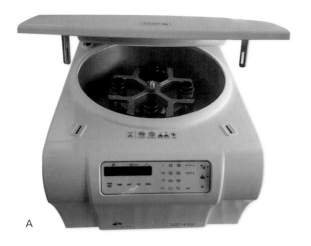
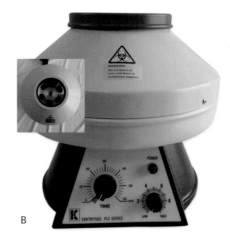

Figure 02 Centrifuge. rotor type (A), Simple (no rotor) type (B).

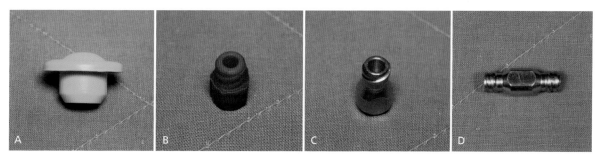

Figure 03 Various kinds of needle adaptor caps and barrel end stopper and a transfer.
A rubber barrel end stopper (A), a disposable needle adaptor cap (B), a stainless steal needle adaptor cap (C) and a stainless steal transfer (D).

end stopper separately to prevent air contact and loss of aspirates during centrifugation. Instruments made of plastics, rubber or stainless steel are being sold in the market (Figure 3). A transfer is used for moving the purified fat from the 10cc Luer-Lok syringe to the 1cc Luer-Slip syringe.

(4) Fat injection

Punch Awl or 18G needle is used to make entry site for fat injection (Figure 4A and 4B). Generally, diameter of 18G (1.2 mm) with the length of 5 cm or 7 cm is most frequently used for fat injection in Korea (Figure 4C). I have used 18G stainless Coleman's cannula type II for all my Safi cases except

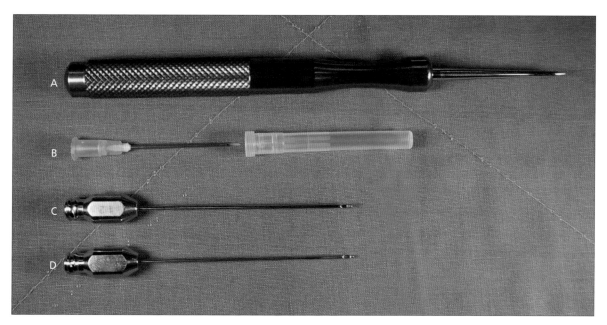

Figure 04 Instruments needed for fat injection.
Awl (A), 18G needle (B), injection cannula (18G, 5cm length) (C), and injection cannula (19G, 5cm length) (D).

using 19G cannula only for correction of upper sunken eyelid in rare cases (Figure 4D). Personally, I prefer to use flexible stainless cannulas, which can be bent manually because it can easily approach to all areas of the face without changing other shape of cannulas during the procedure. Additionally, it is also quite economic because there is no need to buy various kinds of cannulas.

(5) Cleaning

It is significant to carefully clean, sterilize, and manage the cannulas which are used for both liposuction and fat injection.

Cannula cleaning is very crucial because remaining fat or oil debris inside of the cannula causes cannula blockage or postoperative inflammation. After surgery, put all of the cannulas into warm water. Next, wash the inside of the cannulas by connecting them to syringe filled with alcohol solution or clean directly using thin brush. Then, sterilize them using ultrasonic cleaner (Figure 5A) or by boiling them in water.

However, fat or oil debris on the inside of the cannula cannot be completely eliminated by these methods. To handle this, easy, convenient and effective method for removing debris inside of the cannula is described as following. Add 15 ml of neutral detergent solution (commonly used for washing clothes)[2] and 13 grams (1 spoon) of baking powder[3] to 1000ml of water and mix them. Then, put cannula into the mixture and boil it for about 20 minutes. This method utilizes detergent effect in disaggregating oil and baking powder effect in neutralizing acid substance and absorbing disaggregated oil. The ingredients used for this method are easily available and effective for cleansing, according to the author's experience. Of course, instead of boiling, it would be more convenient to use an ultrasonic cleaner with these ingredients added.

Generally, the cannula is sterilized in autoclave (Figure 5B) or E.O. gas(ethylene oxide) sterilizer (Figure 5C). One thing to bear in mind is that the cannula can only be used several days after sterilization. The best method is to disinfect the cannula in sterilizer the day before procedure and take it out from the sterilizer on that day. Usage of cannula which has been sterilized more than 24 hours ago should be avoided.

Actually, the ultrasonic cleaner is not an essential instrument. However, if you want to buy it, the length of the cannula should be considered first to select the size of the cleaner. Cannula cleansing brushes is used to remove tiny fat debris, oil, and dust from the internal surface of cannula (Figure 5D). Cleansing stylet is used for pushing intraluminal fat or fibrotic tissues out to prevent blockage of cannula (Figure 5E). Autoclavable cannula tray can be used for packing of all instruments during autoclave sterilization and storage (Figure 5F).

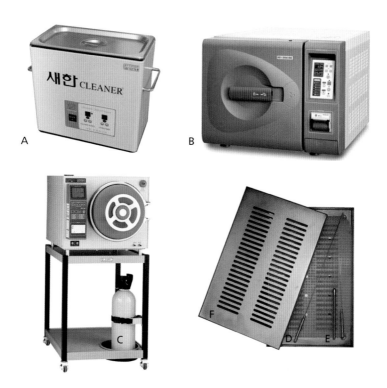

Figure 05 Instruments needed for cleansing and storage.
Ultrasonic cleaner (A), Autoclave sterilizer (B), E.O. gas(ethylene oxide) sterilizer (C), Cannula cleansing brushe (D), Two cleansing stylets (E), and Autoclavable cannula tray (F).

2 Preparation of anesthetic tumescent solution

Generally, Klein's solution is most commonly used for tumescent anesthesia. Essential components of the solution are 2% lidocaine solution (20mg/ml), epinephrine (1mg/ml), 8.4% sodium bicarbonate solution (Bivon®), normal saline solution and etc. Various modifications of Klein's solution can be used at diverse harvesting areas as shown in Table 1[4]. Ringer's lactate solution with dextrose water can be used as a substitute for 1000ml of normal saline solution.

3 Liposuction for harvest

1) Determining donor site and designing

Fat can be harvested from any regions as shown in Figure 6[5]. However, the preferred areas of donor sites in facial fat grafting are shown in Table 2.

Table 01 The Klein's and the modified Klein's tumescent solutions to different areas.

	Lidocaine(mg/L)	Epinephrine(mg/L)	Bicarbonate(mEq/L)
Basic	500	0.5	10
Hips; lateral, medial; anterior thigh; knees	700~750	0.65	10
Back; male flank; arms	1000	0.65~1.0	10
Female abdomen(medial)	1000~1250	1.0	10
Male abdomen(medial), male breasts	1250	1.0	10
Abdomen(lateral)	750	0.65	10
Female breasts; chin, cheek, jowls	1500	1.5	10
Facial resurfacing(CO2 laser)	2400	4	20

Table 02 Preferable donor sites for fat harvest

1st choice	Abdomen and lateral thigh
2nd choice	Medial thigh, frank, and love handle
3rd choice	Supra-pubic, anterior thigh, and supra-knee

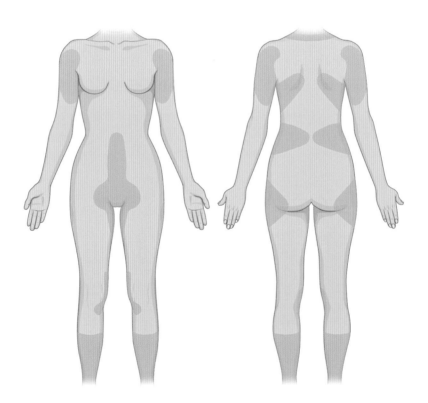

Figure 06 Anatomical regions commonly associated with liposuction.

Designing donor site is not very different from that of general liposuction surgery. But, in many or most cases, it should be noted that the liposuction area for harvesting is considerably limited or smaller than that of general liposuction because the required amount of aspirated fat is about 50 ml or not more than 100 ml. Even if a relatively small fat is harvested, the design should be thoroughly considered to make a smooth line (contour) with surrounding areas. Entry site depends on the location of the donor site and the surgeon's position and scar exposure should be considered as well.

2) Entry site

After the skin is desensitized with 2% lidocaine and epinephrine solution (1:100,000). The doctor makes a tiny incision, usually 3-6mm with No.11 or No. 15 blade. To avoid cutting the entry site too deep or much, use pierce-like incision (stab-like incision) method which holds the blade 0.5~0.7cm from the tip with fingertips as in Figure 7.

3) Infiltration of tumescent solution

I love to use a 25 cm long infiltration cannula with the diameter of 15G (1.8 mm). Many surgeons who perform the tumescent technique inject 1 ml of fluid for each 1 cm^3 of the expected fat harvest[6]. However, I sometimes use up to 2cc of tumescent solution for pain-sensitive patients. When injecting tumescent, it is injected into the middle layer of subcutaneous fat firstly and then into the superficial layer. It should be injected into deeper layer doubtlessly when the fat is harvested from deeper layer due to fat inadequacy. In particular, when injecting into the deeper layer, muscle fascia should not be touched. To decrease pain during liposuction, it is recommended to inject tumescent into the area of 1.5~2 cm outside the designed line. Liposuction is recommended after waiting for minimum 10 minutes or after waiting long enough for 30 minutes.

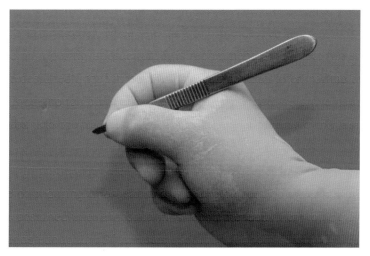

Figure 07 The method of holding a blade to make the entry site incision for liposuction in a safe manner.

Tumescent injection should be carefully performed with attention to following precautions. First, excessive injection should be avoided because adipocytes may be damaged due to direct pressure of tumescent. Second, when tumescent solution is suddenly injected in huge volume and with high pressure, it may develop a lake in the tissue and eventually liposuction may not be carried out evenly and sufficiently. Third, pressing or massaging with surgeon's hands to evenly distribute the injected tumescent must be avoided because it promotes damages to mature adipocytes.

4) Liposuction method and cautions

Generally, liposuction for fat grafting mainly follows traditional liposuction procedure. Considerations for liposuction are as follows.

First, focus on air volume inside syringe during the liposuction. It should be frequently checked if the air volume of the syringe is too much due to the excessive pulling back of the plunger during liposuction, or due to considerable air coming into the syringe from outside. Proper intra-luminal pressure of the syringe during liposuction is shown in Figure 8[6].

Second, the cannula should be moved back and forth within its entire length which is from the entry site to the marking line. When you want to harvest fat from the very next segment, direction of the cannula should be changed near the entry site as shown in Figure 9A. When moving to the next seg-

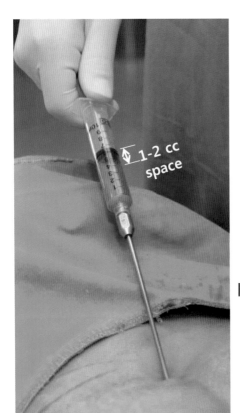

Figure 08 Proper negative pressure during syringe liposuction for fat harvest. To do this, the plunger of the syringe should be gently manipulated to provide about 1 or 2 cc of negative pressure space in the barrel of the syringe while the cannula (length of 25cm and diameter of 3mm) connected to the 10 cc Luer-Lock syringe is pushed through the harvest site. The high vacuum (more than 2cc) may damage the harvested fat cells during harvest procedure.

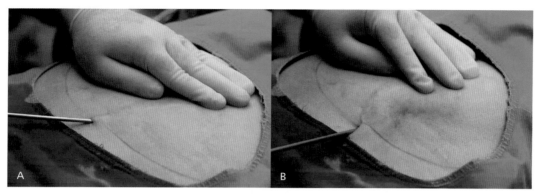

Figure 09 The basic technique of easy cannula movement for liposuction. Cannula moving to next area near the entry site (A), Cannula moving to next area at the middle part of the targeting area for liposuction (B).

ment during suctioning at the middle part of the targeting area, movement of the cannula is restricted due to formation of artificial fold near the entry site. Therefore, sensing of the tip of the cannula becomes dull and suctioning may not be successful as shown in Figure 9B. Sometimes the area near the entry site would be over-suctioned due to the entire cannula movement and repeated pass. For this reason, the cannula movement and suction pressure near the entry site should be minimized.

Third, liposuction should not be repeatedly operated on a single same area. Fat should be evenly suctioned by regularly moving left to the right or right to the left; this should be performed while being involved with the second point mentioned above.

Fourth, minimum force should be used on fingers, hand and arm holding the syringe. The syringe should be moved according to the exact feeling from the tip of the cannula that which layer and location the cannula are at that time.

Fifth, the role of the left hand is considerably important in assistance. It is because the left hand must feel the location of cannula during liposuction and it participates in an important assisting role when cannula should be moved to deeper or more superficial layer for liposuction as in Figure 10.

Left hand pushes skin towards the entry site (approach for deep liposuction, Figure 10A), pulls skin away from entry site (approach for superficial liposuction, Figure 10B), pinches the skin or subcutaneous tissue up with thumb and fingers (approach for deep liposuction, Figure 10C), and touches or presses gently with palm (approach for superficial liposuction and checking the location of the cannula, Figure 10D). These assisting actions are very substantial for facilitating suction by making easy and precise cannula movement depending on depth and location. However, surgeons should be careful not to press the fat inflated with tumescent when pinching the skin and subcutaneous fat up with fingers.

Sixth, skin may be damaged by friction of the entry site during suction. Thus, as in Figure 11, by not pressing the entry site's skin, hold the cannula and move carefully. The damage of entry site cannot be avoided when large amount of fat is harvested. Followings are methods can be used for prevention. The free oil, which is taken from the centrifugation at the early stage of liposuction, can be used as

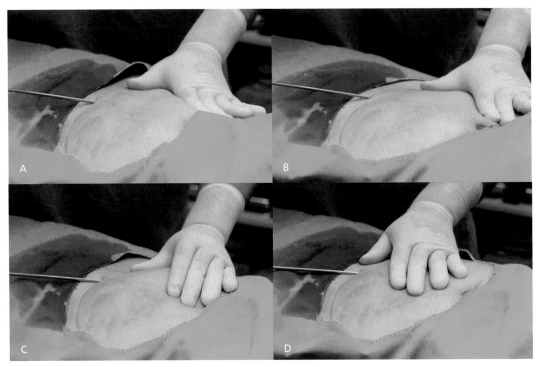

Figure 10 How to approach to superficial or deep layer for liposuction,Liposuction for deep layer (A,C), Liposuction for superficial layer (B,D).

lubricant to be dropped to the cannula's outer surface and the entry site. Wound protector inserted into the entry site is commonly used to avoid friction, but it can enlarge the incision of the entry site.

Seventh, during the liposuction, the color of the aspirates should be always checked. If bleeding occurs, stop the suction and move to other segments to avoid blood contamination. If bleeding is in-

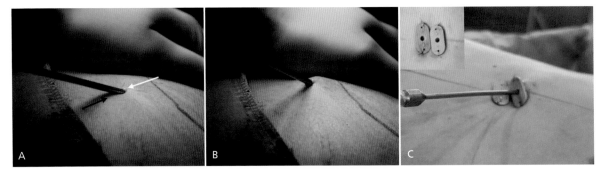

Figure 11 Suction technique for the prevention of superficial burn from the repetitive friction of the cannula against the skin margins (especially lower edge) of the incision site. Pressing or friction on the lower edge of the incision by cannula movement (A). Lift up the cannula more to minimize the pressure or friction on the lower edge of the incision (B). The wound protector is inserted into the entry site (C). White and black arrows indicate the upper and lower edge of the incision respectively.

tense or patient complains of pain, more tumescent should be injected or press the area for a moment. In order to prevent blood contamination, there is a method of designing the suction area as in Figure 12. However, the method can cause irregularity after the procedure, so the cannula should be moved smoothly when moving to next segment.

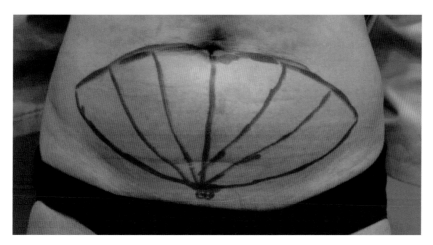

Figure 12 Preoperative marking of the segmental liposuction for prevention of blood contaminated aspirates. In case of bleeding during suction at one segment, liposuction should be performed at other or next segment. However, it is important to pay attention to avoid the formation of irregularities between segments.

Eighth, the boundary between the suctioned area and the non-suctioned area should be smooth without thickness difference when touched by hands. Borderline between the two areas should be checked whether it is natural or not.

Ninth, if any depressed area occurs due to excessive suction on a particular area, it is recommended to inject fat again to that area as soon as the suction finishes.

Tenth, debridement and subdermal suture are recommended for prevention of scar and wound dehiscence. Nylon 6.0 is suitable for suturing. As in Figure 13, reversed vertical mattress suture is recommended and the suture can be removed 7-10 days after.

No critical side effects will occur if the precautions mentioned above are well followed. But even with regional suction for fat grafting, complications are same with those of general liposuction. Especially, surgeon should be very careful on preventing expected complications such as irregularities, unevenness, skin necrosis, hyperpigmentation, and etc.

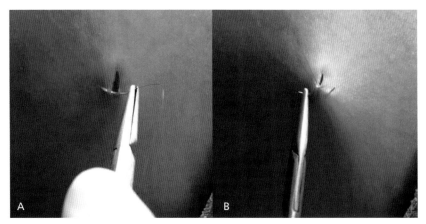

Figure 13 Reversed vertical mattress suture is used to close the entry site. First step (A). Second step (B).

4 Fat purification

1) Washing and centrifugation

When excessive blood has flowed into the fat aspirates, it is recommended to wash the fat inside the syringe. Insert the syringe containing fat aspirates into a syringe rack for 3-5 minutes to precipitate. After pushing out the lower layer of tumescent solution contaminated by blood, mix with 5% dextrose water or Ringer's lactate solution, and then precipitate it again or centrifuge. Generally, the fat aspirate is centrifuged at 1200-1280g for 3 minutes.

2) Elimination of free oil

After centrifugation, free oil, the yellow liquid at the uppermost layer in the syringe should be eliminated. Because free oil is one the reasons for causing inflammation when injected into body; hence, it should be eliminated as much as possible. Free oil and contaminated upper fat layer can be removed by holding the syringe diagonally and just pour the contaminated layer out. Besides, the remained oil should be absorbed and wiped by wet gauze or oil cleansing tissue (e.g. Codman neuropads).

I would like to introduce an interesting method as shown in Figure 14, where the contaminated layer is removed by absorption, by using appropriately cut paper towels (kitchen towels) which were sterilized, rolled up and put in centrifuged syringe. This method is used by Australian cosmetic surgeon Longin Zureck[8]. Precaution should be taken for not putting all parts of the oil removing-pad and gauze into the fat.

3) Separation and recharge

After eliminating free oil in the upper layer, discharge the lower infranatant fraction which contains

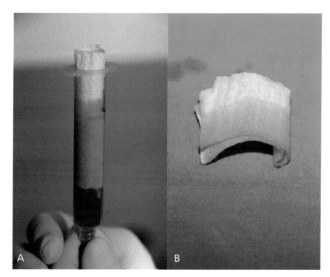

Figure 14 Dr. Longin's technique for removal of free oil from the centrifuged fat aspirates using a paper towel. The free oil is absorbed quickly into the rolled up paper towel (A). The used paper towel contains the free oil (B).

blood and tumescent anesthetics. Then, recharge fat from 10cc Luer-Lok syringe to 1cc syringe by a connecting transfer tube and use it for grafting.

5 Practical guide for preparations

The content is written for the purpose of practical guide for nurses to prepare fat grafting conveniently and easily.

1) Solutions

(1) Basic concept
① Concentration
  (i) Normally concentration of the solution is designated by the percentage (%) of the solute's weight (gram) in 100ml of solution, e.g. 0.5% of Bupivacaine or 1% of Lidocaine (1%=1g/100mL=1000mg/100mL=10mg/mL).
  (ii) Fast calculation is possible with standard of 1% equals to 10mg/ml.
    e.g. 0.5% of Bupivacaine = 5mg/mL, 2% of Lidocaine = 20mg/mL
② Dilution
  Dilution requires the thorough mixing of a small, accurately measured sample with a large volume of sterile water, saline or other appropriate liquid called the diluent or a dilution blank. For

ease of calculation, dilutions are done in multiples of 10 or 100. For example the dilution of 1 mL into 9 mL is written 1/10 or 10^{-1} and can be called as 1:10 dilution.

(i) When doing very high dilutions, e.g., drug added to anesthetic, dilution degree is designated as like 1:10,000 or 1:100,000.

e.g. 1:200,000 means 1mg per 200mL (i.e., 0.0005%)

(ii) Dilution examples of drug use in small volume are seen in Table 3.

(iii) Example of making 2% of lidocaine + 1:100,000 Epinephrine solution

-> Mix together the 2% of lidocaine 19.8ml + 0.2ml Epinephrine (1mg/ml)

(2) 3 kinds of anesthetic solutions for fat grafting

① Solution A is used for skin infiltration and composed of 2% lidocaine and epinephrine (1:100,000)

② Solution B is used for body liposuction as a modified Klein's solution.

H/S or N/S	:	500ml
2% Lidocaine (400mg/20ml)	:	20cc
Epinephrine (1mg/1ml)	:	0.5cc
8.4% Sodium hydrogen carbonate (Bivon®)	:	5cc

③ Solution C is used for facial liposuction and fat grafting as my modification of modified Klein's solution, which is mixed together in the 2:8 ratio of Solution A (2 ml) and Solution B (8 ml).

2) Instruments and the other materials

Spread sterilized operation towel on operating assistance table and arrange instruments as in Figure 15.

3) Preparation of patient

(1) Designing

① Escort the patient to locker room and let him or her wear the patient gown.

② After washing his or her face, ask the patient to put on a hair band and take photographs.

③ Prepare essential objects for design such as a marking pen and etc.

④ After design process, move the patient to the operation room and then prepare for sterilization.

Table 03 Dilution examples of drug use in small volume.

Solution Volume	1:100,000 (1mg/100mL)	1:200,000 (1mg/200mL)
1mL	0.01mg	0.005mg
5mL	0.05mg	0.025mg
20ml	0.2mg	0.1mg

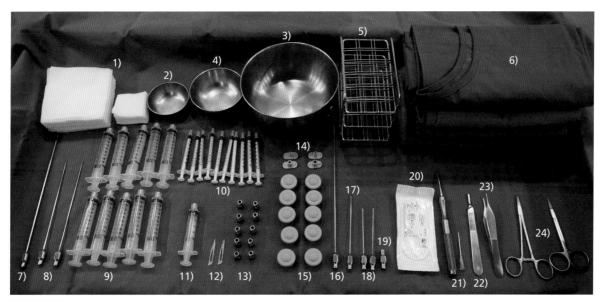

Figure 15 Instruments and their arrangement for fat grafting and liposuction.

Instruments	No.	Instruments	No.
1) Gauze (4x4), (2x2)	10,10	13) Syringe needle adapter cap	10
2) Small bowl for solution A	1	14) Wond protector	4
3) Large bowl for solution B	1	15) Syringe barrel end stopper	10
4) Small bowl for solution C	1	16) Infiltration cannula for tumescent anesthesia (body) (15G×20.0cm)	1
5) Syringe rack	1	17) Infiltration cannula for tumescent anesthesia (face) (18G×9.0cm)	1
6) Operation towel for face and body	8	18) Fat injection cannula (19Gx7.0cm, 18Gx7.0cm)	1, 1
7) Liposuction cannula (Body) (3.0mm×20.0cm)	1	19) Transfer	1
8) Liposuction cannula (face) (1.6 and 1.8mm ×15.0cm)	1, 1	20) Suture material (Nylon 6-0)	1
9) 10cc Luer-Slip disposable syringe	10	21) 18G needle or awl	1
10) 1cc Luer-Lok disposable syringe	10	22) Scalpel handle	1
11)) 5cc Luer-Slip disposable syringe for skin desensitization	1	23) Adson teeth forceps	1
12) Blade No.11 and 15	1	24) Needle holder, Iris scissor	1, 1

(2) Preparation of sedation

① Before or after designing, prepare an intravenous route for fluid supply and connect it to 500ml of normal saline solution.

② Prepare oxygen supply (3-5L/min) as it might be needed before or during sedation.

③ Before the surgery, inject antibiotics into connected i.v. line. It is recommended to inject glycopyrrolate (Robinul® 0.2mg/ml, 0.004mg/kg, muscle injected) as anticholinergic 30 minutes before sedation, to decrease secretion during the sedation.

④ Attach patient monitoring devices which are necessary for sedation, monitor blood pressure, pulse, respiratory rate, and oxygen saturation rate, and record them on operation chart.

(3) Disinfection

① Ask the patient to lie down on the operation table.

② For donor site, uses 10% povidone iodide solution (butadiene®) to sterilize areas broader than the designed areas and sterilize every area that is vulnerable to contamination during surgery. Especially, the region of the entry sites should be thoroughly sterilized.

③ Put a towel or hair band to the patient's head to fix his or her hair in order not to fall down during the surgery.

④ Apply antibiotic ointment to protect the corneas of the eyes, asks the patient to close his or her eyes and put gauzes on the patient's eyes. Secure them with disposable paper plasters to avoid blinking.

⑤ Sterilize the patient's face with 0.2% Benzalkonium chloride (zephanon®) or povidone iodide solution. Sterilization should be performed on every area, including nasal prong, which is possible to contacts during surgery.

⑥ Cover body areas, except the donor site for fat harvest and recipient site for fat injection, with operating towels.

4) Fat Harvest

(1) Injection of tumescent solution into donor site and face

① Prepare 5 or 10cc syringe containing solution A (2% lidocaine and epinephrine (1:100,000)) in order to anesthetize the entry sites.

② Prepare a Luer-Lok 10cc syringe with tumescent solution B for donor site anesthesia and attach a cannula (15G×25cm) for injection. Wait for 10 minutes in minimum or up to 30 minutes after injection. Regional tumescent anesthesia on the face is performed while waiting.

③ Prepare tumescent solution C for facial anesthesia. Generally, 20-30cc is prepared for facial anesthesia. When liposuction for both the face and neck area are conducted, prepare an additional 100 ml of the solution C.

④ Prepare a 18G needle which is used to make entry sites on the face. Attach an injection cannula (18G×9cm) to a 10cc Luer-Lok syringe filled with tumescent solution B for face.

⑤ After tumescent solution is injected into the patient's face, liposuction for donor site is performed.

(2) Liposuction for the donor site

For fat harvest from donor site, attach a cannula (3.0mm x 20.0cm) to 10cc Luer-Lok syringe for injection. Cannula contamination should always be careful during liposuction.

(3) Fat separation and centrifuge

① Hold the syringe containing fat aspirates upright, put a needle adaptor cap on the tip of the syringe, separates the piston from the syringe carefully, and then covers the barrel shield hole with a barrel end stopper (Figure 16A).

② If the fat aspirate is contaminated with large amount of blood, fill Hartman's solution when extra space is available in syringe. Or else, let the syringe stays upright for 3-5 minutes in a syringe rack and then throw the lower blood contaminated layer away, refill with Hartman solution, let it stays upright for another 3-5 minutes, and then throw it away again.

③ For balanced loading of the centrifuge rotor, equalize the fat aspirates' volume in every syringe (Figure 16A). When there is lesser volume, equalize them by adding Hartman's solution or additional fat aspirates.

④ When syringes containing fat are placed in a centrifuge, they should be in perfect symmetry as displayed in Figure 17. Rotor, sleeve, and sleeve rack in the centrifuge should be sterilized in advance. Even though fixed rotors are harder to be sterilized, they must be sterilized at least by using alcohol. Centrifugation speed and time are 1280g and 3 minutes. Noise during centrifugation means imbalance of fat volume, so stop the centrifuge and check the fat volume

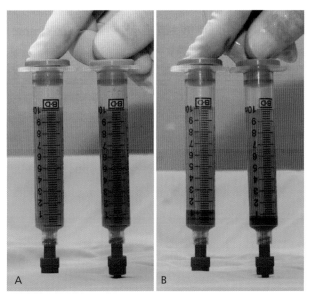

Figure 16　Autologus fat aspirates before (A) and after centrifugation (B).

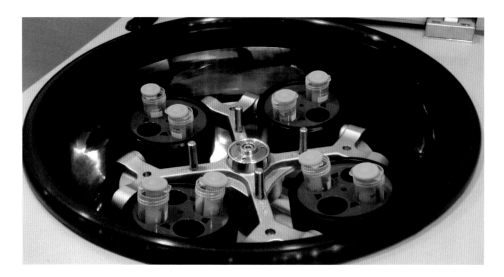

Figure 17 The syringes should be placed into a centrifuge with symmetrical position. The recommended centrifugation is at 1280xg for 3 minutes.

balance. During centrifugation, prepare suture stitch (Nylon 6-0), needle holder, forceps, and scissors for wound closing of entry site.

(4) Purification after centrifuge

① After the centrifugation, take out the syringes containing fat aspirates from the centrifuge and remove the uppermost free oil from the barrel. The easiest way to remove the free oil is shown in Figure 18. Tilt the barrel of the syringe to pour away the free oil. Next, wipe out the remaining oil which is still remaining on the uppermost fat layer and inside wall of the barrel by using the gauze. Please pay attention not to let the fiber pieces of the gauze fall into the barrel.

② After the oil is removed, the needle adaptor cap can be removed from the threaded tip of Luer-Lok syringe. The lower aqueous component will be expelled out of the syringe spontaneously.

③ Install the plunger in the barrel again and attach a transfer to the tip of 10cc Luer-Lok syringe packed with purified fat. Next, press the plunger to check whether the fat has totally filled the transfer. Then, connect this to a 1cc Luer-Slip syringe as shown in Figure 19. The plunger should be completely pushed ahead to avoid formation of air bubbles.

④ When moving the fat through the transfer, do not push with too much pressure. Push the plunger of 10cc syringe while pulling the plunger of 1cc syringe. The pressure should be minimized to prevent damage to the fat.

⑤ It is recommended to charge only 0.7-0.8cc in a 1cc Luer-Slip syringe. If air enters into the charged syringe, turn the 1cc syringe upside down and move in spraying manner towards the

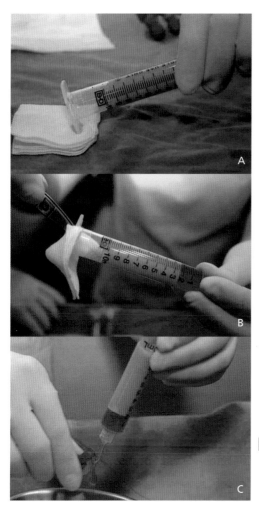

Figure 18 Removal of the upper oil and the lower infranatant solution. Pour the upper oil by tilting a syringe (A), Wipe out the remaining oil in the lumen of barrel (B), and throw out the lower serosanguineous solution (C).

space to push intraluminal air out of the syringe. Next, attach a cannula (18 or 19G × 0.7cm) for injection.

⑥ Prepare a suture fiber (Nylon 6-0, 7-0) for the entry site immediately after fat grafting.

6 Postoperative care

① Clean the face with gauze soaked in normal saline solution. Dry after sterilizing with povidone iodide solution in suture area, and put Steri-Strip™ from 3M™ Company[9].

② In the case of facial liposuction performed simultaneously, put on facial band, which position should be corrected accordingly so that fat grafted area is not pressed.

③ Clean the liposuctioned area with gauze soaked in normal saline solution and put Reston® foam

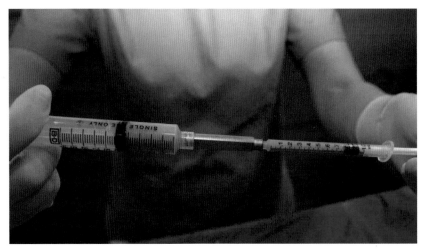

Figure 19 Recharge of fat to a smaller syringe. The purified fat in 10ml Luer-Lok syringe is moved to a 1ml Luer-Slip syringe using a transfer. During this time, you should pay attention to avoid accidental insertion of air bubbles into the barrel of syringe or column of the fat.

after drying. To prevent skin damage, spray Cavilon™ (3M™: no sting barrier film 3346) to the area for Reston® foam application before putting the Reston® foam on. Next, put on 6 inch elastic bandages.

④ Stitch out the facial entry site suture after 3 days and put on Steri-Strip™ for 2 more days. Washing face is possible after this.

⑤ Remove Reston® foam and elastic bandages on the donor site on the next day of the surgery. Put on girdle or maternity belt that can put pressure on the donor site for more than at least 2 weeks.

⑥ In case of dermal suture in the entry site, stitch out after minimum of 7 to 10 days after the procedure. The patient has to take shower with the Steri-Strip™ on for 2 days.

⑦ Take photographs on the last day of the treatment.

Reference

01. http://www.medizone1.co.kr/, Tel. & FAX : +82-2-433-6862, E-mail: y6682@nate.com

02. http://en.wikipedia.org/wiki/Detergent

03. http://en.wikipedia.org/wiki/Baking_powder

04. Klein JA. Tumescent formulation. In Tumescent technique: Tumescent anesthesia & microcannular liposuction. Klein, JA (de) St. Louis, Mosby 2000:187-195.

05. Available at http://www.aestheticsurgery.ie/images/liposuction1.jpg.

06. Kuhbier JW, Weyand B, Radtke C, Vogt PM, Kasper C, Reimers K. Isolation, characterization, differentiation, and application of adipose-derived stem cells. Adv Biochem Eng Biotechnol. 2010;123:55-105. doi: 10.1007/10_2009_24.

07. Coleman SR. Structural Fat Grafting. Quality Medical Publishing, Inc., St. Louis, Mo. 2004;Pp 404.

08. Login Zurek. Personal communication, Sydney Australia. March 2011. http://www.s-lift.com.au/

09. 3M US. Nexcare Steri-Strip Skin Closure". 3m.com. http://www.3m.com/product/information/Nexcare-Steri-Strip-Skin-Closure.html. Retrieved 2011-03-22.

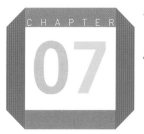

a novel facial fat grafting technique with a concept of volumetric lifting

Anesthesia

1 Sedation anesthesia

1) Introduction

Although there are several methods of anesthesia for facial fat grafting, the sedation for outpatient is preferred because facial fat grafting requires a small incision, relatively less tissue damage and short operation time about 1-2 hours. In order to eliminate or reduce the pain, it is recommended to use analgesics or local anesthetics additionally. Recently, conscious sedation is commonly used along with adequate local or regional anesthesia. Conscious sedation features anxiolytic, sedative, and analgesic effects through using combination of medicines and it features fast onset time and short duration.

In order to do proper anesthesia for facial fat grafting, satisfactory sedation is required to decrease pain caused by precipitate of local anesthetics. And side effects should be prevented as much as possible by using minimal dose of analgesics[1].

2) Sedation

(1) Definition

Sedation refers to the way of suppressing central nervous system by drugs to decrease consciousness. It is the concept including several levels according to the degree[2], from very shallow depth of sedation which responds well to verbal commands and markedly retains protection reflexes to general anesthesia which the conditions of loss of consciousness and reflex, sensation(aponia) and muscle relaxation.

(2) Classification

American Society of Anesthesiologist (ASA) classifies sedation into several types: minimal sedation, moderate sedation/analgesia (=conscious sedation), deep sedation/analgesia and general anesthesia as shown in Table 1[3].

Table 01 Classification of the sedation.

	Minimal Sedation	Moderate Sedation/Analgesia	Deep Sedation/Analgesia	General Anesthesia
Responsiveness	Normal response to verbal stimulation	Purposeful response to verbal op tactile stimulation	Purposeful response after repeated or painful stimulation	Unarousable, even with painful stimulus
Airway	Unaffected	No intervention required	Intervention may be required	Intervention often required
Spontaneous ventilation	Unaffected	Adequate	May be inadequate	Frequently inadequate
Cardiovascular function	Unaffected	Usually maintained	Usually maintained	May be impaired

(3) Purpose of sedation

The purpose of anesthesia for fat grafting is conscious sedation, which makes patient comfort and relaxed during the procedure though avoiding anxiety and decreasing pain. It also allow patient to make cooperative in surgery by easily awakening to verbal commands or physical stimuli from the sleep state and not allow patient remembering surgical procedures[4].

The ideal drug for sedation should be convenient and potent amnesic and anxiolytic with a rapid onset of action, have rare adverse effects and possess a short duration of action, thus allowing the patient to return to normal life immediagely[5]. Nonetheless, it is practically difficult to maintain the ideal condition due to diverse surgery manipulations and pharmaco-dynamic differences in different individual.

3) Guidelines for conscious sedation.

Since the sedation level is unclear, it may suddenly shift to the deeper sedation than the primarily planned level. Hence, surgeon practicing sedation should be aware of patient's response changes according to sedation process, and have the ability to rescue patients induced to deeper sedation. It is also essential to evaluate frequently the patient's reflex and status of consciousness after sedation start.

(1) Contraindication

Sedation should be avoided for patients who cannot lie down straight due to dementia, heart failure, cardiovascular disease, COPD, hiatal hernia, and who may have possibility of aspiration by reflux such as achalasia. It is requires to diagnose whether the patient has a hypovolemia because of high possibility of rapid hemodynamic change. Since decrease of circulating blood volume in body may be intensified due to fasting, even in the case of patients without cardiovascular disorders, prophylactic fluid infusion is conducted before surgery. In my case, 300-500ml of physiological saline is infused for prevention by monitoring dryness of tongue.

(2) Fasting

Fasting is the most critical factor in sedation anesthesia. It must be checked several times right before anesthesia because patients may unconsciously drink coffee or water while waiting for the surgery. Fasting period according to ingested materials is as shown in Table 2 below[3].

Table 02　Minimal fasting periods according to the various ingested materials in anesthesia.

Ingested Material	Minimun Fasting Period+
Clear liquid++	2h
Breast milk	4h
Infant formula	6h
Nonhuman milk+++	6h
Light meal++++	6h

These recommendations apply to healthy patients who are undergoing elective procedures. They are not intended for women on labor. Following the Guidelines does not guarantee a complete gastric emptying has occurred.
+The fasting periods apply to all ages
++Examples of clear liquids include water, fruit juices without pulp, carbonated beverages, clear tea, and black coffee.
+++Since nonhuman milk is similar to solids in gastric emptying time, the amount ingested must be considered when determining an appropriate fasting period.
++++A light meal typically consists of toast and clear liquids. Meals that include fried or fatty foods or meat may prolong gastric emptying time. Both the amount and type of foods ingested must be considered when determining an appropriate fasting period.

(3) Preparation

Following factors should be prepared for the basic examination for sedation and in the case of unintended transition to general anesthesia.

① **Patient assessment**

　(i) Major organ malformation

　(ii) Experience of side effect in previous anesthesia.

　(iii) Drug allergy, present medication, and correlation between medication and anesthetics.

　(iv) Time and type of ingested materials (food or water).

　(v) Alcohol, smoking, drug abuse.

Airway assessment procedures for sedation and analgesia are in Table 3 for reference[3].

Table 03 Airway assessment procedures for sedation and analgesia.

Positive pressure ventilation, with or without tracheal intubation, may be necessary if respiratory compromise develops during sedation-analgesia. This may be more difficult in patients with atypical airway anatomy. In addition, some airway abnormalities may increase the likelihood of airway obstruction during spontaneous ventilation. Some factors that may be associated with difficulty in airway management are:

History	Previous problems with anesthesia or sedation Stridor, snoring, or sleep apnea Advanced rheumatoid arthritis Chromosomal abnormality (e.g., trisomy 21)
Physical Examination	Habitus
	Significant obesity (especially involving the neck and facial structures)
	Head and Neck
	Short neck, limited neck extension, decreased hyoid--mental distance (3 cm in an adult), neck mass, cervical spine disease or trauma, tracheal deviation, dysmorphic facial features (e.g., Pierre-Robin syndrome)
	Mouth
	Small opening (3 cm in an adult); edentulous; protruding incisors; loose or capped teeth; dental appliances; high, arched palate; macroglossia; tonsillar hypertrophy; nonvisible uvula
	Jaw
	Micrognathia, retrognathia, trismus, significant malocclusion

② Basic emergency equipments for sedation, analgesia, and resuscitation

Table 4 shows the equipments and drugs for sedation as recommended by ASA[3]. Table 5 shows the summarized index and descriptions of sedation (anesthesia) and emergency resuscitation equipment in clinic offices.

③ Drugs used in emergency resuscitation

Table 6 shows the reference of drugs used in emergency during sedation (anesthesia)[12,13].

(4) Adverse reactions of sedation

Emergencies that may occur during sedation include airway obstruction, hypoxia, cardiovascular complication due to arrhythmia and etc. Complication incidence increases by prolonged operation time and known cardiovascular diseases[14]. It is important to install monitor devices such as ECG, non-invasive sphygomanometer, pulse oximeter, end tidal capnometry, and etc. And check patients thoroughly and supply constant oxygen.

If airway obstruction outbreaks happen, hypoxia occurs within a few minutes and reflux of gastric contents may be accompanied. Pulmonary edema may befall even when negative pressure in airway

Table 04 Emergency equipment for sedation & analgesia.

Appropriate emergency equipment should be available whenever sedative or analgesic drugs capable of causing cardiorespiratory depression are administered. The lists below should be used as a guide, which should be modified depending on the individual practice circumstances. Items in brackets are recommended when infants or children are sedated.

Intravenous equipment	Gloves Tourniquets Alcohol wipes Sterile gauze pads Intravenous catheters [24-22-gauge] Intravenous tubing [pediatric "microdrip" (60 drops/ml)] Intravenous fluid Assorted needles for drug aspiration, intramuscular injection [intraosseous bone marrow needle] Appropriately sized syringes [1-ml syringes] Tape
Basic airway management equipment	Source of compressed oxygen (tank with regulator or pipeline supply with flowmeter) Source of suction Suction catheters [pediatric suction catheters] Yankauer-type suction Face masks [infant/child] Self-inflating breathing bag-valve set [pediatric] Oral and nasal airways [infant/child-sized] Lubricant

Advanced airway management equipment (for practitioners with intubation skills)	Laryngeal mask airways [pediatric]
	Laryngoscope handles (tested)
	Laryngoscope blades [pediatric]
	Endotracheal tubes
	    Cuffed 6.0, 7.0, 8.0 mm ID
	    [Uncuffed 2.5, 3.0, 3.5, 4.0, 4.5, 5.0, 5.5, 6.0 mm ID]
	Stylet (appropriately sized for endotracheal tubes)

Pharmacologic Antagonists	Naloxone Flumazenil
Emergency medications	Epinephrine Ephedrine Vasopressin Atropine Nitroglycerin (tablets or spray) Amiodarone Lidocaine Glucose, 50% [10 or 25%] Diphenhydramine Hydrocortisone, methylprednisolone, or dexamethasone Diazepam or midazolam

happens even for a short period of time; therefore, it should be immediately solved.

Fully monitor whether the patient respires well voluntarily, or if the airway is obstructed. If it is partially obstructed, perform triple airway maneuver or insert oral airway. If it is totally obstructed, insert oral airway or practice endotracheal intubation immediately if necessary. After the airway is secured, supply oxygen to correct hypoxia. Generally, apnea seldom occurs as long as the airway is secured.

Table 05 Descriptions and photos of anesthesia equipment and emergency resuscitation

Equipment name	Photo	Usage	Ref.
1. Oxygen tank		To provide oxygen in case of emergency	
2. Nasal prong		To provide oxygen in case of emergency	6.
3. AMBU (air-mask-bag-unit)		Usually used in artificial respiration and to provide sufficient oxygen and ventilatory volume	7.
4. Pulse oxymeter		Non-invasive device to measure oxygen saturation of arterial blood	8.
5. Patient Monitors		To monitor patient condition 1) Standard features: EKG, BP, Pulse Rate 2) Advanced features : Standard features: + Resp Rate, Expiratory Co2	9.
6. Infusion pump		To deliver a measured amount of drugs over long periods of time	10.
7. Defibrillator (Bi-phasic)		To treat life -threatening cardiac dysrhythmias and ventricular fibrillation (200J).	11

Especially, peripheral O_2 saturation ratio (SpO_2) should be intensively monitored from the pulse oximeter. Clinically, arterial O_2 saturation ratio(SaO_2) is considered as the same with a SpO_2. As shown Figure 1, normal partial arterial oxygen pressure (PaO_2) is more than 100 mmHg, SaO_2 is more than 95 %, the number of 95 is observed on the display of the pulse oximeter as a SpO_2. Hypoxemia is defined when PaO_2 is dropped under 60 mmHg. When PaO_2 is 60 mmHg and SaO_2 is 90%. 90 on the display of pulse oximeter means an emergent situation as an early state of hypoxia. Therefore, when-

Table 06 Drugs used during emergency of sedation anesthesia

Type	Drug	Dosage	Indication
Antidote	Flumazenil	0.2mg IV over 15 seconds, usual dose 0.3~0.6mg, Maximum dose 1.0mg	Reversal of the sedation effects of benzodiazepines on the CNS
	Naloxone	0.2mg IV over 15 seconds, usual dose 0.3~0.6mg, Maximum dose 1.0mg	Reversal of opoid Recovery of self-ventilation
Emergency medications	Epinephrine	For emergency use (e.g. cardiac arrest) 1mg IV every 3-5minutes	Asthma, urticaria, drug shock, and cardiac arrest
	Ephedrine	5~10mg IV	Control blood pressure at the occurrence of hypotension
	Atropine	0.5mg subcutaneous or intramuscular injection CPR : inject 1mg IV at interval of 3-5minutes Maximum dose 3mg	Bradycardia

ever SaO_2 is dropped under 95%, it should be increased up to 95% with prompt airway management and oxygen supplement. Another thing to care for is change of SaO_2, because it decreases slowly in the interval between 100% and 95%, but drops abruptly after 95%.

If hemodynamic change occurs due to cardiovascular complication, it can be suspected as hypervolemic shock, anaphylactic shock, neurogenic shock or pain shock (by pain). cardiac arrest may

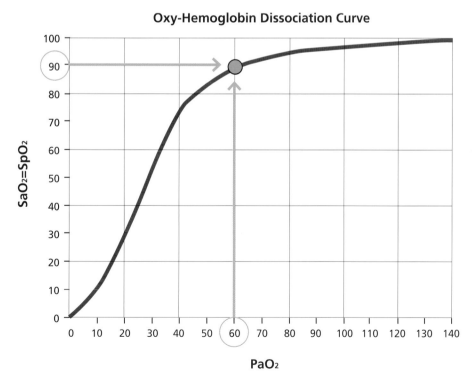

Oxy-Hemoglobin Dissociation Curve

Figure 01 Relationship between SaO_2 and PaO_2.

happen. Supply sufficient intravascular volume and treat with appropriate drugs. Table 7 shows CPR(cardiopulmonary resuscitation) guidelines revised by the American heart association in 2010[15].

The 2010 Guidelines were most notable for the reorientation of the universal sequence from A-B-C (Airway, Breathing, Compressions) to C-A-B (Compressions, Airway, Breathing) to minimize time to initiation of chest compressions. As updated recommendations for the 2015 adult basic life support (BLS) guidelines, there is increased emphasis on the rapid identification of potential cardiac arrest by dispatchers, with immediate provision of CPR instructions to the caller. Recommendations are made for a simultaneous, choreographed approach to performance of chest compressions, airway manage-

Table 07 **American heart association/guidelines for CPR & ECG in 2010.**

Component	Recommendations		
	Adults	Children	Infants
Recognition	Unresponsive (for all ages)		
Recognition	No breathing or no normal breathing (ie, only gasping)	No breathing or only gasping	
Recognition	No pulse palpated within 10 seconds for all ages (Healthcare Providers: HCP)only		
CPR sequence	C-A-B		
Compression rate	At least 100/min		
Compression depth	At least 2 inches (5 cm)	At least 1/3 AP diameter About 2 inches (5 cm)	At least 1/3 AP diameter About 1 inches (4 cm)
Chest wall recoil	Allow complete recoil between compressions HCP rotate compressors every 2 minutes		
Compression interruptions	Minimize interruptions in chest compressions Attempt to limit interrruptions to <10 seconds		
Airway	Head tilt–.chin lift (HCP suspected trauma: jaw thrust)		
Compression-to-ventilation ratio (until advanced airway placed)	30:2 1 or 2 rescuers	30:2 Single rescuer 15:2 2 HCP rescuers	
Ventilations: when rescuer untrained or trained and not proficient	Compressions only		
Ventilations with advanced airway (HCP)	1 breath every 6-8 seconds (8-10 breaths/min) Asynchronous with chest compressions About 1 second per breath Visible chest rise		
Defibrillation	Attach and use AED as soon as available. Minimize interruptions in chest compressions before and after shock; resume CPR beginning with compressions immediately after each shock.		

The 2010 Guidelines were most notable for the reorientation of the universal sequence from A-B-C (Airway, Breathing, Compressions) to C-A-B (Compressions, Airway, Breathing) to minimize time to initiation of chest compressions. As updated recommendations for the 2015 adult basic life support (BLS) guidelines, there is increased emphasis on the rapid identification of potential cardiac arrest by dispatchers, with immediate provision of CPR instructions to the caller. Recommendations are made for a simultaneous, choreographed approach to performance of chest compressions, airway management, rescue breathing, rhythm detection, and shock delivery (if indicated) by an integrated team of highly trained rescuers in applicable settings.

ment, rescue breathing, rhythm detection, and shock delivery (if indicated) by an integrated team of highly trained rescuers in applicable settings.

4) Drugs for sedation

(1) Classification

Since surgical site is face, anesthetics for sedation are intravenous anesthetic rather than inhalation anesthetic. Intravenous anesthetics can be broadly classified into barbiturate derivatives and non-barbiturate derivatives as Table 8. Barbiturate derivatives feature significant sedation and hypnotic effect but have no analgesic effect and poor amnesic effect. Non-barbiturate derivatives feature an excellent amnesic effect but no analgesic effect and various hypnotic effects; so, some drugs of them generally have characteristics which are difficult to be expected as below

Table 08 **Classification and kinds of intravenous anesthetic**

Barbiturate	Thiopental, Thiamylal, Methohexital	
Non-barbiturate	Non-opioid	Benzodiazepines(Diazepam, Lorazepam, Midazolam), Ketamine, Etomidate, Propofol
	Opioids	Morphine, Peperidine, Fentanyl, Sulfentanil, Alfentanil, Remifentanil

First, ketamine features good analgesic and hypnotic effects but has hypnopompic hallucination.

Second, etomidate has good hypnotic effect but no analgesic effect and poor amnesic effect.

Third, propofol features similar characteristics like barbiturates.

Fourth, opioid has superb analgesic effect but poor hypnotic effect and has almost no amnesic effect.

Induction level, onset time, duration time and analgesic effects of generally used intravenous anesthetics are listed in Table 9[13]. Exact induction dose for different level of sedation are lack of references. Therefore, it is recommended to use intravenous anesthetics by referred induction dose and individual's susceptibility differences.

(2) Drugs of benzodiazepine derivatives

Benzodiazepine drugs like diazepam and lorazepma are not used for sedation because of long onset time and duration compared to other drugs. Commonly used midazolam (0.07-0.1mg/kg IM, 0.04~0.05mg/kg IV) is hydrosoluble; it features includes no pain in the muscle or intravenous injection, sedation, antianxiety, oblivion and anticonvulsant characteristics. It has a short onset time and 1-4 hours of half-life and stronger than diazepam by 2-4 times. Its advantages are that it has antidote called flumazenil(Anexate®) and comes back to the normal state immediately from oblivion after anesthesia.

Table 09 Induction level and characteristic of various intravenous anesthetics.

	Induction level (mg/kg)	Onset time (Sec.)	Duration (Min.)	Severity of pain
Thiopental	3~6	<30	5~10	+
Thiamylal	3~6	<30	5~10	+
Methohexital	1~3	<30	5~10	++
Diazepam	0.3~0.6	45~60	15~30	+++
Lorazepam	0.03~0.06	60~120	60~120	++
Midazolam	0.2~0.4	30~60	15~30	0
Ketamine	1~2	45~60	10~20	0
Etomidate	0.2~0.3	15~45	3~12	+++
Propofol	1.5~3.0	15~45	5~10	++

(3) Propofol

① Characteristics

Propofol, 2,6-diisopropylphenol, has clinical attributes that cause it to be a widely used anesthetic and sedative, but it is a difficult compound to formulate in stable aqueous vehicles suitable for routine clinical use.

It is an oil with a slightly yellowish color in its pure form at room temperature, but it freezes at only 19°C. Because of its unique chemistry, poor water miscibility and high lipophilicity, it cannot be administered as aqueous salts compared to the other intravenous anesthetics. The high lipophilicity means that good propofol miscibility can only be achieved in lipophilic substances or organic solvents. Because vehicles for clinical delivery of anesthetics should be evenly disperse the active ingredient in a suitable volume that allows the clinician to administer the drug in a convenient dose size while not inducing side effects, researches about some kind of emulsifiers or surfactants have been done. So far, Propofol soybean oil emulsion formulations have met with considerable success but various side effects according to their formula (pain, hyperlipidemia, allergy, etc.) were still remaining.

Propofol has substantial hypnotic, sedation and amnesic effects with characteristics of short induction time and fast metabolism. Because, it is not accumulated much in the body even with a constant injection, it also has some advantages: fast recovery from anesthesia, little frequencies of postoperative nausea, vomiting, drowsiness and emergency situation. Therefore, it is commonly used as an appropriate drug for anesthesia for outpatients who desire smooth recovery. It is also known to enhance sedation and analgesic and amnesic effects when combined with opioid compared to using alone.

② **Dose**

Generally, induction dose and maintain dose is 1.5~3.0 mg/kg[16]and 25~75μg/kg/min respectively. ED_{50} for loss of consciousness is 1~1.5 mg/kg.

③ **Action and metabolism**

After injection of the induction dose, loss of consciousness occurs within one minute and sedation effect lasts for about 4 minutes and wakes up after 5~10 minutes. Most patients pretreated with opioid show temporary apnea for 30-90 seconds, so it should be carefully monitored. In addition, myoclonus, hiccup, sneeze, and etc. may occur. So oxygen saturation level in blood and airway should be maintained in optimal condition. Induction stage should be carefully observed for the elderly or hypovolemic patients because pulse increases temporarily while mean arterial pressure decreases to about 30% after injection.

Hypovolemic patients generally tend to have higher pulse than normal people and shorter onset time after drug injection. Especially, for the elderly, since compensation is not active, it is safe to inject a 50% of primary induction dose and to monitor the drug's response, and then to inject additional dose when needed.

Respiratory depression occurs due to decreased sensitivity of respiratory drive despite of increased CO_2, especially decreased central inspiratory drive.

On central nervous system, it decreases the intracranial pressure, cerebral perfusion pressure, cerebral metabolic rate, and intraocular pressure but, maintains the brain's normal response to CO_2. In case of bolus injection into vessel at a time, drug concentration shows tendency to decrease rapidly because of redistribution. The drug is mostly metabolized in liver and excreted through kidney, but it is also assumed to be metabolized in organs other than the liver. It is also reported that Propofol metabolism is not greatly influenced by liver or kidney diseases. However, the injection dose should be decreased for the elderly patients because they have decreased redistribution function.

④ **Injection method**

To prevent pain during intravenous injection, choose thicker vein and pretreat with simultaneously injection of lidocaine or fentanyl and decrease drug temperature to 2~4°C. The drug can be used with dilution in 5% dextrose water or physiological saline. The usage concentration is shown below.

i) How to inject by using infusion pump

Use of infusion pump is recommended because it has exact maintenance amount with flexibility in time set up.

(i)Induction dose: 1~2mg/kg

If the patient's total body weight(TBW) is 60kg, the induction dose can be calculated as 60 Kg × 1~2 mg/kg = 60 ~ 120 mg. Since 10mg is contained in 1ml of 1%propofol, 6~12ml of 1% propofol is the induction dose. Appropriate injection dose should be determined by considering the patient›s age and TBW.

(ii)Maintenance dose : 25~75 mcg/kg/min

Conversing maintenance dose from per minute to per hour, maintenance dose is 25~75 mcg/kg/min= 1500~4500 mcg/kg/hr (60 min = 1hr). After conversing mcg to mg, maintenance dose is 1.5~4.5 mg/kg/hr (1000 mcg = 1 mg). If the patient›s TBW is 60kg, the maintenance dose is 90~270 mg/hr. Since 10mg is contained in 1ml of 1%propofol, the final maintenance dose is 9~27 ml/hr.

(iii) Easy calculation for maintenance dose (mg/hr, TBW X 1.5 ~ TBW X 4.5)(Table 10)

e.g.) If TBW is 60kg, maintain dose per hour is 60X1.5 ~ 60X4.5 mg/hr

(In other words, 1% propofol 9~27ml/hr)

Table 10 Easy calculation for the maintenance dose of propofol per 1 hour.

Total body weight (Kg)	Maintenance dose (ml/hour)
40	6 ~ 18
45	6.8 ~ 20
50	7.5 ~ 22.5
55	8.3 ~ 24.8
60	9 ~ 27
65	9.8 ~ 29.3
70	10.5 ~ 31.5

ii) Maintenance dose when not using infusion pump can be identified through below methods.

1% propofol 1ml = propofol 10mg (10mg/ml), 1000mg of propofol is contained in 500ml of diluted solution. That is 1000mg/500ml. Therefore, in 1ml of diluted solution, 2mg of propofol is contained. That is 2mg/ml.

If a patient weight is 60kg, 90~270mg/hr of propofol is needed for sedation. In other words 45~135ml/hr of diluted solution is needed. 20 drops equals to 1ml, so 45~135ml/hr equals to 900~2700 drops/hr of diluted solution. Conversing drops/hr to drops/min, it is 900~2700 drops/hr = 15~45 drops/min(gtt).

⑤ **Cautions**

Caution should be taken as there are some disadvantages like systemic vascular resistance decrease, hypotension caused by direct suppression on cardiac muscle, dose-dependent respiratory depression and pain during injection. Patients who are allergic to egg whites should be careful to allergic reaction. In some cases, it needs adjustment for the drug dose for desired sedation due to diversity of individual's drug susceptibility. Of course, it should be accompanied with intensive patient monitoring.

(4) Ketamine

① Characteristics

Ketamine(50mg/ml: 1 ample) is a lipid soluble drug which passes through blood brain barrier so well that it has excellent analgesic effect on particular regions of the central nervous system. The drug does not depress hemodynamics or respiration, and has broad safety margin by normal pharyngeal reflex and airway maintenance. But, it shows dysphoria such as increased secretion, nightmare and hallucination.

When combined with propofol, it increases sedation effect and easily maintains self-respiration. So, it can provide superb sedation and analgesic effect without hemodynamic change and respiratory depression.

② Action

The drug increases blood pressure and pulse rate from 10 to 50% and increases cerebrospinal fluid and intracranial pressure, but does not produce skeletal muscles relaxation.

③ Dose

Hypnotic effect occurs in blood concentration of 1.5~2.5 mcg/kg/ml, while only analgesic effect occurs in 0.2 mcg/kg/ml. Maintenance dose for sedation and analgesic is 0.2~0.8 mg/kg for intravenous injection over 2~3 minutes or 2~4mg/kg for intramuscular injection.

④ Action and metabolism

Immediately after induction anesthesia, respiration becomes shallow and rapid for a few minutes, but comes back to normal state afterwards. It should be monitored carefully when a great volume is injected to adults because airway obstruction or respiration depression may appear although this seldom happens. The drug injection features dissociated anesthesia that the patients' eyes are opened and seems awake but has no memory or consciousness. There is a disadvantage of continuous hallucination which may happen even after awakening. To solve this problem, diazepam can be used in combination. Recovery time from the drug injection is proportional to net injection dose; thus, if great volume is repeatedly injected for anesthesia maintenance, awakening is delayed.

⑤ Contraindication

It increases intracranial and intraorbital pressures so it should be prohibited to be used to patients who have hypertension, history of cardio-cerebro-vascular disease, increased intracranial pressure state, upper respiratory tract infection, intraorbital surgery, and susceptibility to the drug itself.

(5) Anticholinergic

Anticholinergics include atropine(0.5mg/ml muscle injection), scopolamine(0.3-0.6mg muscle injection), glycopyrrolate (Mobinol® 0.2mg/ml, 0.004mg/kg muscle injection) and etc. They are used for antisialagogue effect, sedation, vomit depression, gastric pH decrease, and prevention of chronotropic baroreflex.

Atropine and glycopyrrolate are commonly used. Glycopyrrolate features twice stronger for saliva secretion depression and triple drug duration time compared to atropine. It decreases gastric pH and volume, prevents superbly brachycardia induced by vagus nerve, and has no action on central nervous system, so it is more commonly used. On the other hand, there are some reports that atropine increase nightmares.

These anticholinergics have side effects on central nerve poisoning, relaxing lower esophagus muscle, pulse alteration, pupil dilation, body temperature increase, drying of oral cavity and airway, physiological rigor mortis increase, and etc.

Therefore, it should be used carefully for patients with hyperthermia, dehydration, tachycardia, hyperthyroidism, angle closure glaucoma, asthma, respiratory tract inflammation, and etc.

(6) Combined injection

Single drug cannot satisfy every condition; thus, two or three drugs are used in combination for decreasing side effects caused by overuse of a single, as well as increasing sedation and analgesic effects. It is usually composed of combination of sedative and analgesic. The following three methods are commonly used practically.

① Midazolam + Fentanyl

② Midazolam + Propofol + Ketamine

③ Propofol + Ketamine

The combined use of a propofol-ketamine is most commonly used because it is convenient to control and may minimize the need for supplemental opioid analgesics. And they have different actions in central nervous system; propofol counterbalances the action of ketamine which causes an increase in blood pressure, an increase in intracranial pressure and hallucination, while ketamine possesses strong analgesic properties. Nevertheless, it may be complicated to diagnose the reasons why unexpected symptoms occur sometimes when using combination of drugs. Therefore, sufficient knowledge and experiences for each drug and combined drugs are required. If the experience and knowledge of combination anesthesia is little, it is suggested that single drug is mainly used and the other drug is administered as an adjuvant for the safety of the patients.

2 Sensory nerve block

Sensory nerve block is commonly used technique in addition to sedation and local infiltration anesthesia for facial fat grafting.

1) Introduction

(1) Definition

Sensory nerve block is a way to attenuate pain temporarily by injecting anesthetics into nerves or their periphery.

(2) Drugs

Most commonly used agents for temporary sensory nerve block are 1% lidocaine and bupivacaine. The onset of action of lidocaine is about 2 to 3 minutes and its duration is about 30 minutes. On the other hand, bupivacaine has longer onset but has 4-6 times longer duration time. Epinephrine (1:100,000) is frequently combined with lidocaine, it provides prolonged duration time by inhibiting absorption of lidocaine.

Dosage of 1% lodocaine hydrochloride for nerve block is approximately 1-3 ml, and 25-27G needle is usually used. Sodium bicarbonate is combined to decrease pain during injection, whereas some doctors prefer to use dilution of lidocaine and epinephrine in the ratio of 1:1000 as a traditional method[17]. Table 11 show the drugs used for sensory nerve block[18,19,20].

(3) Caution

Generally, adverse drug reactions are rare when lidocaine is used as a local anesthetic correctly. But, the procedure of sensory nerve block is contraindicated when patients have allergy to anesthetics, coagulopathy[21], inflammation on infiltrating region, and do not agree with the procedure or not willing to cooperate with the procedure. In addition, most adverse drug reactions associated with this technique is systemic exposure to excessive quantities of lidocaine, mainly results in central nervous system

Table 11 Commonly used local infiltrating anesthetic agents.

Agent	Drug class	Concentration (%)	Onset	Duration	Maximum dose (mg/kg)
Lidocaine(Xylocaine)	Amide	1	Rapid	30 to 60 mins.	4
Mepicacain(Carbocaine)	Amide	1	Moderate	45 mins. to 1.5 hrs.	4
Bupivacacain(Marcaine)	Amide	0.25	Slow	15 to 60 mins.	3
Procaine(Novocaine)	Amide	1.0 to 2.0	Slow	2 to 3 mins.	7
Tetracacain(Pontocaine)	Amide	0.25	Slow	2 to 3 hrs.	1.5
Chloroprocaine(Nasacaine)	Amide	2	Slow	30 mins.	6 to 7

* Dilution is increased in local anesthetics that contain epinephrine.

Table 12 Potential local anesthetic systemic toxicity (LAST).

Central nervous system	Light-headedness Tinnitus Metallic taste Visual disturbances Numbness of the tongue and lips (rarely progressing to muscle twitching) Loss of consciousness Seizures or coma
Cardiovascular system	Decreased ventricular contractility Decreased conduction Loss of vasomotor tone.

(CNS) and cardiovascular effects. Related symptoms are shown in Table 12[22].

To prevent these symptoms, use minimal dose and drug should be checked whether it is injected into blood vessel. More cautions should be paid to bupivacaine (marcaine®) as it can increase the risk of cardiovascular complications[23]. Overdose in pregnant women can be exposed to her fetus and it may cause side effects[24]. And, anesthesia on the neck of pregnant women must be prohibited. Methods to manage these side effects are shown in Table 13[25].

Table 13 Algorythm for the management of local anesthetic systemic toxicity (LAST).

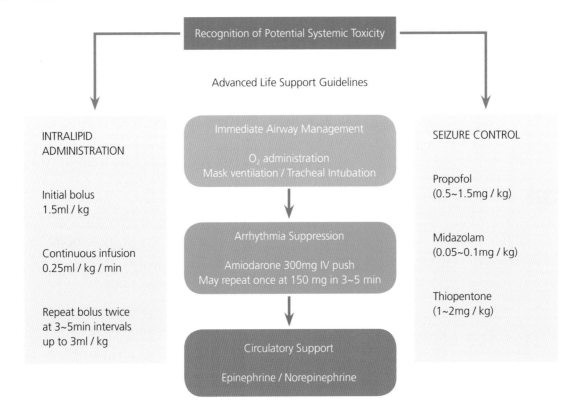

The critical factor for successful sensory nerve block is to detect the target nerves precisely. Hence, it requires many practices to find out the accurate location of nerves and their related anatomical structures on facial surface. The locations of sensory nerves and their sensory distributions are seen in Figure 2.

2) Regions for sensory nerve block

(1) Infraorbital nerve block

Infraorbital foramen opens downward and medially and is located within 1 cm below the inferior orbital rim, which is on the perpendicular line from medial limbus of the cornea[26], but, sometimes is located on a lower region than this. Before the infraorbital nerve exits the foramen, the anterior superior alveolar nerve branches downward from this infraorbital nerve and it supplies sensation of the anterior gingiva and maxillary teeth. However, this branching may be just prior to the foramen or 20 mm behind it. During the block, if an anesthetic is directly injected into the inferior orbital foramen, the gum and teeth become anesthetized from central incisor back to premolar teeth on that side. The sensory of infraorbital nerve can be blocked by approaching through oral cavity or skin.

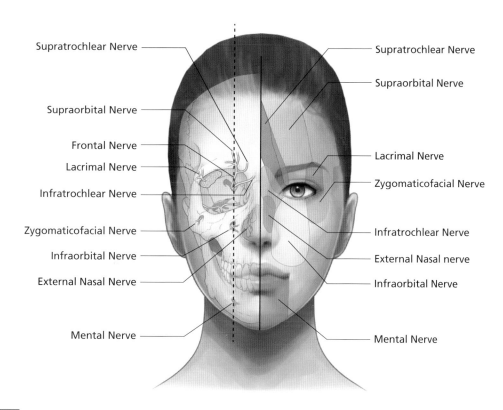

Figure 02　Nerves for the regional block and their areas of anesthesia in face.

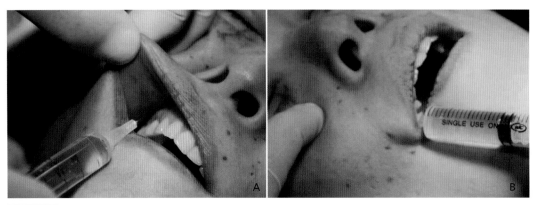

Figure 03 Intraoral approach method for the infraorbital nerve block.

Approach through oral cavity is as follows. With your 3rd finger on the infraorbital foramen, the finger should be moved downwards until a shallow depression is felt. Use thumb and index finger to retract the lip exposing the muco-buccal fold as shown in Figure 3A. The needle should be inserted in a parallel line with supraorbital notch, medial limbus of the cornea, and infraorbital notch and second bicuspid tooth at a sufficient distance (5 mm) from the labial plate to pass over the canine fossa. The needle should be guided with the help of the 3rd finger which was placed on the infraorbital foramen as shown in Figure 3B. Make sure that the needle did not penetrate more than 2 cm and use the 3rd finger to prevent the needle from entering the orbital cavity. Approximately 2-3 cc of local anesthetic solution is deposited and third finger is used to hold the needle in position until the end. Aspirate just before the injection, if negative, 2-3 ml of anesthetic is infiltrated.

There are 3 ways to block the nerve through skin.

First, mark the location of inferior orbital foramen on skin and sterilize it with povidone iodine (Betadine®). Next, insert the needle through skin, pass through subcutaneous fatty layer, and penetrate levator lavii superioris muscle as shown in Figure 4A. Since the nerve is very close to facial vessels, combined administration of epinephrine needs to be avoided and intravascular injection must be checked[27].

There is another method of anesthesia. Place 2nd finger on upper margin of inferior orbital rim, from the direction on the upper part of the patient's head, and move the needle towards inferior orbital foramen in the line of medial limbus of the cornea as in Figure 4B.

The last method is that the needle is inserted into a point in the center of an imaginary V which is defined by the nasolabial fold and the alar base inset as in Figure 5A. Holding the needle like a pen and the index finger of the opposite hand is placed on the infraorbital rim as in Figure 5B. It is directed upward and laterally to a point 5-7 mm below the infraorbital rim and from a line drawn straight down from the medial limbus[28].

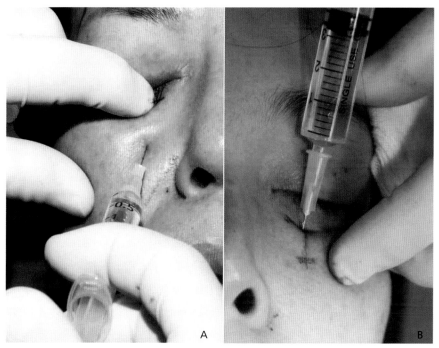

Figure 04 Two techniques for extraoral infraorbital nerve block.

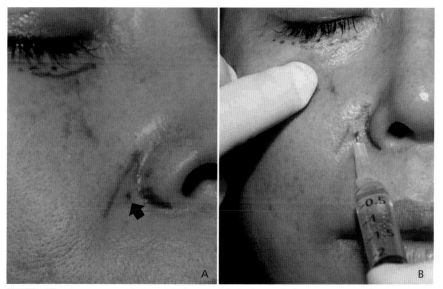

Figure 05 The extraoral infraorbital nerve block through the central area between nasolabial folds and nasal alar.

(2) Mental nerve block

The mental nerve, a branch of the inferior alveolar nerve, exits at the mental foramen which is palpated between the 2nd lower premolar teeth. The mental nerve exits at the foramen as two to three branches or as a group that rapidly divides into three or more branches. Two of the three branches supply the lip and slightly below the vermilion to the labiomental fold and one may supply skin lower down onto the chin. However, sometimes, the third branch may exits from another mental foramen which is separated, or may appear as a branch that runs downward and supplies sensation to the skin and chin below[29,30]. This branching variability may contribute to unsuccessful transcutaneous external block to the mental foramen. Because the mental nerve directly enters the submucosal layer in buccal sulcus near the second premolar teeth and is seen across the mucosa in the area of the lower canine tooth[31]. For the successful anesthesia of whole chin, the mental nerve can be blocked, at the mental foramen or a few centimeters after it leaves the foramen submucosally.

To block it at the foramen, locate the second premolar tooth as shown in Figure 6A. Place the needle tip in the buccal sulcus near the base of the tooth and inject. The nerve, after it leaves the foramen, is covered only by a thin layer of mucosa and perineural sheath. Anesthetics can also be injected into this submucosal layer in the opposite of gingiva lateral to canine[32] as shown in Figure 6B. This mental foramen and submucosal injection are reliable approaches to desensitize the lower lip down to the labiomental fold except the chin pad and the area lateral to it. So, to block the whole chin, it is recommended that an end branch of the mental nerve and the terminal branches of the mylohyoid from inferior alveolar nerve should be blocked because either of these two branches may supply the chin. Immediately after the mental block at foramen as described above, additional anesthetics must be injected in the supraperiosteal plane anterior to and beyond the lower border of the mandible with at least a 1.5-inch length needle as shown in Figure 6.

(3) Supraorbital nerve block

The supraorbital notch is easily palpable at the supraorbital rim just above the medial limbus of the cornea. The supraorbital nerve traverses the lower corrugator muscles and then branches. The medial ascending branches, on the surface of the frontalis, supply sensation to the skin of the forehead medially. The lateral transverse branches, under the frontalis muscle, supply sensation to the lateral forehead[33]. If the lateral forehead is not desensitized with supraorbital nerve block, the surgeon must inject

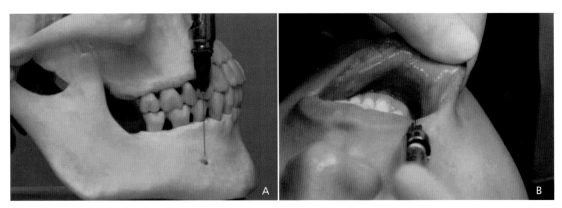

Figure 06 Intraoral technique for the mental nerve block.

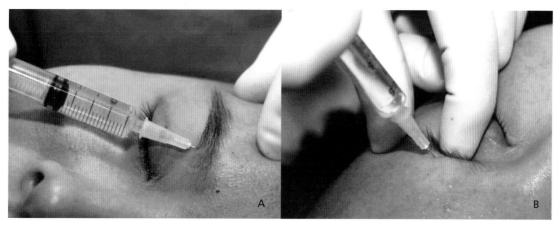

Figure 07 Two techniques for the supraorbital nerve block. The supraorbital notch is easily palpated on the superior rim of the orbit, the needle can be inserted right above and lateral to this notch. A: infrabrow hotizontal approach, B: suprabrow perpendicular approach.

local anesthetic under the frontalis muscle 1 cm above the rim at the zygomaticofrontal suture and proceeds toward the medial eyebrow because the lateral branches sometimes exit an accessory foramen above the rim. The supraorbital nerve block can be done as shown in Figure 7 and 8[34].

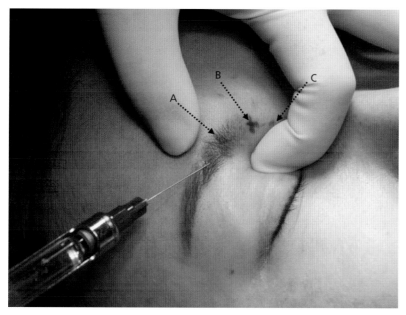

Figure 08 Lateral approach for the supraorbital (A), supratrochlear (B), and infratrochlear (C) nerve block. Pierce the lateral part of the middle third of the eyebrow. Aim the needle at the supraorbital notch. After injecting 1 to 2 cc prior to the notch under the muscle (A), the needle moves medially a few millimeters along the rim, and another cc is injected (B). Finally, another 1 cc is injected as the needle advances toward and touches the nasal bones (C). This approach has a higher risk of peri-orbital ecchymosis, compared to the other approaches.

(4) Supratrochlear nerve block

The supratrochlear nerve supplies sensation to the mid-forehead. It can be found at 0.9-1.0 cm medial to supraorbital notch. This nerve can be blocked by direct anesthetic injection on periosteum of supero-medial orbital rim as shown in Figure 9. And it is also can be blocked as shown in Figure 8B[34].

(5) Infratrochlear nerve block

The infratrochlear nerve of a branch of the nasociliary nerve runs along the medial orbital wall and leaves the orbit below the trochlea. It supplies sensation to the skin in the medial eyelids, the side of the nose above the medial canthus, medial conjuctiva, and lacrimal apparatus. It is blocked as shown in Figure 8 or by injecting 1–2 ml of local anesthetic solution at the junction of the orbit and the nasal bones as shown in Figure 9.

(6) External nasal nerve block

The external nasal nerve (anterior ethmoid branch of the nasociliary nerve) emerges 6–10 mm from the nasal midline at the osseous junction of the inferior portion of the nasal bone[35] and runs under the nasalis transverse muscle to supply sensation to some of the skin of the ala, vestibule, and lip. A external nasal nerve block will supplements nasal anesthesia by providing desensitization over the area of the cartilaginous nasal dorsum and tip. Palpate the nasal midline and feel the end of the nasal bones using the thumb on one side and the index finger on the other. Injecting 1 to 2 cc of anesthetic is sufficient for each side. This block is very useful to avoid painful injection into the nasal tip, therefore, it should be used before any infiltration at the nasal tip.

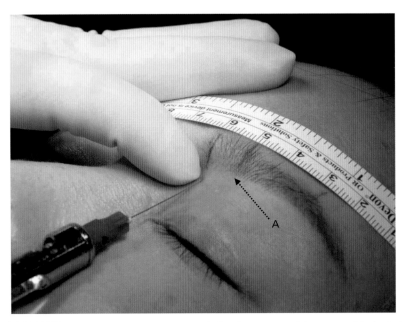

Figure 09 Infrabrow horizontal approach for the supratrochlear nerve block. A shows the supraorbital notch.

(7) Zygomatico-temporal nerve block

The zygomatico-temporal nerve is one of the terminal branches of the maxillary trigeminal nerve and pass through a foramen into the anterior part of the temporal fossa. This foramen is actually located on the posterior concave surface of the lateral orbital rim posterior to the zygoma at the approximate level of the lateral canthus. Sometimes, the foramen is positioned about 1 cm below the level of the canthus. Subsequently, it ascends under the temporalis muscle and pierces temporal fascia located 2.5 cm above the zygomatic arch. The nerve provides sensory innervation to fan-shaped area A posterior to the lateral orbital rim as shown in Figure 10. To block this nerve, from above the patient's head, the surgeon injects anesthetics behind the lateral orbital rim with needle insertion at about 10 to 12 mm behind and just below the palpable zygomatico-frontal suture. By sliding the 1.5-inch needle along the mid-posterior bony wall towards the point about 1 cm below the canthal level, anesthetic can be injected as shown in Figure 10A.

(8) Zygomatico-facial nerve block

This second terminal branch of the zygomatic nerve emerges from one or two foramina on the antero-lateral aspect of the malar bones just lateral to the infraorbital rim. This nerve is often damaged during the mid-face lifting surgery. Anesthetic is infiltrated into a coin-sized (diameter less than 2.0 cm) area just lateral to the junction of the lateral and inferior orbital rim as shown in Figure 10C. When the periorbital nerve

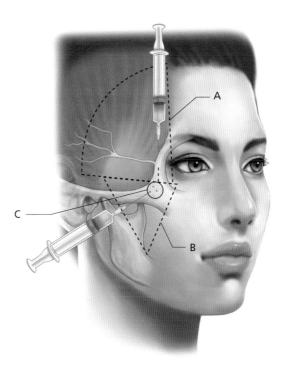

Figure 10 Techniques for the zygomatico-temporal and zygomatic-facial nerve block and their areas of anesthesia (dotted area).

block is performed, either infraorbital or zygomatico-temporal nerve is blocked first, and then zygomatico-facial nerve is done. It is more helpful to decrease pain during this nerve block[28].

(9) Greater auricular nerve block

The great auricular nerve appears at the posterior border of the mid-sternocleidomastoid (SCM) muscle. It passes almost straight upward on the fascial surface of this muscle. The great auricular nerve reaches 6.5 cm down from the external acoustic meatus. The nerve divides into end branches that supply the skin over the parotid and angle of mandible, most of the lower ear, and the skin over the mastoid process. To block this nerve, mark the skin of the upper anterior and posterior SCM borders with two parallel lines. Then, draw a third line between the first two parallel lines directly in mid-muscle. Mark a line of 6.5 cm from the lower border of external acoustic meatus down towards the mid- SCM. Inject a circle of anesthetic (diameter 2.0 cm) onto the muscle fascia. The lower one-third of the ear and the lower post-auricular skin become desensitized.

3) Complications

Complications caused by regional nerve block are as in Table 13[27].

Table 13 Common complications of the regional nerve block

Bleeding
Hematoma formation
Allergic or systemic reaction to anesthetic agent
Infection
Sensory change due to nerve damage
Unintentional injection into artery or vein
Swelling of the injected site
Failure to anesthetize

The most common complications are hemorrhage and hematoma. More attention should be paid to prevent an intravascular injection of anesthetic. In order to prevent this complication, the surgeon should understand the anatomy related to facial nerve block, check the possibility of vascular perforation just before injection, use minimal dose of anesthetics, and check allergic and pathologic history of the patient.

Most of the sensory changes are due to damages by the needle. However, approximately 95% of postoperative sensory changes will resolve within 4-6 weeks and most of these will occur during the first week. About 99% of sensory changes will resolve within the first year. To prevent the complications, the surgeon should avoid inserting the needle perpendicularly towards periosteum, insert the needle parallel to the course of the nerve as far as possible, and use smaller needles (24G) because it causes less nerve injury compared to larger needles (19G), even though the effect of the needle size on severity of nerve injury is controversial.

◼**3** Anesthesia with tumescent solution

1) Areas and methods

I love to use tumescent anesthesia for preauricular, temple, and buccal regions, where are supplied by auriculotemporal, lessor occipital and zygomatoco-temporal, and buccal nerve separately. About 10 ml of tumescent is sufficient for each side of the face. Excessive tumescent injection should be avoided, because it alters osmotic pressure and contributes to prolonged edema, and often confuses the surgeon during determination of precise injection volume. The concentration of lidocaine must be less than 7mg/kg because the face has highly developed vascularity and lidocaine absorption reaches maximum within 15 minutes regardless of whether epinephrine is combined or not[13]. To avoid lidocaine toxicity, small amount of the tumescent should be injected slowly. But, if the injection speed is fast, even though the concentration of the lidocaine is low, toxicity may occur.

2) Complications

The most common complications of tumescent anesthesia are bleeding and edema. To prevent these, cannula should be moved gently and smoothly during the injection and the procedure should be started at least 20-30 minutes after the tumescent injection. It is recommended to use isotonic tumescent solution or infiltrate with small volume of tumescent for prevention of the postoperative edema.

◼**4** Oral sedation and preemptive analgesia

1) Oral conscious sedation

Oral conscious sedation provided prior to the procedure is an excellent choice for patient who has mild to moderate levels of fear[36]. It retains the patient's ability to independently and responds normally to tactile stimulation and verbal command without any impairment of ventilator and cardiovascular function. This means that most patients cannot remember anything associated with the procedure. Additionally, sedation anesthesia, regional nerve block, and local infiltration can then be provided as needed to make the patient even more comfortable. Drugs which can be used for sedation include diazepam, triazolam, zaleplon, lorazepam, and hydroxyzine. Combination of diazepam and acetaminophen are commonly used for oral conscious sedation in my clinic. Depending on the situation, an antibiotic is taken simultaneously. Sometimes, I prefer to use the oral conscious sedation to the patient who performs the fat grafting only under the local and regional anesthesia. Usually, an oral sedative is taken prior to the procedure and the patient should be brought to the patient's home by a designated driver.

2) Preemptive analgesia

The concept of preemptive analgesia was formulated by Crile GW[37]. It has been defined as pretreatment of pain killers before the procedure in order to prevent the establishment of central sensitization caused by incisional injury and inflammatory injuries. It effectively reduces the pain both in the period of procedure and in the initial postoperative period. Whenever I perform the facial fat grafting, I love to inject the pain killer (ex; Diclofenac Sodium or Tramadol HCl) intramuscularly 30 minutes before the procedure.

5 Requirements for recovery and discharge

Risk associated with facial fat grafting is very low, because it is composed of small amount of liposuction and less-invasive fat grafting procedure. Therefore, the requirements for recovery and discharge after the procedure are mainly associated with the recovery from sedation or anesthesia. General requirements for discharge of sedation/anesthesia are as shown in Table 14[13]. When a patient's score is evaluated ≥9, the patient can be discharged.

Table 14 Postanesthesia discharge scoring system (PADS)[38].

Criteria	Points
Vital signs	
Within 20% of preoperative baseline	2
Within 20-40% of preoperative baseline	1
>40% of preoperative base line	0
Activity level	
Steady gait, no dizziness, at preoperative level	2
Requires assistance	1
Unable to ambulate	0
Nausea and vomiting	
Minimal, treated with oral medication	2
Moderate, treated with parenteral medication	1
Continues after repeated medication	0
Pain: minimal or none, acceptable to patient, controlled with oral medication	
Yes	2
No	1
Surgical bleeding	
Minimal: no dressing change required	2
Moderate: up to two dressing changes	1
Severe: three or more dressing changes	0

Reference

01. Baker TJ, Gordon HL. Midazolam(Versed) in ambulatory surgery. Plast Reconstr Surg 1988; 82:244-246.

02. Woodbridge PD. Changing concepts concerning depth of anesthesia. Anesthesiology. 1957;18(4): 536-550.

03. An updated report by the American Society of Anesthesiologists Task Force on Sedation and Analgesia by Non-Anesthesiologists : Practice Guidelines for Sedation and Analgesia by Non-Anesthesiologists. Anesthesiology 2002;96:1004-1017.

04. Irwin MG, Thompson N, Kenny GNC. Patient-maintained propofol sedation: assessment of a target-controlled infusion system. Anesthesia. 1997;52:525-530.

05. Smith I, Monk TG, White PF, Ding Y. Propofol infusion during regional anesthesia: sedative, amnestic, and anxiolytic properties. Anesth Analg. 1994; 79:313-319.

06. Medical land Ltd. www.medicalland.co.kr

07. Rescu-2TM Manufactured by GaleMED, Taiwan.

08. MP-110P Manufactured by MEK, Republic of Korea.

09. MP-800 Manufactured by MEK, Republic of Korea.

10. Agilia Manufactured by Fresenius Kabi, France.

11. CU-HD1S Manufactured by CU medical system, Republic of Korea (HYPERLINK "http://www.cu911.com/" ₩t "_blank"www.cu911.com)

12. Availabel at http://new.kimsonline.co.kr/

13. Korean society of anesthesiologist. Anesthesia and pain management, 2nd edition, Elsvier Korea L.L.C, 2009.

14. Bailey PL, Pace NL, Ashburn MA, Moll JWB, East KA, Stanley TH. Frequent hypoxemia and apnea after sedation with midazolam and fentanyl. Anesthesiology 1990;73:826-830.

15. O'Connor RE, Brady W, Brooks SC, Diercks D, Egan J, Ghaemmaghami C, Menon V, O'Neil BJ, Travers AH, Yannopoulos D,. Part 10: acute coronary syndromes: 2010 American Heart Association Guidelines for Cardiopulmonary Resuscitation and Emergency Cardiovascular Care. Circulation. 2010 Nov 2;122(18 Suppl 3):S787-817. Review. Erratum in: Circulation. 2011 Feb 15;123(6):e238.

16. Kim DH, Kang BJ. Concious sedation using target-controlled infusion with propofol in regional anesthesia patients. Korean Journal of Anesthesiology 2000;38:20-24.

17. Berry FR, Arianayagam C. Regional anesthetic technique for the face. Plast Reconstr Surg. 1999;103(1):329

18. Murphy MF. Local anesthetic agents. Emerg Med Clin North Am. 1988;6:769-776.

19. Philip BK, Covino BG. Local and regional anesthesia. In: Wetchler BV, ed. Anesthesia for ambulatory surgery, 2d ed. Philadelphia: Lippincott, 1991:309-374.

20. Salam GA. Regional anesthesia for office procedures: Part I. Head and neck surgeries Amarican Family Physician. 2004;69(3)3,585-590. Availabel at www.aafp.org/afp.

21. Barash PG, Cullen BF, Stoeling RK. Peripheral nerve blockade. In: Handbook of clinical anesthesia. 2nd Edi. Philadelphia: Lippincott, 1993:238–255.

22. Neal JM, Bernards CM, Butterworth JF 4th, Di Gregorio G, Drasner K, Hejtmanek MR, Mulroy MF, Rosenquist RW, Weinberg GL. ASRA Practice Advisory on Local Anesthetic Systemic Toxicity. Reg Anesth Pain Med. 2010;35:152-161.

23. Tetzlaff JE. The pharmacology of local anesthetics. Anesthesiol Clin North Am. 2000;18:217-233.

24. De Jong RH. Local anesthetics. St. Louis: Mosby, 1994:345-380.

25. Dillane D, Finucane BT. Local anesthetic systemic toxicity : Can J Anesth/J Can Anesth. 2010;57:368-380. DOI 10.1007/s12630-010-9275-7

26. McMinn RMS. Color atlas of head & neck anatomy. Chicago: Year book Medical Publishers,1981.

27. Byrne KM. Infraorbital nerve block. 2010. Available at http://emedicine.medscape.com/article /82660-overview.

28. Zide BM, Swift R. How to block and tackle the face. Plast Reconstr Surg. 1998 Mar;101(3):840-851.

29. Roberts GD, Harris M. Neurapraxia of the mylohyoid nerve and submental analgesia. Br J Oral Surg. 1973. :11(2):110-113.

30. Marinho RO, Tennant CJ. Paresthesia of the cutaneous branch of the mylohyoid nerve after removal of a submandibular salivary gland. J Oral Maxillofac Surg. 1997;55(2):170-171.

31. Katz J (Ed.). Atlas of Regional Anesthesia. Norwalk, Conn. Appleton-Century-Crofts. 1985. Pp.28-29.

32. Haribhakti VV. The dentate adult human mandible: An anatomic basis for surgical decision making. Plast Reconstr Surg. 1996; 97(3):536-541; discussion 542-543.

33. Knize DM. Transpalpebral approach to the corrugator supercilii and procerus muscles. Plast Reconstr Surg 1995;95(1):52-60;discussion 61-62.

34. Knize DM. A study of the supraorbital nerve. Plast Reconstr Surg. 1995;96(3):564-569.

35. Zide BM. Nasal anatomy: The muscles and tip sensation. Aesthetic Plast Surg. 1985;9(3):193-196.

36. American Dental Association guidelines for the use of conscious sedation, deep sedation and general anesthesia for dentists. Chicago: American Dental Association. 2000:1.

37. Crile GW. The kinetic theory of shock and its prevention through anoci-association. Lancet 1913; 185: 7–16.

38. Marshall SI, Chung F. Discharge criteria and complications after ambulatory surgery. Anesth Analg. 1999 Mar;88(3):508-517.

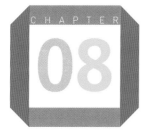

Theory and method of SAFI technique

1 Definition

SAFI (Sequential Autologous Fat Injection) is an innovative way of restoring the patient's face as their original youthful appearances by considering the following factors : the structures for maintaining the facial contour, the facial structural changes by the aging process, and the influence of gravity.

In order to do SAFI, the whole face is divided into several zones, and then autologous fat is injected into each zone and area using a sequential process.

2 Methods of fat grafting

Many different types of artificial fillers, implants, and autologous fat have been used to repair facial wrinkles, folds, and depressions caused by the aging process and to treat partial congenital facial hypoplasia. Among them, autologous fat transfer has been found to be especially beneficial; it uses the patient's own tissue, so it is safer (no adverse immunologic reactions) and more economical (inexpensive) than using artificial fillers. The autologous fat can be harvested easily from parts of the body with unwanted fat. So, it has an additional advantage for body contouring.

In chronological order, the historical background of autologous fat grafting is the following: As early as 1893, Neuber F. reported that he successfully used a free fat graft to fill out a specific area for soft tissue loss on a patient's face[1]. However in 1950, Peer L. reported that successful maintenance of fat graftings occurred in only 50% cases[2]. From then until the 1990's, researchers reported 20-90% survival rates for fat grafting. So many clinicians who were skeptical about fat grafting had been in favor of artificial fillers. However from the 1990's, many more positive results for fat grafting have been reported[3].

In the 1997, Coleman SR. developed a new method of 3 dimensional volume restoration of soft tissue by multiple injections into many different layers of subcutaneous tissue. His techniques have made fat grafting a much more popular procedure than before[4]. He ultimately published 'Structural Fat Grafting' (SFG) in 2004 describing his techniques in detail[5]. He has also authored and co-authored many articles describing his methods of fat grafting, such as 'Facial augmentation with structural fat grafting' in 2006[6].

In 2000, Donofrio LM. developed the technique of multiple small fat injections over the period of 1-2 years in order to reduce the prolonged edema which has proved to be one of the difficulties with Coleman's fat grafting techniques[7]. For this, he has also used the frozen fat in his fat grafting process. And, he had tried to perform the rebalancing technique that the micro-liposuction and the fat grafting done simultaneously on areas of fat hypertrophy and volume depletion respectively.

In 2000, Fournier PF. introduced a lipo-filling technique in hypotrophic malar areas looked like congenital insufficient development of deep structure[8]. It is based on the idea that the facial drooping with atrophied tissue is caused by volume reduction of deep facial tissues. While pointing out the limitations of rhytidectomy based on surface surgery concept, which lifts surface of the facial skin tissue, he suggested the lipofilling would be a good solution for reversing the aging process as volume surgery. Also, he was the first user of syringe-needle unit or syringe cannula unit to completely block contact with air. He also tried to clean the harvested fat to remove the blood effect on it. Finally, he tried molding to shape the grafted fat.

In 2001, Amar RE. an anatomist and plastic surgeon had developed F.A.M.I (Fat Autograft Muscle Injection) method to improve the overall facial aging process. This method injects harvested fat into the facial mimic muscles to increase the bulkiness of aged muscle, restore the elasticity and simultaneously correct regional facial volume depletion of areas such as lip, tear-trough deformity, chin, and perioral regions[9]. This technique was influenced by Coleman method and research results of Guerreroantoe J. et al. regarding increased intramuscular fat survival rate[10] and the relevant anatomy of facial mimic muscles. Compared with the previous methods, this technique had shortened downtime by decreasing edema. However, side effects like bruise, edema, and temporary palpable lumpiness were still appeared. Also, inappropriately named intramuscular fat grafting and technical difficulties were regarded as problems.

As the methods mentioned above, the fat grafting has been evolved from trials of restoring the volume depletion of facial tissue to 3-dimensional change of facial structure, rebalancing technique by simultaneously performed liposuction with lipofilling while considering facial aging process, and functional approach of F.A.M.I. method.

Recently, complementary fat grafting has been used numerously as an adjunctive treatment of conventional rhytidectomy to restore the volume of aged face which cannot be improved by conventional rhytidectomy[11,12]. Thus, fat grafting is doubtlessly the best method to improve facial volume depletion. The current clinical practices are based on Coleman's structural fat grafting method with combinations of other methods of fat grafting.

As one of the advanced and systemic methods of structural fat grafting, SAFI is a concrete way of fat injection, where soft tissue foundation, aging process, and its related anatomical structures are taken into consideration. When SFG is performed, SAFI can offer practical, step by step guidelines for protecting against complication of fat grafting such as sagging and unnatural appearance. SAFI attempted these methods and in a result, it has acquired the concept of volumetric facial lifting

■3 Current problems with autologous fat grafting

There are a number of well-known side effects of autologous fat grafting: bleeding, ecchymosis, irregularities, lumpiness, hardness, and arterial occlusion due to the inappropriate injection technique, variable rates of absorption requiring recurring fat injections, over-correction to prevent reabsorption, and an increase in infection rates due to the use of preserved frozen fat.

However, even if the autologous fat grafts are successfully performed, the unnatural facial contour and the drooping (gravitational ptosis) due to gravitational forces by surrounding tissue are concerned as the newly discovered side effects, which must be taken into consideration while performing the procedure. This phenomena leads to unnatural facial contour with gravitational descent, which mostly occurs if the fat grafting is treated like artificial fillers, where clinicians simply correct volume depletion without consideration of the supporting structures of normal facial contour, the underlying congenital or acquired structural abnormalities, the anatomical functional changes that are part of the aging process, and the influence of the gravitation by the weight of the injected fat.

After fat grafting as a simple volume correction, it seems that the areas of volume depletion have been corrected. However, with a careful inspection on the surroundings or the entire face, it can be observed that the unnatural facial contour including further facial drooping and fat accumulation phenomena which is more likely to occur in the elderly.

4 Survival rate and the ideal method of autologus fat grafting

Fat grafting and artificial fillers are the most common methods to restore the facial volume depletion. However, it is also an undeniable fact that current fat grafting has some negative aspects, because not only the clinicians, but also the patients have lack of confidence in the survival rate and longevity, including anxiety for the possible side effects.

Recently, to increase the survival rate and longevity, adipose-derived stem cells (ADSCs) and platelet rich plasma(PRP)[13,14] became to be more popular, and more positive research results on these technique have been published[15,16]. However, more researches are still required for making a successful survival and longevity of injected fat and reducing the side effects. Especially, even though the manual syringe injection techniques for the fat placement are important basic steps, the hand skills were often neglected.

However, it is obvious that the finely tuned manual dexterity of an experienced clinician during fat grafting is a primary factor in minimizing trauma to the surrounding tissues and increasing the survival rate. Several syringe grip techniques have been well known, but for better results, it is necessary to do more research for a new ideal syringe grip technique. An experienced clinician with an ideal syringe grip technique is an expert in judging where and how to make injections and therefore knows how to reduce the occurrence of bruising, bleeding, irregularities and lumpiness. The differences between the ability of the injection skill of clinicians affect surgical outcome, such as survival rate of grafted fat and the incidence of complications in fat grafting.

And, in spite of high survival rate, it cannot be a successful result if the face looks unnatural and droopy due to the weight of transferred fat. Therefore, a successful result should show a correction of the volume depletion without any drooping signs. Moreover, the most ideal fat grafting method would give a lifted facial appearance with a volume increase.

5 SAFI method's hypothesis

As mentioned in the definition, the SAFI method is based on the following hypothesis.

1) Hypothesis using local approach method.

(1) The concept of the skin lifting and fixation-like effect as the supplementary phenomena of volume icrease

As seen in Figure 1, skin lifting is achieved as the volume is increased. C, the midpoint between A and B on the surface of the skin is tensed, resulting in shortened distance between A and B.

As seen in the Figure 2, the loss of elasticity can be seen in the volume depleted area (A) due to aging. It is also more likely to move and droop due to gravitational effect. At this time, fat grafting into whole layer and areas surrounding the retaining ligament will result in increased volume with tenser

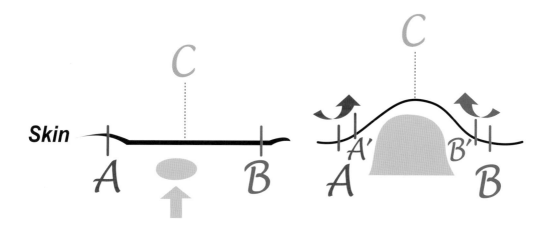

Figure 01   Basic concept of volumetric skin lifting effect. A and B are supposed to be certain points on the facial skin. C is the midway point between A and B. Autologous fat should be injected into under the skin, and then both point A and B are pulled toward the center (C) as the volume of the injected fat is increased. The positions of A and B can be shifted to A' and B'. Finally, the distances between (A-C) and (B-C) should become shorter after injection. It is suggested that this concept is called volumetric skin lifting phenomenon.

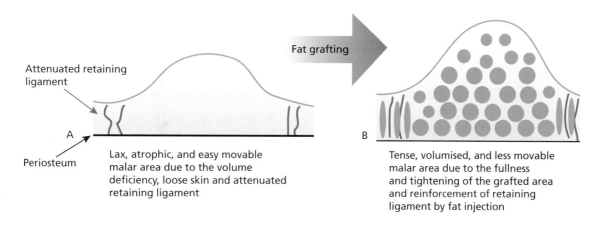

Figure 02   Basic concept of volumetric fixation-like effect. The lax and movable appearance of some facial area can be changed into tense and less movable appearance that seems to be attached or fixed to the bone. This volumetric fixation-like effect is due to the fullness and tightening of the grafted area by autologous fat grafting.

skin surface and reduction in movement. It makes the area as a fixed state (B); the author defined it as a fixation-like effect.

The SAFI method has been developed using these two concepts. However, these concepts are not applicable when too much or too little volume is injected, or in situation where skin elasticity is significantly deceased.

(2) The relevant vectors in tissue surrounding the fat injected area

Figure 3 is a schematic explanation of the possible potential vectors between the injected fat and the surrounding tissue when the fat is grafted under the concept of Figure 1 and 2.

(3) Prevention of droopiness by using different amounts of injected fat in various areas.

If the design and planning for the fat grafting are completed in standing position while the actual procedure is carried out in lying down position, the final result will be evaluated in the standing position. When the patient changes from lying down position to standing up position, the injected fat might droop and therefore the injected area might not look as it was intended to look.

Figure 4A is a diagram that shows how standing up affects drooping of the injected fat and the surrounding tissues after fat grafting, only proportional amount of the fat injected into the depressed area in lying position.

To prevent what is shown in Figure 4A and achieve what is shown in Figure 4B, a greater amount

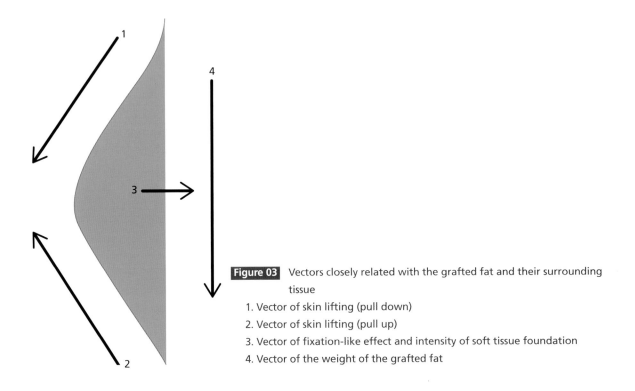

Figure 03 Vectors closely related with the grafted fat and their surrounding tissue
1. Vector of skin lifting (pull down)
2. Vector of skin lifting (pull up)
3. Vector of fixation-like effect and intensity of soft tissue foundation
4. Vector of the weight of the grafted fat

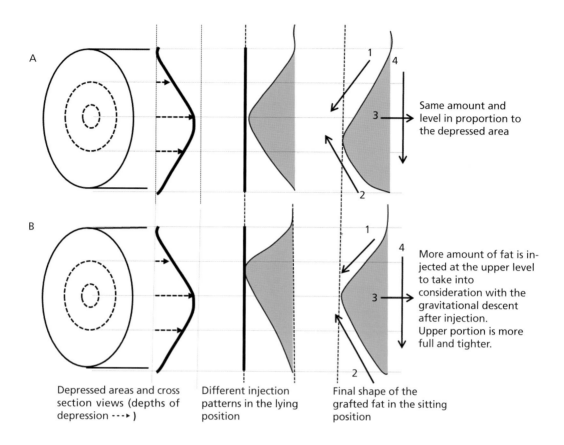

A

Same amount and level in proportion to the depressed area

B

More amount of fat is injected at the upper level to take into consideration with the gravitational descent after injection. Upper portion is more full and tighter.

Depressed areas and cross section views (depths of depression ---►)

Different injection patterns in the lying position

Final shape of the grafted fat in the sitting position

Figure 04 Predictable shapes of the grafted fat and their surrounding tissue can be changed according to the injection level and amount (upper portion: more, lower portion: less) in the lying position.

of fat is injected into the superior part of the depressed area and a lesser amount into the inferior part. Figure 4 shows the degree of droopiness and the shape which results when variable amounts of fat are injected into different levels, even though the vectors are identical in both cases.

(4) Change of the descent according to depth of placement, shape and amount of injected fat, and injection equence

During the fat grafting, the depth of placement is very important. Because the bone has a function to support the soft issue, so the injected fat is further from the bone, the skeletal support of the bone is reduced and the soft tissue foundation become weaker. This means that there is higher possibility of soft tissue descent when the fat is injected further from the bone. As seen in Figure 5 and, when the same amount of fat is injected into same region but different in depth, it can be predicted that the descent phenomenon of Figure 5B is less than that of Figure 5C.

As seen in Figure 6A, when inject a greater amount of fat into the deep layer firstly (1, 2, 3 and 4) and gradually reduce the amount of injected fat sequentially from the deep to the superficial layer; it is more likely to bring out not only the augmentation of soft tissue, but also lesser sagging or descent

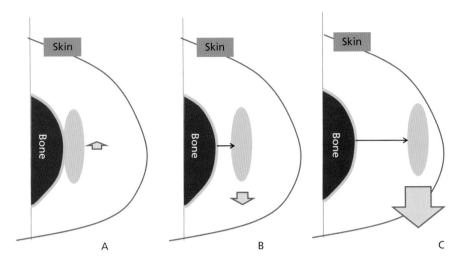

Figure 05 The effect of the placement of fat (depth) on the gravitational descent under the assumption that there are 3 regions of the same soft tissue foundation (A, B, and C). Let us suppose that the same amount fat is injected into the soft tissue with different depth of placement. The zero distance means that the fat is injected under and just above the periosteum. The fat injection of distance zero makes effect like the bone larger and increase skeletal support for the soft tissue. The shorter the distance between bone and injected fat, the stronger the skeletal support. Therefore, the deeper the fat is injected into the face, the lesser the injected fat to descent inferiorly. (A) zero distance, (B) shorter distance, and (C) longer distance.

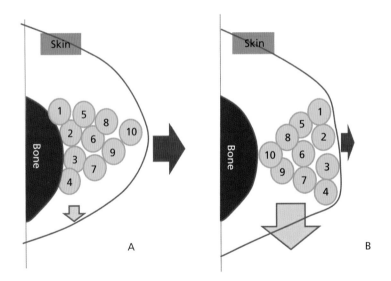

Figure 06 The close relationship with the shape of injected fat, the injection sequence, and incidence of gravitational descent. The more deeply implanted fat does not easily descent inferiorly (A). If the fat injected into superficial layer firstly, the anterior projection will not be enough and the incidence of gravitational descent will also be increased (B). The numbers from 1 to 10 show the injection sequence. Red arrows mean the extent of anterior projection.

phenomenon. However, as seen in Figure 6B, first of all, when a greater amount of fat is injected into the superficial layer (1, 2, 3 and 4), it is augmented temporarily in the early stage of injection. But, it might become flat or even more depressed surface with hardness. In this case, even if additional fat is injected into deeper layer, it might be less successful than expected. I think it is because of decreased skin elasticity due to the fullness of the superficial layer in the early stage of fat injection. Also, as the hypothesis of Figure 5, the descent phenomenon will get worse.

Therefore, in order to augment the soft tissue by injecting fat, it is recommended to implement the following basic principles.

Firstly, inject fat from the deep layer to the superficial layer.

Secondly, inject a greater amount of fat into the deep layer; inject a lesser amount of fat as getting closer to the superficial layer.

However, the amount of injection according to the depth is subjected to be adjusted differently because the structure of each facial volume deficiency areas and their causes of occurrence are distinguished from each area of face. Still, there are no objective evidences for the three concepts ((1), (2), (3), and (4)) mentioned above. They are hypothesis and analogy concepts based on the author's experience. Hence, additional researches are necessary for objective verification.

2) The concept and principle for systemic approach

There is important structural and functional co-relation of the aging and soft tissue foundation between 2 or more facial deficient areas which are in contact or located nearby. So, facial fat grafting should be performed under consideration of facial aging with its related changes of anatomical structures and soft tissue foundation. To achieve this, a consistent and a systematic sequence of fat injection into the whole face are necessary.

(1) Facial soft tissue foundation (STF), facial countour, and aging

Facial aging involves in aging of the whole tissue–from bony framework to skin. This process progresses systemically and progressively by gravitational effect mainly. With age, the facial soft tissue contour undergoes big change. The most remarkable one is the facial contour change of oval or inverted triangular shape to pentagonal or triangular figure due to the antero-inferior drooping of soft tissue.

The facial soft tissue contour is formed and maintained by variable ligamentous fixations which connect skin, subcutaneous fat, and muscle, and hold them to the bony skeleton. There are some important factors which affect the facial contour. The intrinsic factors are the shape of skeleton, location and shape of facial mimic muscle, position and amount of fat layers, thickness and elasticity of skin, and the presence of varying ligamentous fixation which links and fixes them. The extrinsic factors are gravitational effect and overuse of facial mimic muscle.

Among the intrinsic factors, skeleton and ligamentous fixation play important roles in maintenance of facial contour. The ligamentous fixation forms soft tissue foundation. Different facial zones have different STF. This is because the varying areas have different constituents with different factors affecting STF. Based on this concept, I divided face into 3 zones as shown in Figure 7.

First, the strongest zone of STF in maintaining soft tissue contour is marked red in Figure 7A. The bottom of this zone is composed of zygomatic and maxillary bone and firmly supported by true retaining ligaments. This zone has a relatively thick skin, where the fibrous septa separate superficial fat layer into compartments that abut each other. The deep subcutaneous layer is made up of suborbicularis oculi fat and prezygomatic fat which is strongly attached to the zygomatic bone. Three strong true type retaining ligaments are the orbital ligament, orbital retaining ligament, and zygomatic retaining ligament. These ligaments strongly connect the soft tissues of this zone to the bones. Also, the buccal-maxillary retaining ligament which forms the anterior border of this zone supports superior part of the nasolabial fold.

Second, the second strongest zone of STF is the lateral cheek area marked blue in Figure 7B, which is the posterior part of anterior border of masseter muscle. This zone forms lateral wall of oral cavity, consists of subcutaneous fat, parotid gland, masseter muscle, and platysma muscle, and is supported

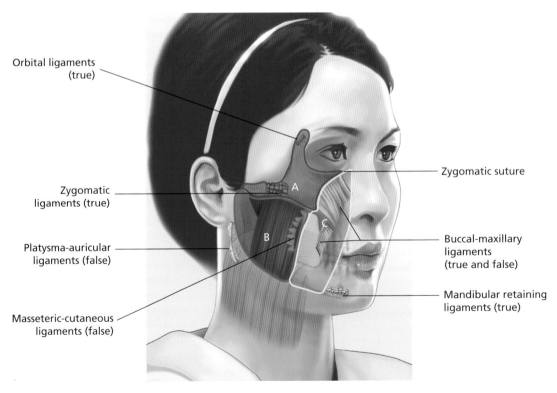

Figure 07 Dr. Safi's 3 facial zones according to the different facial soft tissue foundation (STF).
A red colored zone indicates strongest STF, a blue colored zone indicates second strongest STF, and a yellow colored zone indicates weakest STF.

by mandible and zygomatic bone. The SMAS (superficial muscular aponeurotic system) is well developed, and the superior part is connected to the zygomatic bone, which is important for maintaining the soft tissue contour. So, the long superficial subcutaneous fat compartments which are arranged perpendicularly are very well developed. However, the deep subcutaneous fat layer is almost undeveloped. As the false type retaining ligament, the platysma-auricular ligament runs both perpendicularly and horizontally, while the masseteric cutaneous ligament is only arranged perpendicularly to support the soft tissue in this zone.

Third, the weakest zone of STF forms the antero-lateral wall of oral cavity which is marked yellow in Figure 7C. This zone is formed as thick membranous soft tissue. But, it is separated with maxilla, mandible, and teeth and is hung to the maxillary bone. Therefore, the soft tissue foundation of this zone is very weak. The facial mimic muscles of this zone are thin and actively moving. Most of them run obliquely in an antero-inferior direction. In this zone, the SMAS becomes thinner as it gets closer to the mid-face and fused with facial mimic muscle and skin. Also, the subcutaneous fat layer of the nasolabial folds are the densest among the facial zones and abundantly packed with adipocytes, while others are scarcely packed with loosely connected fibrous septa from superficial fascia to skin, resulting in high motility. Moreover, buccal fat pad of the deep subcutaneous fat layer shows significant reduction in size with development and aging.

The true buccal-maxillary ligament extend to connect the maxillary bone to the superior part of nasolabial folds, whereas the most attenuated and weak ligament called the false buccal-maxillary ligament support the inferior portion of the fold in an oblique direction. Also, the jowls are indirectly supported by the posterosuperiorly positioned masseteric cutaneous ligament. The strong mandibular retaining ligament supports the most antero-inferior region of this zone. This zone abuts two aesthetic units of the lip and nose including philtrum medially. These units have almost no or less sub-dermal movement because there is no superficial fat and the fibrous septa are directly connected to the skin.

If it is supposed that there are situations affecting facial aging, the changes of three zones will be significantly different. It can be speculated that the difference of constituents of soft tissue, soft tissue foundation, and motility of mimic muscle on each zone and additional gravitational influence will be the key factors of facial aging, especially for the vector of drooping and the amount of volume depletion.

Considering these characteristics, it can be concluded that the zone of weakest soft tissue foundation and highest motility will initially droop, while the strongest zone of soft tissue foundation will droop relatively little and slowly. Also, the drooping of the weakest zone can be affected by anterior protrusion of mid face, nose, mouth, and chin as well as strong support of mandibualr ligament. I think that the characteristics mentioned above are helpful to understand the antero–inferior facial drooping phenomenon with aging.

(2) Approach of fat grafting according to different STF

Why is STF important in fat grafting? It is because the result of the grafting could be different according to the characteristics of target area has different STF zones even if same amount of fat is injected. Also, it could be further affected by the physical development and aging of face.

As in Figure 8, let us suppose that the anterior appearance of facial depression area is A, and cross-section view is B. This figure is an expectation of how the injected fat and the surroundings would look like in two different zones — one with the weakest STF (Figure 8D), and the other with the strongest STF (Figure 8E) — after fat grafting in lying position while designing in standing position on the facial depression areas. It demonstrates the possibility of different drooping appearances in different STF zones even though same amount and shape of fat is supposed to be grafted. It also suggests that the STF can significantly affect aging and the outcome of fat grafting.

3) Why should we inject fat sequentially?

As shown in Figure 9, if a surgeon tries to inject fat into two areas that abut each other, which area should be injected first? Before answering, we should analyze these two areas first. For example, suppose that the lateral cheek depression area or lateral part of submalar hollow as area (a), anterior part of submalar hollow or jowl as area (b), and masseteric cutaneous retaining ligament as area (c).

The followings are is a summary of my opinion.

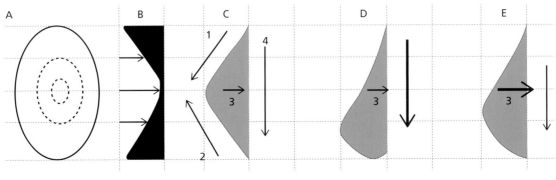

Design of the depressed area, anterior (A) and cross section view(B) →

(C) Same amount of the fat is injected in proportion to the depressed area in the lying position

Final shapes of the grafted fat in the sitting position influenced by the weight of the grafted fat and the different zones of the soft tissue foundation(STF)

(D) Weaker STF zone with less fixation-like effect and more ptotic

(E) Stronger STF zone with more fixation-like effect and less ptotic

Figure 08 The shapes of the grafted fat and their surrounding tissue can be changed according to the different zones of soft tissue foundation.

1. Vector of skin lifting (pull down)
2. Vector of skin lifting (pull up)
3. Vector of fixation-like effect and intensity soft tissue foundation
4. Vector of the weight of the grafted fat

- First, area (a) is postero-superiorly positioned, while area (b) is antero-inferiorly situated.
- Second, area (a) has higher soft tissue foundation, fixation-like effect, and skin elasticity than area (b).
- Third, the direction of the soft tissue drooping occurs from area (a) to (b) on aging.
- Forth, the depression occurs due to the combination of volume depletion and drooping in area (b). However, the main cause is volume depletion in area (a).
- Fifth, as aging progresses, area (c) will become attenuated and will fall towards antero-inferior direction

Then, as in Figure 9B and 9C, what sort of results can be expected when the sequence of fat grafting is different?

In case of Figure 9C, If the same amount of fat which is required in Figure 9A (b) was grafted into b" first, drooping of b" will be more severe since this area has the weakest STF with the smallest fixation-like effect. Due to the drooping of b", both a" and c" will be fallen into antero-inferior direc-

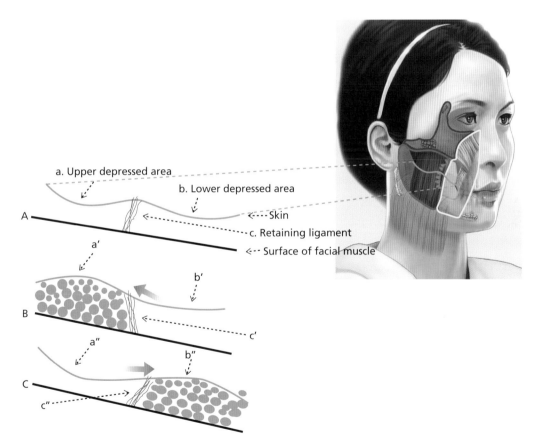

Figure 09 2 possible injection sequences in facial fat grafting into two depressed facial areas which abut to each other. Schematic crossection view of 2 depressed areas which fat is injected (A), one sequence that the fat is injected first into the upper depressed area (a') (B), and the other sequence that the fat is injected first into the lower depressed area (b") (C). Reds arrows show the direction of the skin lifting.

tion, and the skin tension of a" will be increased and eventually volume depletion will occur. Then, it is more likely not to result in sufficient volume recovery and expected facial contour eventhough the same amount of fat as Figure 9B (a') is grafted into the a". Because of this, relatively more fat is likely to be injected into a". Consequently, the risk of unnatural contour with drooping may be more increased in Figure 9C than 9B.

However, if the fat is injected to a' first, as seen Figure 9B, the soft tissue of b' and c' will be postero-superiorly lifted. The skin tension in b' will be more tightened and volume of b' will be decreased. Especially, it should be noticed that the drooping and depression of b' can be partially improved by preferential fat graft to a'. At this state, when the same amount of fat is injected into b' as b", the drooping due to the weight of injected fat will be prevented and natural cotour can be achieved. Consequently, sufficient amount of fat can be injected into b' without any risk of drooping. In most cases, more natural contour without drooping might be appeared with smaller amount fat injection than that of we expected.

When the fat is grafted into B (c') and C (c") in both cases, will the soft tissue foundation be more solid by strengthening of the retaining ligament? The retaining ligament is known as one of the major structures for maintaining the soft tissue foundations of the face. However, with aging, its moprphology will be changed as described in Chapter 2. Eventually, the soft tissue foundations become weakened and it can also be responsible for laxity of face. Fortunately, autologous fat can be injected into intra and peri-ligamental space, so, it can help to strengthen the attenuated retaining ligament. This will provide more solid soft tissue foundations.

From the above two kinds of injection sequences, it is suggested that the fat should be sequentially injected from a' to b' as shown in the sequence B. This sequence is exactly one of the most important concepts of SAFI technique. My opinion, a necessity of regular sequence in facial fat grafting, comes from the hypothesis where facial structures, soft tissue foundation, aging and influence of gravity are taken into consideration. If this concept of sequence is applied to fat grafting of whole face, it would be a reasonable approach to perform fat grafting sequentially from superolateraly positioned positioned area to anteroinferiorly positioned positioned area.

4) Evidence of volumetric face lifting by fat grafting

A 55 year-old man in Figure 10 visited my clinic for improvement of deep nasolabial folds. He had deep nasolabial folds with mid-face volume depletion and under-developed malar bone. The dotted areas of Figure 10B are for fat grafting. Autologus fat grafting was performed sequentially to palpebro-malar grooves, malar eminence, tear trough deformities, and mid-cheek furrows. It was performed only once without additional injections within 6 months. Also, no fat was injected to the depressed portion of nasolabial folds

Figure 10C is taken immediately after fat grafting. Significant reduction in nasolabial volume is

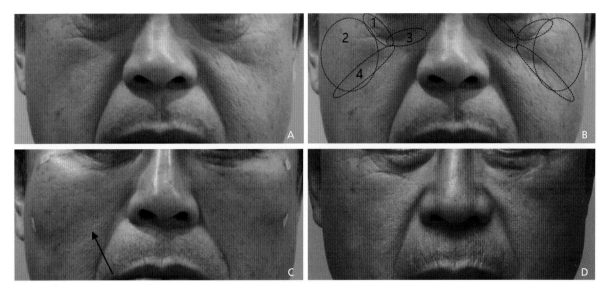

Figure 10 Evidence of the volumetric face lift using only sequential autologous fat injection (SAFI) technique. A 55 year-old man with deep nasolabial folds caused by small malars with soft tissue volume deficiencies in the lower lid and the mid- face. After the injection, the volume of these areas was improved considerably and the deep nasolabial folds were significantly softened (C and D). Preoperative view (A), Preoperative markings (B), Immediately after fat grafting (C), and 6 months after fat grafting (D). The numbers (1, 2, 3 and 4) mean the area of palpebro-malar groove, malar eminence, tear trough deformity, and mid-cheek furrow. Black arrow indicates the actual volume loss caused by volumetric face lifting.

caused by tightend skin tension as a result of the increased volume in these 4 areas. In the 6 months of postoperative view, Figure 10D shows siginificant improvement of nasolabial folds when compared to the preoperative view, Figure 10A. The result obtained above shows the possibility and actual result of volumetric face lifting produced by improvement of skeletal support by fat grafting to flat, small malar eminence and followed by sequential fat grafting to the other areas.

5) The meaning and feasibility of the overall systemic approach

Almost all of the current practice of fat grafting uses the local approach of directly injecting fat into wrinkles and depressed areas only. However, SAFI method is a systemic approach of fat grafting to the sites related with the cause and the process of aging as well as the results of aging such as wrinkles and depressions. It is necessary to analyse the whole facial aging process for this systemic approach. .

For instance, we suppose that mid-cheek groove or malar hypotrophy is associated with a patient who wants improvement of deep nasolabial folds by fat grafting. Generally, almost all surgeon will try to inject fat directly only into the depressed portion of the nasolabial folds. This is just a local approach like a simple artificial filler injection technique without consideration of the mutual relationships between volume depletion of the postero-superior zone and cause of deep nasolabial folds.

Because the deep naoslabial folds are not only formed by the reduction in the soft tissue of the depressed portion of the nasolabial folds but affected by all of these various factors: size of malar bone, volume of malar fat, the skeletal remodeling of orbital rim, laxity of facial ligaments, the subcutaneous fat loss in the mid-face such as the deep mid-cheek furrows, presence of maxillary retrusion, premaxillary hypoplasia, the hypertrophy of the nasolabial fat, and influence of gravity. So, it is not logical to graft fat only into the depressed portion of the nasolabial folds without considering all of the above factors.

Of course, good result can be achieved only by the simple injection method if the nasolabial folds are not severely affected by aging and structural abnormality. However, as in most cases, more reasonable approach would be needed to graft fat firstly into the postero-superior areas which causes deep nasolabial folds, and then followed by fat injection into the depressed portion of nasolabial folds. Sometimes, liposuction of nasolabial folds fat is needed if it is hypertrophied and more protruded than the malar fat.

6) Indication of the SAFI method

SAFI is good to apply to every fat grafting. However, specific indications are listed as below.

- First, prevention of gravitational descent due to the weight of grafted fat.
- Second, simultaneous achievement of sufficient facial volume recovery and lifting effect.
- Third, improvement of skeletal contour and increase skeletal support for the soft tissue.
- Fourth, improvement of soft tissue contour of whole face.
- Fifth, facial liposuction for achieving natural facial contour without any drooping.

▄▄ 6 The naming of SAFI

The phrase "Autologous fat graft induced-lifting" has been named since the first workshop, conducted by me in 23th September 2006, for lifting appearance after the procedure as in Figure 11A. Since the 9th workshop (Figure 11B) which was held in 20th October 2007, it was named "Sequential autologous fat injection: SAFI" under the basic principle that fat grafting should be performed in a certain sequence by considering the aging of whole face.

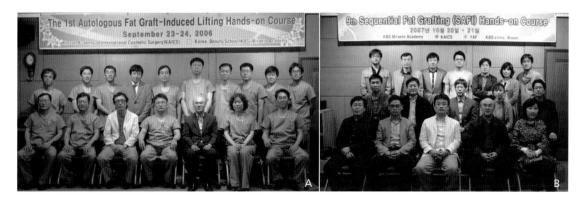

Figure 11 Naming of SAFI from the two commemorative photographs.

■7 SAFI lines, zones, sequence of fat grafting, and entry sites

In the early days of my fat grafting experience, I injected fat into areas located in the supero-lateral part of face first and then inject into areas located in the infero-medial part without any standard line for determining the injection of sequence. At that time, I had felt the necessity of a systemic and academic approach, so I had tried to connect structures which play major roles in maintaining facial contour and aging process. Interestingly, I found that the lines were running perpendicular to the direction of the soft tissue sagging and the face could be divided into 5 zones (Table 1). So, I decided to use these lines as strict standard for my fat grafting and named them SAFI lines (Figure 12 and 13).

1) SAFI lines and zones of face and temporal region

(1) SAFI lines of face and temporal region

SAFI line 1 means the most postero-superior border of face and temporal hollow. This line starts

Table 01 5 Zones for the SAFI technique

Zone	Boundary
I	Area within 5cm from the hair line as a temporal scalp portion including euryon above the SAFI line 1
II	Area between the SAFI line 1 and 2
III	Area between the SAFI line 2 and 3
IV	Area between the SAFI line 3 and 4
V	Area below the SAFI line 4

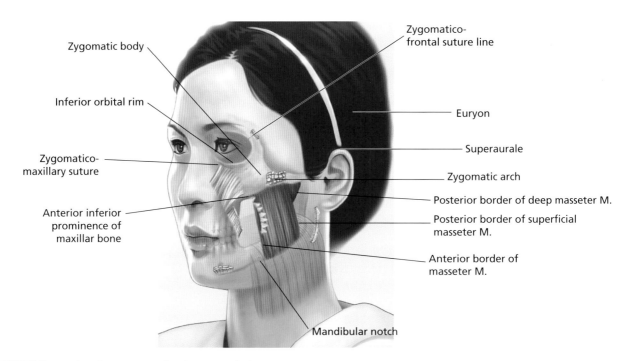

Figure 12   Facial surface anatomy for the SAFI technique.

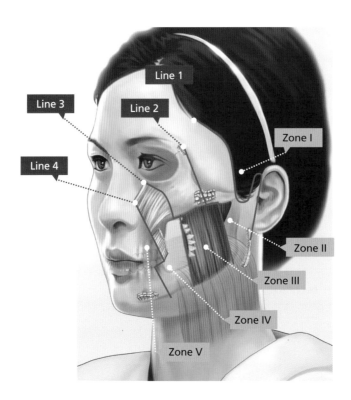

Figure 13   4 SAFI lines and 5 zones for SAFI technique.

at the meeting point of superior temporal line and the hairline. Along the temporal hair line, it is connected down to anterior auricular border. With the surgeon standing at the side of the patient, SAFI line 1 is drawn after confirming the structures.

SAFI line 2 and 3 are the imaginary lines connecting the characteristic sites of structures running perpendicular to the direction of the facial soft tissue sagging. They also consider the functional and structural characteristics of the facial tissues such as facial skeleton, bony suture, retaining ligament, muscle and fat. Therefore, these lines have the meaning of defense line against the antero-inferiorly drooping vectors.

SAFI line 2 links the orbital ligament, the posterior border of the orbital process of the zygomatic bone, the connecting part of zygomatic body and arch involving zygomatic retaining ligament, and the posterior border of the superficial masseter muscle. With the surgeon standing at the side of the patient, SAFI line 2 is drawn after confirming the structures.

SAFI line 3 links the zygomatico-maxillary suture that can be touched in the mid or medial 1/3 part of inferior orbital rim, the anterior inferior prominence of maxilla bone in the lateral and inferior tip of this suture, and the anterior border of superficial masseter muscle which is just below this projection. With the surgeon standing in front and looking at the patient's face, SAFI line 3 is drawn after confirming the structures.

SAFI line 4 is an imaginary line connecting the nasolabial fold to the labiomental fold. These two folds appear as striking features of aging at the middle part of the face. With the surgeon standing in front and looking at the patient's face, SAFI line 4 is drawn after confirming the structus.

(2) Zones
The face is devided into 5 zones by 4 SAFI lines as shown in Figure 13 and Table 1.

(3) Areas
The areas belong to each zone can be divided into the following two areas (Figure 14).
• First, the areas where patients want to improve, such as deep wrinkles, grooves, folds and depressions.
• Second, the other areas which are not complained by the patient but are necessary to be corrected to improve skeletal support, strengthen soft tissue foundation, and achieve a natural contour.

These areas can be represented diversely from the differences in bone structures related to ethnicity or race, the concept of beauty, age, development, aging status, and patient's expectation. The average amount and placement of fat in each area are shown in Table 2.

Recently, concept of subcutaneous fat compartments of face are found out. It would be helpful to perform SAFI by understanding the structural relationships as shown in Figure 15.

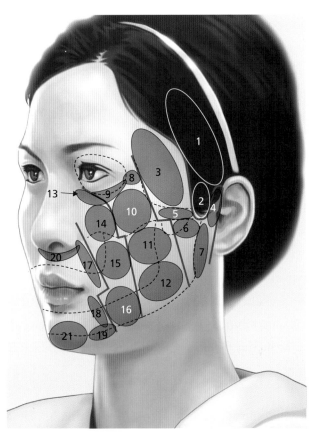

Figure 14 Schematic drawing of anatomical relationships between SAFI lines, possible injection areas and related structures including bones, muscles and ligaments. Black colored numbers (3, 6, 7, 8, 9, 11, 12, 13, 14, 15, 17, 18, 19, 20, and 21) are the area where most of the patients want to perform fat grafting. White colored numbers (1, 2, 4, 5, 10, and 16) are the areas that the physician should inject fat to make natural facial contour without sagging, even though patients do not want to perform fat grafting in those areas. Numbers inside the circles (1-21) mean the sequence of fat injection.

2) Fat injection sequence of the face and temporal area

Fat grafting for the face and the temporal area should be performed systematically as described below (Figure 15).

① Fat injection should be performed in the sequence of zone I, II, III, IV and V.

② Fat injection should be performed from postero-superior area to antero-inferior area within the same zone

③ Fat injection should be performed in the sequence of deep, middle, and superficial layer within an area. Figure 5 and 6 explains the reason why we should follow this injection sequence of fat grafting.

④ Additionally, if an area is large, it can be further divided into 2 or 3 subareas and fat can be sequentially injected into these subareas from postero-superiorly to antero-inferiorly in the same area as shown in area 10 of Figure 19.

Table 02 The definition, placement, and injectable volume of each SAFI areas.

Zone	Area	Area and subarea	Purpose	Placement	Volume*
I	1	Temporal scalp area within 5cm from the hair line	Volume augmentation and strengthen soft tissue foundations	Supraperiosteal layer, the space between superficial temporal fascia (STF) and deep temporal fascia (DTF) , and subcutaneous superficial fat layer.	2.0~3.0
	2	Side burn and its posterior temporal area		Inferior temporal septum	1.0~2.0
II	3	Temporal hollow	Strengthen soft tissue foundations	Orbital ligament and inferior temporal septum	2.0~4.0
			Augmentation	Subcutaneous superficial fat layer, and the space between STF and DTF	
	4	Preauricular area	Augmentation	sub-SMAS and superficial fat layer	2.0~3.0
	5	Zygomatic arch	Strengthen soft tissue foundations	Zygomatic retaining ligament	0.5~1.5
			Augmentation	Subcutaneous superficial fat layer	
	6	Lateral cheek depression	Augmentation	Deep lateral cheek fat, SMAS**, and subcutaneous superficial fat layer	1.0~2.0
	7	Parotid gland area	Augmentation	Subcutaneous superficial fat layer	1.0~2.0
III	8	Lateral canthal area	Augmentation	above the periosteum and under the orbicularis oculi muscle	0.5~1.0
	9	Palpebro-malar groove (lateral Z deformity)	Strong skeletal support and augmentation	Under the orbital retaining ligament, on the periosteum of anterior area to arcuate marginalis, above the orbital retaining ligament, and SOOF***.	0.5~1.5
	10	Malar eminence (flat, small malar)	Strong skeletal support and augmentation	Supra-periosteal layer(pre-zygomatic space), SOOF, and superficial fat layer	1.0~4.0
			Strengthen soft tissue foundations	Zygomatic ligaments and bucco- maxillary retaining ligament	
	11	Lateral subareas of sub-malar hollow	Augmentation	Lateral part of deep medial fat, buccal extension of buccal fat, SMAS, and superficial fat layer	2.0~4.0
			Strengthen soft tissue foundations	Masseteric cutaneous ligament	
	12	Lower part of the masseter muscle	Augmentation	Masseter muscle and subcutaneous fat layer	1.0~2.5
IV	13	Tear trough deformity	Strong skeletal support, and augmentation	Above the periosteum of the inferior orbital rim, under orbital retaining and buccal-maxillary ligament, SOOF and preorbital subcutaneous superficial fat layer	1.0~2.0
	14	Mid-cheek furrow	Strong skeletal support and augmentation	Buccal-maxillary ligaments, above the periosteum and under the lip levator muscles (deep medial cheek fat, a part of SOOF), and superficial medial cheek fat.	2.0~4.0
	15	Anterior subarea of sub-malar hollow	Strong skeletal support, Strengthen soft tissue foundations, and fullness	Supraperiosteal layer of zygomatic and maxillary bone, masseteric cutaneous ligament, and atrophied buccal extenbsion of buccal fat pad, lateral part of deep medial fat, and superficial medial cheek fat	2.0~6.0
			Augmentation	Peripheral of buccal fat pad, under the bucco-maxillary ligament and lip elevator muscles, and the subcutaneous superficial fat layer	
	16	Jowl (hypoplasia)		Deep and superficial fat layer	1.0~2.0
V	17	Nasolabial fold	Augmentation.	Whole layer of depressed part	1.0~2.0
	18	Labio-mandibular fold (Marionette line)	Augmentation.	Whole layer of depressed part of the folds	1.0~2.0
	19	Pre-jowl sulcus	Augmentation	On the periosteum of mandibular bone, and deep and superficial fat	1,0~2.0
	20	Pre-maxillary and upper lip area	Strong skeletal support and augmentation	On the periosteum of the pyriform area and deep fat	1,0~2.0
	21	Small chin	Strong skeletal support and augmentation	On the periosteum of mandible, deep and submental fat layer, and superficial fat layer.	2.0~5.0
Total injectable volume					26.5~57.5

Volume*: Injectable fat (ml/one side face), SMAS** : superficial muscular aponeurotic system, SOOF*** : suborbicularis oculi fat

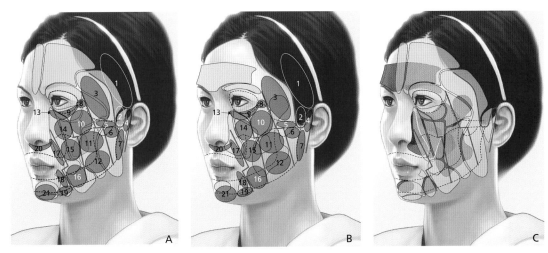

Figure 15 Two schematic drawings showing the anatomical relationships between subcutaneous fat compartments, SAFI lines, and possible injection areas(A, B, and C). Yellow colored-areas indicate superficial fat compartments (A). white gray, white blue, and violet-colored areas indicate deep fat compartments (B). Black circles indicate possible areas for fat grafting, and 4 red colored lines are SAFI lines. White colored numbers (1, 2, 4, 5, 10, and 16) are the areas that the physician should inject fat to make natural facial contour without sagging, even though patients do not want to perform fat grafting in those areas.

3) Entry site and direction of the injection

The selection criteria for injection in entry sites of the face and the temporal area are as follows:

- First, select the easiest and most comfortable site in the target area. Especially, fat injection over the periosteum needs to be performed parallel to the bony surface. Therefore, the relationship in location, morphology of soft tissue, and surgeon's location should be taken into consideration.
- Second, select the optimum site which enables fat to be injected parallel to the advancing direction to minimize damages to the blood vessels and nerves surrounding tissues.
- Third, select entry sites which are not visible considering chances of scar formation.
- Fourth, avoid using the intranasal and intraoral entry sites since they have high risk of infections.

Figure 16 represents the location of entry sites, injectable areas via each entry site, and advancing direction of cannula on performing SAFI. The arrows from each entry site indicate the direction of cannula and available area. However, the selection of the entry sites can vary a lot according to the patients and preferable posture or convenience of the physician.

Points of attention for selecting entry sites are as follows.

- First, area 13 and 14 for the entry site superior to tear trough (A of Figure 16) requires caution due to high risk of bleeding. Thus, beginners are recommended to use the other entry site located within area 10 (C of Figure 16).
- Second, it is quite hard to advance cannula from entry site next to corner of the mouth (B of Figure 16) towards area 15 or 16 because of vertically running several subcutaneous septums in superfi-

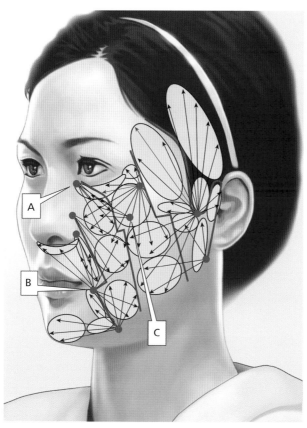

Figure 16 The entry sites (•) and the directions to the target (→) for the SAFI technique. An entry site superior to tear trough (A), an entry site next to the corner of mouth (B), and an entry site within the area 10 (C).

cial fat layer and collapsed buccal fat pad in deep fat layer (refer to Figure 3 and 4 of Chapter 1). If excessive force is applied when the cannula is advanced, there is a high risk of bleeding.

- Third, the cannula should be moved with caution and not to touch eyeball when the entry sites around the eye is used for orbital fat grafting.

- Fourth, the hole of entry site should be made by 18G needle and sutured with No. 6.0 or 7.0 nylon. The sutures are removed 3 days after the procedure.

8 Practice of SAFI method in facial and temporal region

1) Sequence of design

Design should be done under the following sequence.

- First, mark the 2nd, 3rd and 4th SAFI lines on the skin surface while palpating the facial structure manually by hands. The SAFI line 1 does not have to be marked practically.

- Second, mark the areas that need to be corrected by fat grafting.
- Third, mark the entry sites for each area.

2) Practice of SAFI and points of caution for facial and temporal region.

(1) Area 1 and 2 in Zone I

There is a high risk of bleeding due to damage of superficial temporal vessels in these areas as well as the area 3. Also, they require cautions because the temporal branch of the facial nerve runs through these areas. Thus, it is good to understand the course of the temporal vessels, and the cannula should be used in parallel to the vessel's direction with the most delicate manner without applying unnecessary force when injecting tumescent fluid or fat. Especially, if the cannula cannot be moved further during the injection, stop advancing it and advance smoothly by rolling the body of syringe with using thumb and index finger. Additionally, the surgeon's posture, the location of patient's face, the grip, and strength put on syringe are the important factors for bleeding.

If bleeding occurs, the procedure should be paused and manual compression is needed for at least 3 minutes until the bleeding stop. Tumesent anesthesia to these areas is helpful to reduce bleeding. It is highly recommedded that fat grafting should be started at least 10~20 minutes after the tumescent injection. Generally, i do not enjoy intramuscular fat grafting in these areas except in case of severe temporalis atrophy.

(2) Areas 3, 4, 5, 6 and 7 in Zone II

The area 3, temporal hollow is one of the most common sites of fat grafting. The most depressed part of this area is the region located just posterior to orbital process of the frontal bone, because this region is affected by strong closing or frowning of the eyes (Figure 17). This area can be divided into superior and inferior subarea by inferior temporal septum. Fat should be sequentially injected into the superior subarea, the inferior temporal septum for reinforcement, and then the inferior subarea. When the cannula passes through the temporal septum, the surgeon can feel the resistance, which can be felt much larger in inferior subarea than superior. When injecting into the inferior subarea, more caution is required to prevent damage to the middle temporal vein and frontal branches of facial nerve. During the precedure, the cannula should be injected parallel to the vessels and nerves. Also, advancement with excessive force or excessive amount of injection should be avoided. Fat can be injected into the supraperiosteal layer, the space between superficial and deep temporal fascia, and subcutaneous layer. Most importantly, it must be only injected when cannula is drawn back.

In area 4, the preauricular area is characterized by skin laxity and wrinkles due to aging. Only sim-

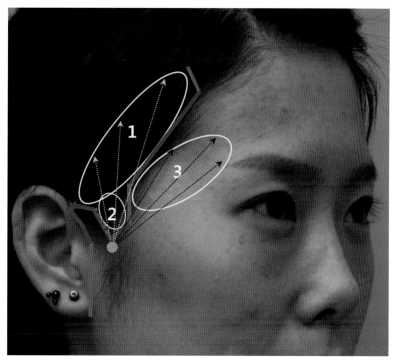

Figure 17 SAFI line 1 (red line), area 1 and 2 of Zone I, and area 3 of Zone II. Possible entry site (blue circle) and directions of injection (dotted arrows)

ple fat injection can bring very good outcome in this area. The skin is relatively thin and the subcutaneous tissue is quiet stiff, but fat survival rate is quite good (Figure 18). When the infra-lobular entry site is used for this area, pay attention to avoid intravascular injection because the course of superficial temporal vessel is same as the direction of injection.

In area 5, flattened or asymmetrical zygomatic arch can be improved by fat grafting. In this area, it can be performed in whole layer from supraperiosteal to subcutaneous fat layer. However, the frontal branch of the facial nerve is passing through the central part of this area; thus, it is recommended that fat is injected into subcutaneous layer rather than directly into the supraperiosteal layer. As described in the Chapter 1, there are groups of zygomatic retaining ligament near the area just in front of the junction of zygomatic body and anterior third of zygomatic arch. The reinforcement of this ligament and their surroundings by fat grafting has a very important meaning. Patients must be informed that this area can be compressed when sleeping in lateral posture after the procedure (Figure 18).

In area 6, the lateral cheek depression has a dimpled appearance just inferior to the middle and the anterior third of the zygomatic arch. It can be easily seen in women in their 30-40s with well-developed cheek bone and high usage of masseter muscle. The floor consists of deep masseter muscle originated from the medial surface of the zygomatic arch. It is mainly caused by absence of superficial masseter muscle and decreased volume of lateral cheek. Also, it is not easy to advance the cannula in between superior surface of masseter muscle fascia and inferior part of the zygomatic arch due to well-developed fibrous tissue. So, for these reasons, this area is harder to be recovered by fat grafting compared to other areas. If hyper-corrected, it may become stiff and flattened, and sometimes looks more depressed than surroundings (Figure 18). Therefore, not only the depressed area but also the causing factors of the surroundings need to be corrected with fat gafting. And the fat should be sequentially injected from deep layer (above the muscle fascia) to superficial layer and it is also important to follow the hypothesis of Figure 6. Besides, it is crucial to inform about the necessity of additional procedures to patients, since it is hard to be corrected by a single procedure.

Area 7 is the parotid gland region. When fat is injected into this area, the utmost care is needed to prevent the damage of the gland. Fat should be injected into the space between parotico-masseteric fascia and skin. It is also performed to strengthen plastysma-auricular ligament.

(3) Areas 8, 9, 10, 11 and 12 in Zone II

Area 8 is lateral canthal depression. It is caused by reduction in thickness of skin and subcutaneous tissues due to overuse of lateral orbicularis oculi and lip elevator muscle, and also affected by the skeletal change of inferolateral orbital limb and reduction in thickness of lateral orbital thickening.

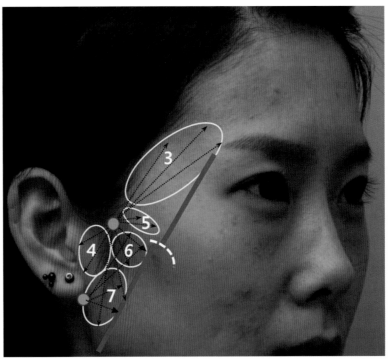

Figure 18 SAFI line 2 (red line), area 3, 4, 5, 6 and 7 of Zone II. Possible entry sites (blue circle) and directions of injection (black dotted arrows)

Under the orbicularis oculi muscle and above the periosteum is the preferable site of fat injection, but, the subcutaneous and intramuscular layer is not recommended. Fat grafting to the orbital ligament can be performed simultaneously through the same entry site. This ligament can be easily attenuated when eyebrow depressor muscle and frontalis muscle have been excessively used. Botulinum toxin is recommended to patients with a lot of movements of these muscles. It can be performed to strengthen the ligament and increase volume of superior ortital rim for strong skeletal support. The proper placement is at the supraperiosteal layer (Figure 19). Cautions should be taken that the cannula will not poke or irritate the orbit during fat grafting. To be safe, put non-dominant hand's finger on the border of orbital rim to prevent poking the orbit. This caution should be applied to area 8, 9, 10, and 14.

Area 9 is called a palpebro-malar groove[17]. Deepening and widening of this groove are caused by the bone loss in infero-lateral orbital rim (lateral trough deformity), weakening of orbital retaining ligament, laxity of orbicularis oculi muscle, and SOOF (suborbicularis oculi fat) loss (Figure 19). Only small amount of fat can improve the groove. Hyper-correction should be approached with cautions since it may exaggerate malar mound and orbital fat protrusion. Please be aware that the complete volume recovery of the groove would not give a natural look.

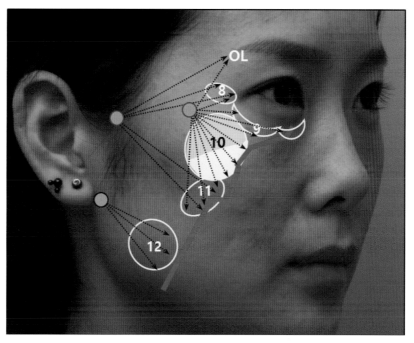

Figure 19 SAFI line 3 (red line), area 8, 9, 10, 11 and 12 of Zone III. Area 10 can be devided into 2 subareas (deep yellow and bright yellow). Fats should be injected into the deep yellow area first and then the bright yellow area. Possible entry sites (blue circle), and directions of injection (black dotted arrows), and OL (orbital ligament) are shown.

Area 10 is a malar eminence (Figure 19). Two malar eminences together with the chin is the main frame of beauty triangle which mimics the shape of an inverted triangle. Malar mounds refer to skin and fat that bulge from the malar eminance. Age-related changes of the midface, such as ptosis and volume loss of the midfacial soft tissue, may contribute to the formation of malar mounds. As shown in Figure 20, the flat and small malar eminence with poor skeletal support is one of the major causes of mid-face sagging with deep nasolabial folds. It may also contribute to the formation of sagging jowl.

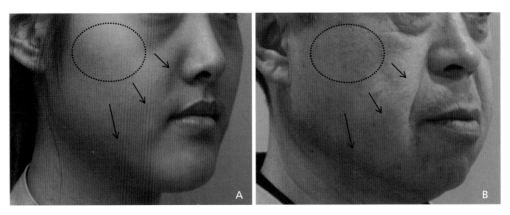

Figure 20 Clinical manifestations of the poor skeletal support due to small and flat cheek bone. Black circle means flat malar and arrows means sagging of soft tissue with deep nasolabial folds and developed jowls. 22-year-old young woman having older appearance than that of her real age (A), 55-year-old man having older appearance than that of his real age (B).

Malar of beautiful face has strong soft tissue foundation. Therefore, fat grafting to the small and flat malar has significant meaning because the loss volume can be restored and the poor skeletal support also can be improved by the hypothesis of "the moss covered stone" as mentioned in Figure 12 of Chap 2. The small and flat malar can be changed into tense and less movable, fixed like appearance due to the fullness and tightening by fat grafting. At the same time, the skin of the antero-inferior regions such as mid-cheek furrows and nasolabial folds get stretched to this malar area, the skin tension of mid-cheek furrow is increased, and the nasolabial folds get softened. The result of this procedure has additional effects; it reduces drooping phenomenon due to the weight of the injected fat and reduces the amount of fat required when the fat is sequentially injected as mentioned in Figure 9.

However, if malar edema is present, in principle, fat grafting is not recommended since it can cause a negative effect. But, when small malar occurs in conjunction with malar edema, fat can be injected only into just above periosteal layer and superficial fat layer, not deep fat layer, because most of the malar edema is caused by insufficient lymphatic circulation of deep fat layer. Subcutaneous liposuction or lipolysis can also be performed in the case of malar mounds due to excessive soft tissue. However, this is not recommended to patients accompanied with systemic disease or severe malar edema.

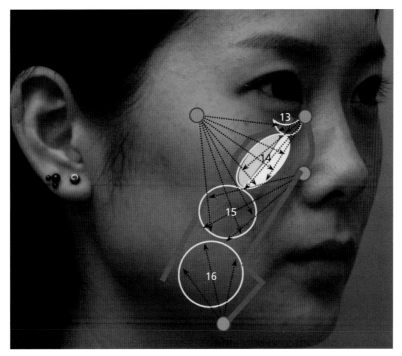

Figure 21 SAFI line III & IV (Red line), area 13, 14, 15 and 16 of Zone IV. Possible entry sites (blue circle) and directions of injection (black dotted arrows). Based on the junction of concave-convex maxillary bone, the area 14 can be divided into 2 subareas (deep yellow colored concave subarea and bright yellow colored convex subareas). The fat should be injected into deep yellow area first and then bright yellow area.

Area 11 is the lateral part of the submalar hollow. The submalar hollow is divided artificially into two areas, medial and lateral part by SAFI line 4. Among the two, the lateral area occasionally extends laterally to the depression of upper-part of the masseter muscle and to the lateral cheek depression (Figure 18). The slight depression of this area is an essential for natural contour of face. But, severe depression needs to be restored. It is because the volume loss of this area is one of the important factors related to mid-face sagging due to the loss of superficial and deep portion of buccal extension of posterior buccal fat pad. All of these details will be explained in area 15.

Area 12 is the inferior part of the masseter muscle. Many asian women, under the influence of physiognomy, do not prefer the hypertrophy of mandible and masseter muscle. Thus, fat grafting is unlikely to be performed into this area. However, with botulinum toxin injection to reduce masseter muscle, it rapidly atrophies and occasionally worsens lateral cheek depression, jowl drooping, and perioral wrinkles. Especially, even lateral cheek may seem to be severely depressed if botulinum toxin is injected to the middle part of masseter muscle. This can be corrected with fat grafting. However, moderate hypertrophy of masseter muscle and mandible are the symbols of youth in westerners, so fat grafting is common to be performed for volume increasing at this area (Figure 19).

(4) Area 13, 14, 15 and 16 in Zone V

Area 13 is called the tear trough[20]. The skin of tear trough is very thin with no subcutaneous fat and overlays the preseptal oculi muscle. The skin inferior to tear trough (cheek skin), in contrast, is thicker and is separated from the underlying orbicularis muscle by well-developed subcutaneous fat compartments. Also, both the oribicularis oculi muscle and orbital retaining ligament are strongly attached to inferior orbital rim (Figure 22 and 23). Tear trough deformity[21] is an undesirable appearance of tear trough by aging characterized by flaccid skin with dark circle, protrusion of orbital fat, resorption of infra-orbital orbital rim (or maxillary retrusion expressed as medial suborbital hypoplasia[22]), and soft tissue drooping of mid-face by aging[23,24].

Many complicated factors affect this area. Therefore, we can distinguish the causes by using the following simple physical examinations (Figure 22)

① Eyelid region: Confirm the protruded orbital fat by palpating inferior orbital rim with tip of finger. If the orbital fat has been confirmed, it is due to flaccid and attenuated septum and orbicularis oculi muscle. It leads to a more anterior projection of the infraorbital subcutaneous fat with a relative deepening of the tear trough deformity.

② Orbital rim region: Check the presence and symmetry of maxillary retrusion and the contour of orbital rim by touching the bone using finger. It provides a direct evidence of characteristic sunken of the tear trough deformity.

③ Mid-cheek region: The depression of upper mid-face caused by sagging and volume loss of subcutaneous fats (nasolabial fat, medial cheek, and SOOF)[23], weakening of orbital retaining ligament, and skeletal remodeling of maxillar bone. These descending factors contribute to the hollowness of the tear trough deformity.

④ Skin pigmentation: Pigmentation that is usually found in this area is ADM (acquired dermal melanosis), Ota nevus, or melasma. If it is melasma, it does not extend into orbital rim. In the

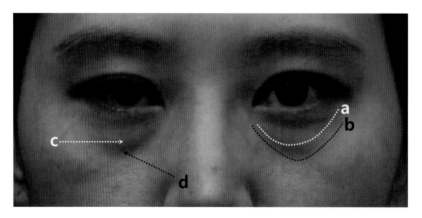

Figure 22 Surface anatomy of the junctional area of lower lid and mid-cheek; Orbital rim (a), lid-cheek junction (b), protruded orbital fat (c), and dark circle (d).

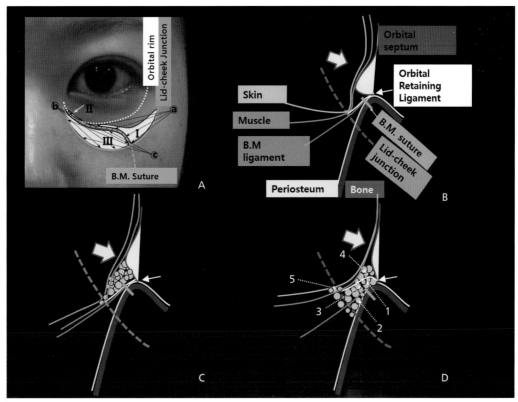

Figure 23 SAFI technique for volume restoration and strong skeletal support of area 13 (tear trough, II and III) and area 9 (palpebromalar fold, I). Fat should be injected sequentially I, II and III through the entry sites (a and b or a and c) (A), The cross section view shows the protruded orbital fat and surrounding structures (B), When fat is placed mainly at SOOF layer without direct attaching to bone, the fat cannot increase skeletal support sufficiently and may have a high risk of movable lumps with less improvement of orbital fat protrusion (C). However, if the fat is placed at appropriate layers following sequential injection, the skeletal support can be increased significantly and may have low risk of movable lumps with improvement of orbital fat (D). Number of 1, 2, 3, 4, and 5 indicate sequence of fat injection. Muscle (Orbicularis Oculi Muscle), B.M. (Bucco-maxillary) ligament, and B.M. (Bucco-Maxillary) suture.

case of ADM, it does not invade medial canthal region towards the nose. Also, the development of microscopic angiogenesis is the characteristic for melasma.

The causes should be analyzed beforehand because the orbit and cheek of different facial aesthetic units abut each other and they concurrently affect aging process of tear trough. And then, it should be decided which of the two surgeries, fat grafting or fat grafting with lower blepharoplasty, is more efficient.

Whatever surgery you choose, the fat can be placed over the periosteum of the inferior orbital rim (1), beneath bucco-maxillary ligament (2), beneath the orbital retaining and lip levator muscle (3), and into medial SOOF (4), and then nasolabial and middle cheek fat (5) as shown in Figure 23D.

The survival rate of this area is relatively pretty good. But, some doctors may be afraid of performing fat injection to this area, because unexpected possible complications such as fibrotic lump and irregularity are fairly common. My method that considers placement and injection sequence to prevent these complications is explained in Figure 23C and D in detail. Additionally, when performing SAFI, it should be noted that overcorrection is avoided. I would like to introduce the endpoint of injection to prevent overcorrection from my personal experience. It is a status that looks like a little bit hypo-corrected in supine position. At that time, you can feel the softness like surrounding soft tissue when pressed with finger and natural surface contour without any protruding when the patient laughs can be observed. In addition, it is also recommended to limit facial expression, use less fibrotic fat, inject fat less than 2mm thick, and apply PRP or ADSCs, and so on.

Area 14 is the mid-cheek furrow also called Indian fold. This area forms italic y appearance from the combination of lid-cheek junction, palpebromalar groove, and tear trough deformity due to aging of the low eyelid and mid-cheek area (Figure 24).

The superficial subcutaneous fat layer of this area is consisted of nasolabial fold fat and medial cheek fat which adjacent to each other and form a slope. The deep fat layer is made up of deep medial cheek fat and proximity of SOOF that abuts to each other. The connection between zygomatic bone

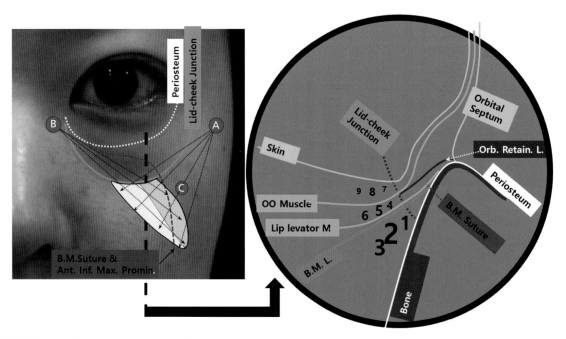

Figure 24 SAFI for area 14 (mid-cheek furrow). It is important to sequentially inject fat deep to bucco-maxillary liga-ments and under the lip elevator muscles (correspond to deep medial cheek fat, 1-4). And, the fat should be injected into SOOF layer (5-6) and finally into superficial medial cheek fat (8-9). But, in the area lateral to B.M suture line, fat should be mainly injected right above the supraperiosteal layer (prezygomatic fat) with mini-mal injection into SOOF and malar mound fat because facial nerves travel within the SOOF and prolonged edema is a major cause of malar mound fat grafting. The different size of numbers (1-9) means relative amount of injected fat. O.O. (Orbicularis Oculi) Muscle, B.M.L. (Bucco-maxillary Ligament), L.L.M. (Lip Levator Muscle), B.M. (Bucco-Maxillary) suture.

and maxillary bone are switched entirely from convex to concave shape. Particularly, knowing the fact of this area develops from concaved surface of maxillary bone in the medial side of zygomatic-maxillary suture is very important to understand the depression of this area (Refer to Figure 37 and 38 of Chapter 1).

Bony change and soft tissue depression of this area is closely related with bone resorption by aging shown in Figure 6 of Chapter 2. Repetitive lip elevation (laughing) may also be one of the important factors for the development of depression and drooping of this area due to the postero-superior shifting of soft tissue above nasolabial folds by contraction of lip elevator muscles. There is high possibility of crashing soft tissue with bones around the zygomatico-maxillary suture and attenuation of the surrounding retaining ligaments (Figure 25). It is important to perform fat injection sequentially into from supraperiosteal layer of maxillary bone, deep medial cheek fat, below of buccal-maxillary retaining ligaments and lip levator muscle, medial SOOF, and finally to superficial medial cheek fat (Figure 24). During the procedure, observe the change in nasolabial folds by injecting fat into mid-cheek furrows with SAFI method as mentioned above. The softening of nasolabial folds while the volume increases in this area can be observed.

Many doctors have had experiences of unsatisfied patients who had performed artificial filler or fat grafting to improve this area. Most of the cases were only injecting fat into the subcutaneous fat layer and superior part of deep fat layer, or injecting artificial filler only to the superior part of subcutaneous

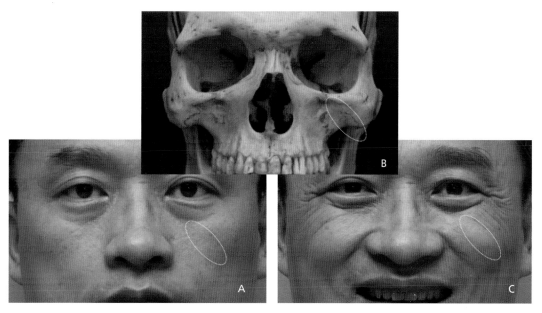

Figure 25 A possible cause of soft tissue loss in the mid-cheek furrow by repetitive facial expresssion. When laughing, the contraction of both muscles of lip elevators and orbiculari oris cause postero-inferior shifting of the naso-labial folds and result in crush of soft tissue of mid-cheek furrow due to repetitive pressure. The crushed area leads to volume depletion of the soft tissue with drooping. The resting status (A), corresponding area of the mid-cheek area in skeleton (B), and the laughing status (c).

fat layer and dermal layer. These results reflect the importance of adequate depth, amount, and order of injection in grafting (Refer to Figure 6).

Area 15 is the anterior part of submalar hollow. The depression of this area exaggerates the prominence of the zygomatic bone and exacerbates the development and drooping of jowl. Sometimes, the area is connected with area 14, mid-cheek furrow (Figure 26).

This area can be affected diversely by various factors such as the atrophy or pseudo-ptosis of buccal fat pad caused by growth or aging, weakening of masseteric–cutaneous retaining ligaments, and resorption of the premaxillary bone due to orthodontic and implant procedures. There is a significant asymmetry of this area between right and left face. Thus, the dimension of surrounding bone and soft tissue, difference of facial expression, and the difference of right and left dentition and loss of teeth need to be observed carefully. Also, factors that can cause side-effects in this area such as jowl can become bigger and droopy with exacerbating labio-mandibular folds should be remembered.

It is strongly recommended to divide the area 15 into 2 subareas because the area has the weakest soft tissue foundation and high risk of sagging due to the weight of the grafted fat. Basic approach is as follows. Using entry site A, fat is injected into the supraperiosteal layer of zygoma and maxillary bone of 11 and 15 area to increase skeletal support (refer to Figure 12 of Chapter 2), into intra- and peripheral region of masseteric cutaneous ligament for strengthening and tightening, and into the atrophied anterior and intermediate lobe of buccal fat pad for greater fullness. Using entry site B, fat is in-

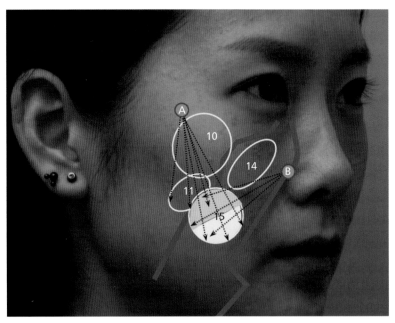

Figure 26 Area 15 and its surrounding areas, 10, 11 and 14. This area can be divided into two subareas (deep yellow and bright yellow). The fat should be injected into the deep yellow subarea first and then the bright yellow subarea sequentially. In all cases, fat grafting for the area 15 should be performed after enough improvement of volume depletion in areas 10, 11 and 14.

jected into peripheral of buccal fat pad and deep medial cheek fat under the buccomaxillary ligament and lip elevator muscles, and then into the superficial medial cheek fat through entry site A and B.

Area 16 is the jowl area which is postero-superiorly positioned to labiomandibular fold. It is characterized by sagging appearance due to fullness and looseness of lower cheek or jowl. Sometimes, it looks more pronounced in the case of small chin with deep prejowl sulcus. The development of this area is the evidence of rectangular or trapezoidal face which is the characteristic of aged face. It can be primarily treated by liposuction. On the other hand, fat grafting also can be performed to patients who have flattened or depressed appearance of the jowl. For reference, in many cases, patients who have sunken cheek demand for full cheeks that resembling their oral cavity is filled with air with their mouth closed during the consultation. Area 11, 15, 16, and 17 get volume increased by this behavior. Even so, if the fat graft is performed only to these areas, the final outcome will be very unnatural.

Liposuction or fat grafting to this area can cause side effect such as antero-inferior drooping. To prevent this, it is need that precise understanding of the status of the postero-superior areas (area 4, 5, 6, 7, 10, 11, and 15) and acquiring pre-estimate ability to prognose changes in soft tissue contour followed by liposuction or fat grfting. For example, drooping due to volume depletion of the postero-superior areas can contribute to the volume increase of jowl. If this is not severe, fat grafting only to the postero-superior areas can reduce the volume of this area. But, when excessive jowl is accompanied with volume loss of the postero-superior areas, liposuction-induced drooping can be prevented with this sequence of procedure, liposuction of jowl first and then fat grafting to these areas. Be aware that not all cases of this above approach can prevent liposuction-induced drooping phenomenon. Effects cannot be expected in patients with thin skin, lack of elasticity, or loose skin which is an indication of rhitydectomy. The characteristics of jows have been explained in detail in anatomy and aging of Chapter 1 and 2. Remember that this is the area where patients complain the most that their "cheek has been drooped" or "moved lower" after fat grafting or liposuction.

(5) Areas 17, 18, 19, 20, and 21 in Zone V

Area 17 is the nasolabial fold which is composed of the folded (augmented) part laterally and the depressed part medially. Let us feel and remember the depressed part and folded part of nasolabial folds by palpation. Then, palpate area 17 again when area 10 is lifted in postero-superior direction by your finger. The feeling should be significantly different in these two cases (Figure 27). The interesting fact is when palpating the nasolabial fold after fat injection into postero-superior areas of nasolabial folds (such as area 10 and 14), the feeling is very similar to that of area 10 lifted in postero-superior direction by finger. This phenomenon suggests the possibility of softening the nasolabial fold by previously performed fat grafting into the postero-superior areas.

It will lead to not only an unoptimal aesthetic result but also an unexpected result such as "a more

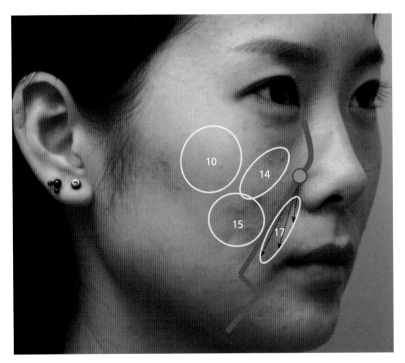

Figure 27   SAFI line V and area 17 and its superolateral areas 10, 14, and 15.

prominent expansion of lateral folded part of nasolabial fold" when injecting fat only to the depressed part of nasolabial fold, such as the medial part of deep medial cheek fat and fat of Ristow's space, in the patient who has a chief complaints on prominent nasolabial fold. This phenomenon can be seen in postoperative photos, not only with the fat grafting but also with various artificial filler injection for the softening of the nasolabial fold. Within a few weeks, patients would complain that "not effective on the depressed part of the fold but became bigger only on the lateral folded part of the fold", and trust can be lost as the consequence.

From the above facts, we are able to recognize that the formation of a proment nasolabial fold is not only caused by a prominent fold itself but also affected by several interesting hypotheses of mid-face aging process such as pseudoptosis theory, compartmental migration and intra-compartmental shift hypothesis, and bony remodeling theory as mentioned in Chapter 2. Additionally, it can also be affected by the tethering effect of fascial dermal insertions at the nasolabial fold. Therefore, when per-forming fat grafting to soften a prominent nasolabial fold, a multifaceted approach considering all the factors need to be carried out. For example, for the correction of prominent nasolabial fold caused by under-developed zygomatic or maxillary bone (e.g. maxillary retrusion), not only a fat grafting should be peformed additionally to reinforce the under-developed bony framework, but also a selective li-posuction for reduction of nasolabial fold fat compartment. At this moment, sequence of procedures is very important. Liposuction should be performed first followed by fat grafting. The fascial dermal insertions of the fold can also be detached by dissector cannula during the liposuction. The fat is sequentially injected into area 10, 14, and 15 for volumetric lifting and then injected into area 17 for volume restoration. The volume augmentation of deep medial cheek fat and Ristow's space alone is not considered as a reasonable approach to soften a prominent nasolabial fold perfectly because it cannot improve the multiple factors such as inferior volume shift within the nasolabial fat, sagging of the nasolabial fat, and atrophy of the superficial medial cheek fat.

It is quite common that "deep nasolabial folds" is the chief complaint of many patients. Among them, many wants to improve or flatten the nasolabial folds like in their 20's and 30's. This is wrong expectation of patients that the perfect correction of deep nasolabial folds would make them look younger. Therefore, it is more important for the patients to understand and recognize what is the naturally youthful look of the nasolabial folds. Practically, improvement of deep nasolabial folds in middle or old aged patient is more obvious not in upper 1/3 but middle and lower 1/3 of the folds because aging mostly happen in lower 2/3 of the folds. In conclusion, this area is not a simple fold; it is rather dynamic folds formed by movements of facial mimic muscles and aging. Therefore, it is more logical to have diverse approaches to soften the folds rather than just simply filling up the depressed area.

Area 18 is the labio-mandibular fold or Marionnate line. The fold exists in between corner of the mouth and mandible, and forms the anterior border of jowl. This is a dynamic fold where only one third is visible when there is no facial movement. However, its whole length appears with the usage of mimic muscle. Especially, it is developed more in individuals with excessive use of depressor angular oris muscle[27]. Also, with aging, it is caused by depression of mandibular bony resorption around mandubular ligament, decreased volume in the lateral edge of labiomandibular fat, and jowl sagging caused by increased volume in the inferior portion of jowl fat and antero-inferior protrusion (or prolapsed) of the buccal fat (Figure 28).

The natural result of fat grafting in this area can be achieved by filling the area to look like a little bit depressed when there is no motion of facial expression muscles. Sometimes, it would be helpful to soften the fold by injecting fat into area 15 and area 16 in patient with involutional face. For patient with moderately developed jowl, grafting of the areas (4,5,6,7,10,14, and 15) and labiomandibular fat after liposuction of jowl fat and/or subcutaneous part of the buccal extension of the buccal fat pad can bring more natural appearance. However, additional surgical face lifting sometimes should be performed for patients with highly developed jowl because this area has the weakest soft tissue foundation.

Area 19 of the prejowl sulcus frequently appears in the form of united with the labiomadibular fold. When fat grafting, fat should be sequentially injected into whole layer from supraperiosteal layer to superficial fat layer because main causes are volume loss of labiomandibular fat compartment, mandibular bone resorption, and retraction of mandibular retaining ligament. In case of severe retractive

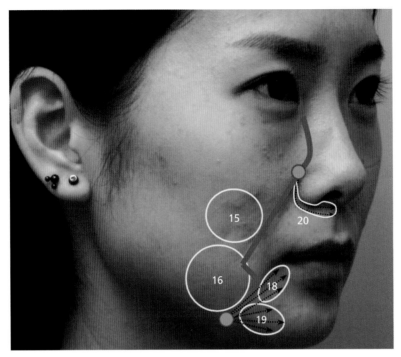

Figure 28 Area 18 and 19 and their superolateral areas 15 and 16.

depression, it would also be helpful to release cutaneous insertions of the depressor anguli oris muscle and mandibular ligament. Overcorrection is not recommended because it can make the jowls look bigger and chin looks smaller than they actually are. Bear in mind that shallow depression and smooth transition are needed for natural look (Figure 28).

Area 20 is the premaxillary and the upper lip area. Resorption of bone, volume loss and laxity of soft tissue due to aging contribute to droopy nasal tip flaccid philtrum, and sagging of upper lip. Fat injection above perioseum of the pyriform for the support of lateral crura, into deep layer of philtrum and upper lip for volume recovery can help in improving signs of aging. However, careful approach is necessary because excessive fat injection into philtrum and upper lip might result in protruded mouth (Figure 28).

Area 21 is chin area. Microgenia is the condition of abnormal smallness of the chin, causing the mouth to look protruded. It can occur in anyone, but is often a sign of Down's syndrome[28]. Microgenia patients cannot close their mouths well due to poor skeletal support and this causes exposure of lower teeth. So, most of the patients tend to use excessive contraction of the mentalis muscle to close their mouth. This is the main cause of chin wrinkles, mentalis dimpling (also known as peau d'orange Chin dimpling[29]) and loss of fat pad behind mentalis muscle. In addition, microgenia usually is accompanied by double chin and is one of the causes of blunted cervicomental angle.

Osteotomy, allograft augmentation, implantation of Goretex or silicone, artificial fillers injection and fat grafting are recommended for improving microgenia. If it is not severe and the patient does not want artificial materials such as filler or implants, then fat grafting is worth a try.

However, it is important to make sure that the patient understands that there might be a need to carry out 2-3 additional surgeries and that fat grafting has lower satisfaction result compared to osteotomy and augmentation with allograft implants. In addition, fat grafting is highly recommended as an adjunctive treatment for correction of problems like asymmetric and under correction after osteotomy and implantation. It is also used to make soft and natural contour between the chin and the face.

If fat grafting is planned to be performed at the chin area, it is essential to weaken the mentalis by using botulinum toxin about 2-3 weeks before the procedure. The basic method of fat grafting for chin augmentation is shown in Figure 29. It should be performed differently according to the status of chin such as short chin, long chin and retruded chin. Artificial fillers also can be injected using the same method as fat grafting. In the case of short chin, inject more fat at the lower part of chin to make the chin look longer (B). In the case of long chin, inject more fat at the anterior part of chin to protrude the chin anteriorly (A). In the case of retruded chin, fat grafting is required in these two parts (A and B).

The unnatural look of Witch's chin is often seen as an unexpected complication after filler or fat grafting. To prevent this sagging appearance, it is highly recommended to apply SAFI technique as shown in Figure 29. The chin area is divided into 2-3 smaller area to apply the SAFI technique. Then, the injection must be performed according to the following sequence; from the upper area to the lower

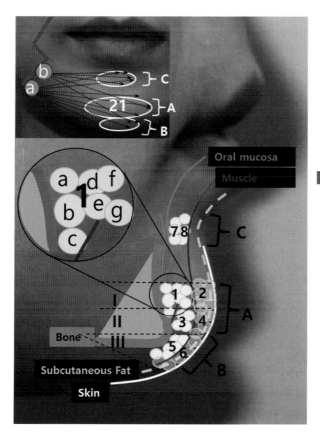

Figure 29 Sequential injection for chin augmentation with artificial filler or fat.

I, II, and III means subareas of area 21 (chin area). The subarea I is a region from level of fornix to upper 1/2 of anterior projection of chin, the subarea II is a region of lower 1/2 of anterior projection of chin, and the subarea III is a region of antero-inferior projection of chin. Region A is for anterior projection in patients with long or retruded chin, Region B is for lengthening in patients with short or retruded chin. Region C is for improvement of mentolabial sulcus and acute labiomental angle. The possible entry sites for injection are expressed as a and b.

area (From I to III), and sequentially from deep layer to superficial layer of each area (From 1 to 2, from 3 to 4, and from a to g). In addition, entire natural contour can be obtained by injection at area of fat pad behind mentalis muscle and subcutaneous layer (C) to soften mental crease and increase labiomental angle. In particular, it is recommended to be careful not to enter the oral cxavity when passing through the oral mucosa during fat grafting in this area.

For softening of the mentolabial sulcus, it is reliable that the fat is only injected into the deep submental fat compartment to decrease the concavity of the labiomental angle as shown in Figure 29. The fat should be injected just above the periosteum (7) and then injected into the deep submental fat compartment (8) underneath the mentalis. However, if the fat is injected beneath the sulcus and into the subcutaneous chin fat layer which is inferior to the sulcus, it would increase the concavity of the angle because there is no fat layer with fibrotic tissues from surrounding muscles underneath the sulcus.

9 Fat grafting of sunken upper eyelid

Fat grafting is often performed to improve sunken upper eyelid. However, utmost care is needed because serious side effects can occur occasionally as shown in Figure 30. I also approach this area with extra care compared to other parts of the face. I will describe the technique in detail since side effects of this procedure happen in many patients recently.

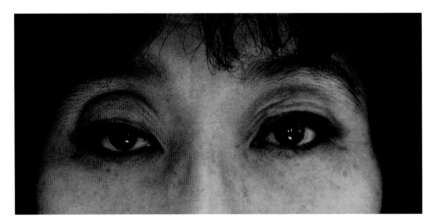

Figure 30 A case of complication of fat grafting for the correction of sunken eye. Right eyelid shows the iatrogenic severe ptosis by the weight of the grafted fat and the incomplete improvement of sunken eye. Left eyelid also show the iatrogenic mild ptosis with irregularities and multiple double fold lines.

1) Definition and causes

Sunken upper eyelid seems to be depressed in the area between upper eyelid and eyebrow. As in Figure 31, it is due to the shortage of the amount of fat in front and behind the orbital septum (Figure 31B) or the displacement of orbital fat which is attached to the levator aponeurosis by tearing or detachment of levator aponeurosis from tarsal (Figure 31C). Also, these two factors can happen simultaneously. However, in majority cases of sunken upper eyelid, it is more often related to the connection problem of the tarsal plate and levator aponeurosis than just simple depletion of fat[30].

There are acquired and congenital causes for this condition[31]. Congenital causes are depletion of collagen and elastin of connective tissue and skin, and decrease of subcutaneous fat due to aging process. And the acquired causes are excessive removal of orbital fat or damage to orbital septum[32], injury of levator aponeurosis, and excessive excision of orbicularis oculi muscles or SOOF during upper blepharoplasty.

2) Application of fat grafting to sunken upper eyelid

The first examination that should be performed to the patient with sunken upper eyelid before fat grafting is checking the presence of lid ptosis. As shown in Figure 32 and 33, the fat grafting procedure should be performed to the patient within the normal range of MRD_1 (margin reflex distance 1). With the presence of mild ptosis, the procedure should be carefully performed. It must not be performed to patients with moderate ptosis. These criteria should be applied more strictly to seniors, and more detailed examinations are required.

Also, sunken upper eyelid are manifestation of the main sign of masked blepharoptosis with almost normal function of the palpebral levator muscle but incomplete connection between the muscle

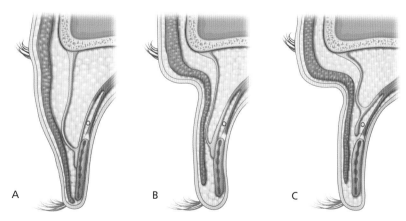

A   B   C

Figure 31 Causes of sunken eye.

A. Cross sectional anatomy of normal upper eyelid.

B. Volume deficiency of both preseptal fat and septal fat or one of them.

C. Detached or weakened levator aponeurosis from tarsus, allows orbital fat to move backwards into the orbit.

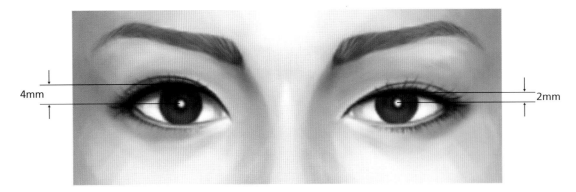

Figure 32 MRD1 is a distance between center lid margin and corneal reflex, it is a quantitative measurement of ptosis, and its normal range is 3-4 mm.

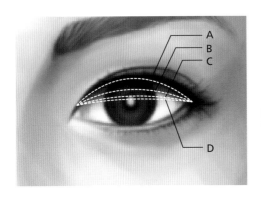

Figure 33 Classification of the eyelid ptosis.
A : Normal eyelid (between 3-4mm)
B : Mild ptosis (between 2-3mm)
C : Moderate Ptosis (between 1-2mm)
D : Severe Ptosis (below 1mm)

and tarsal plate. Especially, presence of eyelid ptosis should be examined prior to the procedure with patients who do not seem to have eyelid ptosis, but have the habit of lifting up their eyebrows when looking up because they have high possibility of the presence of masked blepharoptosis. The degree of ptosis should be measured by blocking the effect of the forehead while opening eyes.

Fat grafting to the patients with lid ptosis or masked blepharoptosis will worsen the symptom of the ptosis. Levator shortening or advancement surgery is the first choice to improve sunken eyelid. However, if the eyelid is still sunken in spite of the levator shortening surgery, fat grafting can be performed to the depleted area for more perfect correction. This should be a fundamental principle for the correction of sunken eyelid.

There is no objective method to measure the deficiency of soft tissue volume (esp. fat) of the upper lid. But there is an indirect method to find the need of fat grafting by pressing smoothly the lower eyelid region in direct ahead gaze without using frontalis[28]. If the upper eyelid region does not swell up as expected, it informs that fat grafting is needed, and vice versa.

3) Effect of aging and facial expression on sunken eyelids

In addition to the cause of sunken eyelid as pointed out above, sunken eyelid is also affected by aging of the eyebrow region. Particularly, brow ptosis is known to be caused by secondary effect of gravitation and reduction of subcutaneous fat layer. On the other hand, the soft tissue change corresponding to skeletal remodeling of superior orbital rim has also been studied as well.

Recently, Rober B. Shaw, Jr et al. suggested that aging change of skeletons around orbital rim makes the overall expansion of the orbits and the rolling of soft tissue into the orbits and dynamic change is one of the major causes of not only brow ptosis and lateral orbital hooding but also protrusion of orbital fat, deep upper eyelid sulcus, enophthalmos, and sunken eyelid[33].

According to this study, the direct and indirect effects of brow ptosis on sunken upper eyelid cannot be excluded. Moreover, most of the patients with sunken upper eyelid are associated with brow ptosis in elder patients, so it is reasonable to correct these two at the same time.

Also, excessive use of mimic muscles is closely related with sunken eyelids. Often lifting up and frowning eyebrows reduces the soft tissue of this area. Because the signs are found not only in the area above and below the eyebrows but also in the medial part of the eyebrows, the changes are also considered in fat grafting.

4) Fat grafting methods currently used

Previously used fat grafting concepts to improve sunken upper eyelid are based on volume restoration only for the sunken area and the fat was injected above the aponeurosis and orbital septum[34], below the orbicularis oculi muscle[31], or periosteum of upper orbital rim and preseptal plane[35] after marking the depressed area. Recently, it was reported that fat was grafted into all these layers of sunken area using special gun[36].

These simple approaches are only for increasing the volume of the depressed area and seem to be insufficient in considering the influence on aging of bones and surrounding tissues. Of course, good results can be expected in small amount of fat grafting to mild cases. However, if the defect is severe, more prudent approach needs to be considered since there are always possibilities of affecting the opening and closing of eyelids by the weight of injected fat.

5) Therapeuetic principle for sunken eyelid.

Assessing the exact causes of sunken eyelid is the basic principle of correcting upper sunken eyelid. If it is related to the function or structural deformity between levator aponeurosis and tarsal plate, the primary thing is to correct this problem such as eyelid ptosis. The followings are some principle for correction of sunken upper eyelid by fat grafting.

First, understand the fine anatomical structures between the upper eyelid and the eyebrow.

Second, fine, delicate, and skilled injection technique should be preceded.

Third, do not inject into upper eyelid structure which interfere the opening and closing of eye movement.

Fourth, never perform hyper-correction.

Fifth, the presence of temporal hollow, depression of medial eyebrow, and suprabrow depression that are caused by the overuse of eyebrow depressore and frontalis muscle must be corrected by fat grafting first.

And sixth, in the case of protruded eyeball appearance with hypoplasia of the frontal bone and its superior orbital rim must also be corrected by fat grafting first.

6) Fat grafting on sunken eyelid with SAFI technique

(1) Design

Make the patient looks straight forward in a sitting posture and then mark the depressed area in both open and closed eye state. The markers should be sectioned orbicularis oculi into 3 zones, the eye brow area, the preorbital area, and the preseptal area as shown in Figure 34.

(2) Anesthesia

The entry sites are infiltrated with 2% lidocaine (1:100,000 epinephrine addition) solution and small amount of lidocaine solution (4 times diluted with saline) can be injected into the subcutaneous layer of eyebrow or pre-orbital area.

(3) The major principle of grafting

The main point of SAFI method on sunken eyelid is to correct it without affecting the movement of upper eyelid. The grafting should be performed in the sequence of starting from eyebrow area, preorbital area to preseptal area, and deep to superficial layer within each area under the basic principle of SAFI method (Figure 34D).

① Fat grafting to eyebrow area above the superior orbital retaining ligament (Zone I)

Eyebrow area is also covered by preorbital orbicularis muscle. Fat is injected into whole layer of depressed part of eyebrows sequentially from deep to superficial layer. In this area, the superior orbital retaining ligament is attached at 2-3mm above the superior orbital rim. The fat should be injected sequentially into whole layer from superior area of this ligament(1-3). This is to increase skeletal support of supra-orbital rim and to restore the subcutaneous fat.

② Fat grafting to the area of pre-orbital orbicularis muscle below the superior orbital retaining ligament (Zone II)

Fat should be injected sequentially into whole layer from the superior orbital retaining ligament to

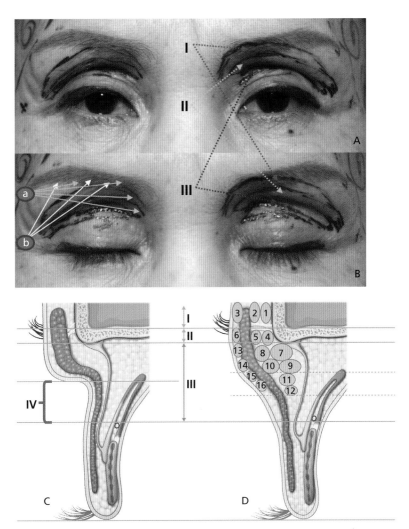

Figure 34 The preoperative markings and injection sequence for the sunken eyelids. Zone I: the eyebrow area above superior orbital retaining ligament, Zone II: the area of pre-orbital orbicularis oculi muscle below the superior orbital retaining ligament, and Zone III: the area of pre-septal orbicularis oculi muscle, and Zone IV: actual sunken area. Open eyelid state (A), closed eyelid state (B), before fat grafting (C), and after sequential autologous fat injection (D). ⓐ, ⓑ: entry sites for injection. Arrows with straight lines (yellow and white colored) show the directions of fat injection.

the inferior edge of the orbital rim (4-6) as shown in Figure 34D. It can be observed that some skin is tightened and the eyelid is less sunken after the fat injection. It is caused by volumetric lifting which the concept is introduced in Figure 12 of Chapter 2 and Figure 9 and 10 of this Chapter. In order to minimize the effects on upper eyelid movements, fat grafting with the concept of roof tile on the rafter (Figure 35) should be performed at the border area of II and III, which are areas 4, 5, 7, and 8.

③ Fat grafting to the area of preseptal orbicularis oculi muscle (Zone III)

Fat is injected from the lower edge of superior orbital rim to the area below, like the edges of Korean tiled-roof slips on the rafters(7-12). It should be put in gradational manner from superior orbital

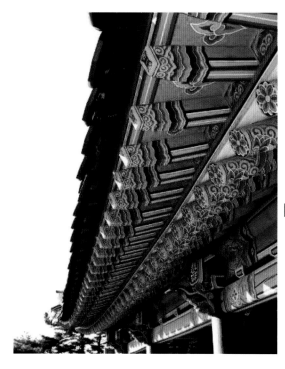

Figure 35 The eaves of traditional Korean tiled-roof house: the edges of tiled roof project out longer than the rafters of the eaves. This picture is for analogy of the concept that the rafters may be compared to the superior orbital rim and projected tiled-roofs may be compared to the implanting way of fat attaching from the upper part of the superior orbital rim to orbital area via the lower part of periosteum of the superor orbital rim without stopping.

rim. Inject fat mainly into ROOF (retro-orbicularis oculi fat) layer and fibrofatty connective tissue behind the orbicularis oculi muscle. Despite fat grafting into these above areas, if there is still skin laxity with a shallow sunken, a small amount of fat can be carefully injected into subcutaneous layer(13-16).

7) Prohibitions and requirments

Cautions needed for this area is to observe the change of upper eyelid movement and sunken area in both open and close status of eyelids while injecting.

Patient must not feel the weight while opening the eyes. Thus, inject fat only up to the point that the sunken disappears. After the procedrue, smooth skin surface without lumps and stiffness should be expected. Especially, it should be avoided that the depleted area looks more swollen and lumped than normal contour when the eyes are closed.

Tensed skin with swollen up appearance of sunken area is the sign of hyper-correction. Of course, edema should be considered at this moment, but performing additional grafting after hypo-correction is better than hyper-correction. Especially, fat grafting into subcutaneous fat layer must not precede other layers as shown in 7-12 of Figure 34D.

The fat amount required differs depend on patients. Generally, 1.0 ml-2.0 ml is usually used for one side and over 2.0 ml is not recommended. However, more than 3-5 ml can be used for additional fat grafting to supra-brow or lower forehead areas. Fat grafting to sunken upper eyelid requires the most delicate and experienced techniques among all of the areas of facial fat grafting. Therefore, it is recommended to conduct fat grafting to this area only after sufficient experience in other facial areas.

8) Contraindication

Do not perform fat grafting to patients with myasthenia, oculomotor nerve paralysis, eyelid inflammation and infection.

▮ **10** The principle and practice of SAFI method for forehead fat grafting

1) Introduction

Major signs of forehead aging are wrinkles, depression and sagging. Methods that commonly used to improve signs of aging are the surgical forehead lifting, allograft implant, autologous fat grafting and artificial filler and botulinum toxin injection.

Among these, fat grafting also has been widely used to improve forehead aging. However, forehead fat grafting has low survival rate and less satisfaction for patients compared to other facial areas. This is because structural characteristics of forehead are different from other facial areas. Recently, excessive movements of forehead mimetic muscle have been regarded as the main factor that interferes the survival rate of fat grafting.

2) My application of SAFI technique to forehead fat grafting

Structure and characteristic movement of the frontalis muscle is one of the main causes of wrinkles and depressions at forehead, as described in Figure 18 and 19 of Chapter 1. Also, there is almost no subcutaneous fat layer in the superior 1/3~1/2 region of the forehead. This area is very stiff since it has well developed fibrous connective tissue band in the area between skin and frontalis muscle fascia. However, the inferior 1/3~1/2 region is easy to move because it has relatively well developed subcutaneous fat layer with presence of galeal fat pad and galeal sliding space. Due to these characteristics, the depression and wrinkles are mostly present in the inferior 1/3~1/2 region. Moreover, the secondary contraction of frontalis muscle will inhibit the survival of grafted fat. For these reasons, I have assumed that physical stress can be reduced on the grafted fat if the secondary contraction is decreased even though the primary contraction of frontalis muscle is still continued.

In order to reduce secondary contraction, I have tried to apply SAFI technique on forehead fat grafting. Fat was first injected into area above frontal hair line beneath galea aponeurosis and frontalis muscle as shown in Figure 36. Patients have more satisfaction, and the overall contour has great improvement than only injecting fat to the depressed area of the central forehead. I have been performing forehead fat grafting with this method. I also analyzed objectively on the relationship between the

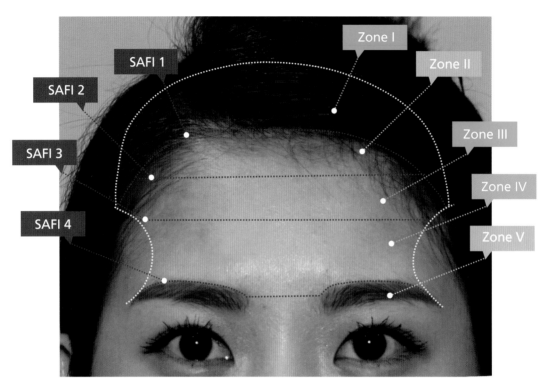

Figure 36 The 4 safi lines and 5 zones of the forehead.

hypothesis and final outcome.

3) SAFI lines and zones of forehead

Four SAFI lines based on the structures related to the morphology and aging of forehead are set as shown in Figure 36 and Table 3. The forehead is divided into five zones with these lines as reference.

4) SAFI method of forehead fat grafting

The five zones of sequential fat grafting are described in Table 4. Sequence of fat grafing is from zone I to V.

When fat grafting to zone I, canular shoud be touched on bone directly.

Table 03 Dr Kang's forehead SAFI lines

Line	Definition
1	Frontal hair line between Rt and Lt superior temporal line
2	Horizontal line connecting transversely on the uppermost margin of the forehead eminence
3	Horizontal line connecting transversely on the lowermost margin of the forehead eminence
4	Horizontal line which is connecting the upper margin of both eyebrows

Table 04 The boundary of SAFI zones, and the placement and injectable volume in each forehead zones.

Zone	Boundary	Purpose	Placement	Volume*
I	Area above 7 cm from the frontal hair line (SAFI line 1)	Tightening of frontalis muscle	Subgaleal space	6-8
II	Area between the SAFI line 1 and 2	Anterior projection and volumetric lifting	Subgaleal space and Superficial fat layer	2-4
III	Area between the SAFI line 2 and 3	Anterior projection and volumetric lifting	Subgaleal space and Superficial fat layer	2-4
IV	Area between the SAFI line 3 and 4	Volume recovery and Strong skeletal support	Supraperiosteal layer or subgaleal plane space, Intramuscular, Galeal fat pad, Subcutaneous superficial fat layer	3-6
V	Brow area below the SAFI line 4	Volume recovery and strong skeletal support	Supraperiosteal layer or subgaleal space, Glabella fat pad, brow fat pad(ROOF), Superficial fat layer	2-4
Total injectable volume				15-26

It is quiet hard to move the cannula and to inject fat evenly in Zone II and III, because the subcutaneous layer are relatively thin, dense and stiff. Thus, be cautious to avoid unexpected complications such as lump and irregularity in these zones.

Ideal fat grafting in zone III is to improve volume depletion and preserve the natural appearance of the frontal eminence. However, age differences in point of view of beauty also can not be ignored. Currently, trend in Korea prefer more projected and rounded mid-forehead.

Zone IV includes the most part of depressed area in the forehead. Sequential fat grafting from zone I to III tightens soft tissues of zone IV with a concept of volumetric lifting. Remarkable volume deficiency is frequently seen in patients who have active facial expression of corrugator and frontalis muscle and it may contribute to brow ptosis. Sufficient volume recovery also can prevent gravitational descent due to weight of grafted fat into zone V. But, if fat is injected only into subcutaneous layer or more fat is injected into this layer than the deep fat layer, the brow ptosis may become severe as shown in Figure 6 of this Chapter.

In Zone V, contour and position of both brows should be observed carefully. Sequential fat grafting to the lateral brow for volume restoration after supraperiosteal fat grafting for strong skeletal supporting is essential to achieve natural looking eyebrow without brow ptosis. The irregularities and lumps can occur frequently in forehead fat grafting. Molding the irregular areas is often performed for smooth and even surface. However, please bear in mind that these complications cannot perfectly improved by molding. It would be better to prevent these complications with fine and elegant injection technique.

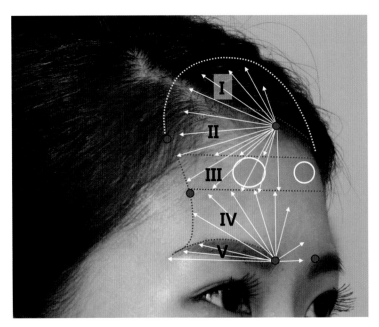

Figure 37 Possible entry sites and directions of injection. Blue circles are the possible entry sites and white arrows show the directions of injection. Two white circles express the frontal eminences.

The available entry sites and directions of injection are shown in Figure 37. After infiltrating lidocaine solution into the entry sites, 18G syringe needle is used to make an opening hole. All entry sites must be sutured with 6.0 or 7.0 nylon. The sutures can be removed after 3 days. Occasionally, if deep horizontal forehead wrinkles are present in zone IV, selection of other entry site along the wrinkles is needed.

01. Neuber F. Fat transplantation Chir Kongr Verhandl Dsch Gesellsch Chir 2266,1893.

02. Peer. L. Loss of Weight and volume in human fat grafts. Plast Reconstr Surg, 1950-5:217.

03. Ersek RA, Chang P, Salisbury MA. Lypolayering of autologous fat: an improved technique with promising results. Plast Reconstr Surg; 1998;101(3):820-826

04. Coleman SR. Facial recontouring with lipostructure. Clin Plast Surg, 1997;24(2):347-367.

05. Coleman SR. Structural Fat Grafting. Quality Medical Publishing, Inc. St Louis, Mo. 2004; Pp404.

06. Coleman SR. Facial augmentation with structural fat grafting. Clin Plast Surg, 2006;33(4):567-577.

07. Donofrio LM. Fat distribution: a morphologic study of the aging face. Dermatol Surg, 2000;26(12):1107-1112

08. Fournier PF. Fat grafting: my technique. Dermatol Surg, 2000 Dec;26(12):1117-28. Comment in Dermatol Surg, 2003;29(8):898

09. Amar RE. Adipocyte microfiltration in the face or tissue restructuration with fat tissue graft. Ann Chir Plast Esthet. 1999;44(6):593-608

10. Guerrerosantos J, Gonzalez-Mendoza A, Masmela Y, Gonzalez MA, Dias P :Long term survival of free grafts in muscle: an experimental study in rats. Aesthetic Plast Surg, 1996:20(5):403-408

11. Swanson E. Malar augmentation assessed by magnetic resonance imaging in patients after facelift and fat injection. Plast Recostr Surg, 2010;126(4) Supplement p32.

12. Samuel M Lam, et al. Complementary fat grafting. Philadelphia Lippicot Williams and Wilkins 2007.

13. Nakamura S, Ishihara M, Takiwawa M, Murakami K, Kishimoto S, Yanagibayasgi S, Kubo S, Yamamoto N, Kiyosawa T, Platelet-rich plasma (PRP) promotes survival of fat-grafts in rats. Ann Plast Surg, 2010;65(1):101-106.

14. Cervelli V, Palia L, Pascali M, De Angelis B, Curcio BC, Gentile P, Autologous platelet-rich plasma mixed with purified fat graft in Aesthetic Plastic Surg. 2009;33(5):716-721. Epub 2009 Jul 9.

15. Yoshimura K, Sato K, Aoi N, Kurita M, Hirohi T, Harii K. Cell-assisted lipotransfer for cosmetic breast augmentation: supportive use of adiposed-derived stem/stromal cells. Aesthetic Plast Surg 2008;32(1):48-55 discussion 56-7. Epub 2007 Sep 1.

16. Matsumoto D, Sato K, Gonda K, Takaki Y, Shigeura T, Sato T, Aiba-Kojima E, Iizuka F, Inoue K, Suga H, Yoshimura K. Cell-assisted lipotransfer: Supportive use of human adipose derived cells for sift tissue augmentation with lipoinjection. Tissue Eng. 2006;12(12):3375- 3382.

17. Mendelson BC, Muzaffer AR, Adams WP Jr. Surgical anatomy of the Midcheek and malar mounds. Plast Reconstr Surg, 2002;110:885-896; discussion 897-911

18. Stuzin JM. Restoring facial shape in face lifting: the role of skeletal support in facial analysis and midface soft-tissue repositioning. Plast Reconstr Surg. 2007;119(1):362-376; discussion 377-378 Nasojugal fold.

19. Loeb R. Fat pad sliding and fat grafting for levelling lid depression. Clin Plast Surg. 1981;8(4):756-776.

20. Flowers RS. Tear trough implants for correction of tear trough deformity. Clin Plast Surg 1993;20(2):403-415.

21. Haddock NT, Saadeh PB, Boutros S, Thorne CH. The tear trough and lip/cheek junction: anatomy and implications for surgical correction. Plast Reconstr Surg. 2009:123(4)1332-40; discussion 1341-1342.

22. Michael Mercandetti et al. Rhinoplasty, maxillary augmentation: Available at http://emedicine.medscape.com/article/1292328-overview.

23. Freeman M5. Transconjunctival sub-orbicularis oculi fat (SOOF) pad lift blepharoplasty. Arch Facial Plast Surg. 2000;2(1):16-21. Comment in Arch Facial Plast Surg 2000;2(1):22.

24. Hirmand H. Anatomy and nonsurgical correction of the tear trough deformity. Plast Reconstr Surg. 2010;125(2)699-708.

25. Rohrich RJ, Pessa JE, Ristow B. The youthful cheek and the deep medial fat compartment. Plast Reconstr Surg 2008;121(6):2107-2112.

26. Pessa JE, Zadoo VP, Mutimer KL, Haffner C, Yuan C, DeWitt AL, Garza JR. Relative maxillary retrusion as a natural consequence of aging: Combining skeletal and soft-tissue changes into an integrated model of midfacial aging: Plast Reconst Surg. 1998:102(1):205-212.

27. Pessa JE, Ganza PA, Love VM, Zadoo VP, Garza JR. The anatomy of the labiomandibular fold. Plastic Reconstr Surg. 1998;101(2):482-486.

28. Lemperle G, Radu D. Facial plastic surgery in children with Down's syndrome. Plast Reconstr Surg. 1980 Sep;66(3):337-745.

29. Carruthers J, Fagien S, Matarasso SL; Botox Consensus Group.,Consensus recommendations on the use of botulinum toxin type a in facial aesthetics. Plast Reconstr Surg. 2004 Nov;114(6 Suppl):1S-22S.

30. Park IH, Park DH: Cosmetic Surgery I(korean version) koonja 2004, p76.

31. Park DH, Paik BS, Nahai F et al. Costmetic and reconstructive oculoplastic surgery. Seoul, Goonja Ltd 2009;297-301.

32. 32. Lee Y, Kwon S, Hwang K. Correction of sunken and/or multiply folded upper eyelid by fascia-fat graft. Plast Reconstr Surg. 2001;107(1):15-19.

33. Shaw RB, Katzel EB, Koltz PF, Yaremchuk MJ, Girotto JA, Kahn DM, Langstein HN. Aging of the facial skeleton: Aesthetic implications and rejuventation strategies. Plast Reconstr Surg. 2011;127(1):374-383. Comment in Plast Reconstr Surg. 2011;127(1):384-385.

34. Park JI, Touriumi DM. Revision double eyelid operation. In Park JI (eds). Asian facial cosmetic surgery. Philadelphia, Saunders. 2007,Pp79.

35. Erik A Hoy, M Brandon Freeman, Rachel Sullivan, Michael Migliori, Patrick Sullivan. Safe and effective autologous fat graft augmentation of the upper lid sulcus: Ab anatomic and clinical approach to rejuvenation. Plast Reconstr Surg. 2010;126(4) Supplement p31-32.

36. Lin TM, Lin TY, Chou CK, Lai CS, Lin SD. Application of microautologous fat transplantation in the correction of sunken upper eyelid. Plast Reconstr Surg Glob Open. 2014 Dec 5;2(11):e259. doi: 10.1097/GOX.0000000000000141. eCollection 2014.

a novel facial fat grafting technique with a concept of volumetric lifting

Ideal syringe grip for fat grafting - Baton grip

1 Introduction

Fat grafting undergoes 3 procedures: harvesting, isolation, and injection. The procedures affect not only the survival rate and durability of the grafted fat but also the occurrence of complications or side effects. Among these procedures, especially, the injection is the procedure of directly grafting the isolated fat into the patient's face through the doctor's hands. Thus, there are big differences in outcome according to the operating doctor's injection techniques, anatomical knowledge and aesthetical sensibility.

The factors affecting the injection procedure are listed below.

- First, the procedure is affected by cannula: the thickness, the size of the bore, the state of the commissure between cannula and syringe, and the speed of the cannula's movements.
- Second, the shape of injected fat varies as follows: linear, round, and continuous or discontinuous.
- Third, the procedure is influenced by the insertion directions: vertical, transverse and cross.
- Fourth, it is influenced by the status of recipient site such as composition of layers, tissue mass, aging, and vascularity.

So far, there have been many studies to achieve high survival rate and longevity for fat grafting. Most of them are focused on the field of sampling and isolating the fat, while the studies on "injection procedure itselt-most influential" are comparatively poor. Furthermore, at latest trend studies based on the survival hypothesis, adipose drived stem cell, stem cell fluid extract, platelet rich plasma, or angiogenetic factor, are more active than studies on separation, isolation, and injection of fat.

Not only edema, hemorrhage, bruise, hematoma, lump, and irregularity, but also embolism and obstruction are well known as complications of fat grafting. And, these complications affect the survival rate and durability of injected fat in patients should not be ignored. Then, what are the causes of these complications? Of course there can be differences between individuals, but, in general, edema or hemorrhage occurs due to pre-tunneling, tumescent anesthesia, and cannula insertion for grafting. Embolism and obstruction are caused by direct fat injection to the vessel. Also, lumpiness or irregularities are caused by unevenly grafted fat. Unfortunately, these side effects or complications occur because of the doctor's hand movements.

I think that the most important factor is "injection method with ideal syringe grip" to prevent above side effects and complications.

2 Various types of syringe grips

Through many books including visual materials, it is emphasized that syringe grip is one of the most important factor make differences in hand movement. Various types of grips are named after the author of the books or the operator in the videos. Figure 1 shows 4 types of syringe grips — Coleman grip[1], Ichida grip[2], Amar grip[3], and Lam grip[4]— and beside these, there is syringe grip for general muscular injection.

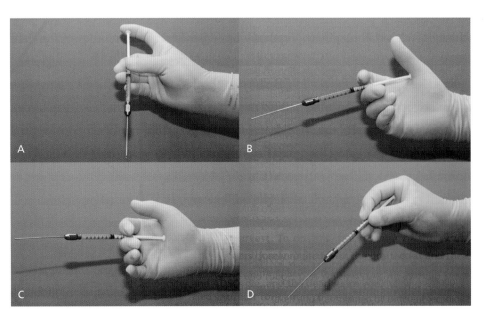

Figure 01　Various types of syringe grips used in fat grafting. Coleman grip (A), Ichida grip (B), Amar grip (C), and Lam grip (D).

▮3▮ Ideal syringe grip

It is not proper to write subjective opinions about the efficiency for each of these syringe grips and hand movements without objective analytical studies. So, the author's subjective view on them are omitted.

However, it is necessary to mention one basic fact. In case of fat grafting while cannula is advancing towards the target area, higher pressure is applied on the fat that is being injected and risk of vascular occlusion is much more increased. Whereas grafting fat while drawing back cannula after approaching the target area lowers the risk of this complication. Considering the composition and motion of hand-finger-syringe, it is important to notice that the syringe grips listed above have the possibility of injecting fat during advancing the cannula toward the target area. Then, what is the most ideal syringe grip to bring successful outcome after fat grafting as well as reducing side effects and complications? The required conditions need to be ideal syringe grip for fat grafting are listed in Table 1.

Table 01   The required conditions need to be ideal syringe grip for fat grafting

(1) Fineness of the injected fat
(2) Accuracy of fat injection into the recipient site
(3) Possibility of adjusting the volume of the fat that is being injected
(4) Possibility of fat injection only during the drawing back of the cannula

For example, it is undeniable that proper grip of the instrument is the most important and fundamental requirement for writing or playing golf. Likewise, to prevent side effects and complication, and to get better outcomes for survival rate or durability of grafted fat, the importance of an ideal syringe grip must be emphasized during the stage of fat injection in fat grafting.

I have developed Baton syringe grip to fulfill most of the requirements in Table 1, and will describe it.

▮4▮ Practice of Baton grip

It is composed of 2 grips as described below. One is "cannula insertion grip" used for moving cannula towards the target area of fat injection, and the other is "fat injection grip" used for fat injection during drawing back of the cannula.

1) Cannula insertion grip

(1) Background

Tissue injury is the major reason for side effects in tissue grafting, even though some doctors emphasize that there is possibility of lifting caused by fibrosis. The author will briefly describe the issues of tissue injury and methods to prevent them.

Facial soft tissues consist of skin, subcutaneous fat, superficial musculo-aponeurotic system (SMAS), mimic muscle, deep fat, deep fat and periosteum. And between them, ligamentous fixations such as retaining ligament, septum, and adhesion are scattered around the face. Each layer is different in elasticity and solidity because the thickness and histological characteristic of each layers are different to the location of facial area.

What will happen if the cannula is inserted quickly with strong force by movements of the whole arm, while moving the cannula cannula in subcutaneous fat along with SMAS? The cannula cannot reach to the target area, passes through quickly, or moves towards the unwanted direction as like skin or deep SMAS. It means that tissue injury is inevitable and the possibility of cannula insertion into non-targeted(or unwanted) site will be increased.

On the other hand, what will happen if the cannula is moved forward inch by inch with weak force using only finger movements and simultaneously feel the resistance of the tissues at the tip of the cannula, while moving the cannula to its target area?

First, cannula can be moved smoothly within the target layer.

Second, since it is easy to figure out the difference in tissue resistance of the forwarded layer, unnecessary motion to penetrate into the target area can be reduced by easily recognizing the shifting between layers and the position of the cannula according to the depth while moving to another layer.

Third, control of the movement of the cannula is easy at the site not only where the bleeding occurs frequently, but also where the movements of the cannula stopped suddenly with unknown factors. Particularly when these situations happen, you can prevent tissue injury like hemorrhage by slowly forwarding and turning the syringe.

Hence, I concluded that the ideal syringe grip to approach the target area with minimizing tissue injury is the "cannula insertion grip" using only weak force from the thumb and index finger's extension and flexion movement.

(2) Definitions

"Cannula insertion grip" consists of flexion grip and extension grip. Figure 2A shows the flexion grip; both the thumb and the interphalangeal joint of index finger are flexed. Barrel of the syringe is positioned between the tip of the thumb and the antero-lateral aspect of the distal interphalangeal joint

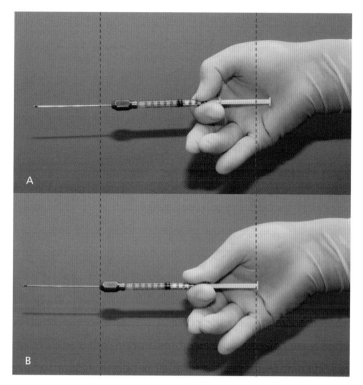

Figure 02 Dr. Kang's cannula insertion grip. Flexion state (A), Extension state (B).

of the index finger. The distal end of little finger is placed on patient's face or periphery of the face. Plunger tip is placed inside of the palm. Figure 2B shows the extension grip; both thumb and index finger are unfolded. Barrel of syringe is positioned between the entire thumb and the antero-lateral aspect of the distal interphalangeal joint of index finger.

(3) Methods

Switch flexion state (Figure 2A) to extension state (Figure 2B) by extending thumb and index finger immediately after the tip of cannula is inserted into the entry site for fat injection. Then, syringe will move forward making the cannula positioned in front to be pushed into the tissue for about 1-2cm. In continuing extension state, relax the interphalangeal joints and push the whole arm to the front smoothly. Then, the interphalangeal joints will be naturally flexed again and switched to flexion state. Hence, grip switching can be performed continuously, naturally and quickly.

When using this grip, other fingers—especially little fingers—are recommended to be placed on patient's face or periphery of the face for supporting the entire fingers and hand it maintains the stability of the procedure during grip movements. Also, take note that entire arm and shoulder, including hand should be fully relaxed and not stressed.

(4) Advantages

Cannula insertion grip uses minimum force formed from the continual extension and flexion movement of the thumb and index finger which have excellent sense and can perform delicate work. Thus, it makes the operator feels tissue resistance easily at the tip of the cannula, and traces position of the cannula, and minimizes tissue injury by quick operation.

2) Fat injection grip

(1) Background

Thumb's flexible first joint allow the special opposition movement that brings the distal thumb pad in direct contact with the distal pads of the other four digits. Opposition is a complex combination of thumb flexion and abduction that also requires the thumb to be rotated 90° about its own axis. It is a delicate hand movement that only humans can do among primates. The tip of thumb and other fingers must meet each other in this movement. Especially, the opposition of thumb and index finger is necessary for delicate finger work.

Generally, what we learn first for handwriting is how to grip the pencil. The difference between neat and scribble writing or quick and slow writing, is mostly depends on how the writer grips the pencil. The characteristics for the ideal pencil grip are holding the pencil with thumb, index finger and middle finger and synchronized balanced movement using these 3 fingers. During this movement, with the pencil as the centre, the motion and force are focused at the tip of the pencil. Neat and quick handwriting is possible using this posture.

I developed a new syringe grip for fat grafting, using the delicate opposition movement of the thumb and index finger, and positioning the plunger tip in the palm. The author named it "Baton grip" as that the shape of the grip is identical to the baton grip of conductor in orchestra (Figure 3).

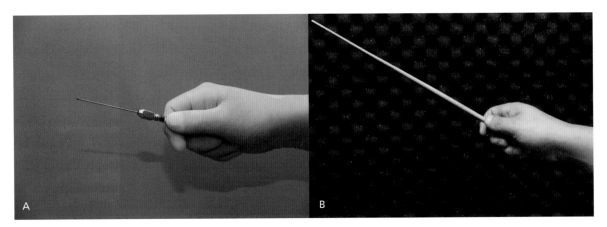

Figure 03 Naming of Baton grip. Image of baton grip (A), Image of syringe grip (B).

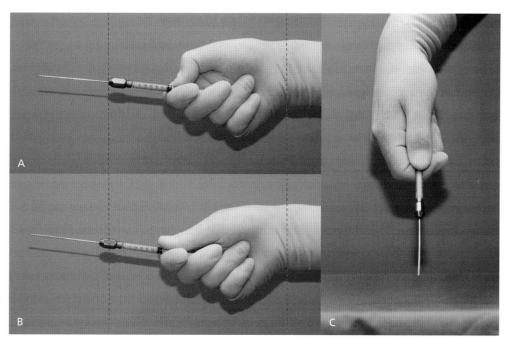

Figure 04 Fundamental position of the baton grip for fat injection. Lateral view of flexion state (A), lateral view of extension state (B), and frontal view of extension state (C)

(2) Definitions

At the end of extension state of cannula insertion grip (Figure 2B), by holding barrel of syringe with anterolateral aspect of the interphalangeal joint of index finger and the anterior tip of thumb (Figure 4A and 4B), the tip of the plunger will meet the starting point of the hypothenar and supported by it. Then, grab the the barrel of the syringe with other fingers like grabbing an egg; this is the basic pose of baton grip.

(3) Methods

After reaching the target area with cannula insertion grip, switch the grip to fat injection grip like Figure 4A and 4B. Switching from insertion grip to fat injection grip can be performed naturally. The pulling force imposed upon the syringe formed by flexion movement of thumb and index finger transferred to the plunger tip supported by the hypothenar and finally fat passes through the cannula, while drawing back cannula with steady speed by using hand and the entire arm. Refer to Table 2 for the movement of joints during the drawing back of the cannula. Right after injecting fat with this method, switch to "cannula insertions grip" and switch flexion state (Figure 2A) to extension state (Figure 2B) by extending thumb and index finger to reach other target area. Then, continuously inject fat by switching again to fat injection grip.

Table 02 The differences between baton grip and modified baton grip in the movement of the wrist, the elbow and the shoulder joint.

Joints	Baton grip	Modified baton grip
Wrist	-	adduction
Elbow	flexion	-
Shoulder	extension	medial rotation

(4) Advantages

The most advantageous characteristic of this method is that the operator can control the amount of fat being injected. This is because the degree of flexion motion of thumb and index finger changes the pulled distance of barrel of the syringe. Furthermore, motion of the fat injection is very natural and easy because the motion of drawing back of the cannula occurs in the same directional property with the movement of both shoulder and elbow joint as described in Table 2.

(5) Disadvantage

It takes significant number of practices and time to be skilled , i.e., follows slow learning curve.

(6) Characteristics

Unique characteristics of baton grip are as follows.

• First, baton grip is based on the opposition movement, which is the most sophisticated movement

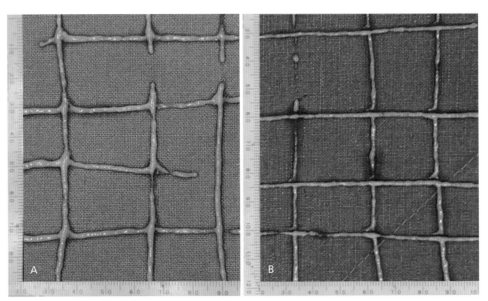

Figure 05 The thread-like fats which are extruded from 2 kinds of cannula with inner diameter of: 15mm (A) and 12mm (B) using the baton grip technique.

can be done by human only.

- Second, the motion of the operator is natural, and the fat is injected easily. This is because the direction of the movements of both drawing back of the cannula by the entire arm and injecting of fat by the flexion of thumb and index finger occur on the same line.

- Third, fat comes out from the cannula in a thread-like shape (Figure 5). Fat passes through the cannula and comes out from the syringe by plunger force generated by the motion of baton grip. Because the cannula is pulled back concurrently with constant speed, the thickness of the thread-like shaped fat is the same as the inner diameter of the cannula. Thus, there is no molding needed to change the shape and position of the injected fat.

- Fourth, it is time-efficient. Highly skilled operator can insert large amount of fat in a short time.

- Fifth, this grip accurately controls the amount of fat being injected, by changing the degree of flexion of the thumb and index finger.

- Sixth, this grip is relatively safe since fat is only injected during drawing back of the cannula.

5 Modified Baton grip

1) Definitions

The operator feels uncomfortable when grafting fat into the left temporal region, nasolabial fold, or jowl from left side of the patient. At this time, the modified Kim's javelin grip[5] can be used to ease injection by changing the operator's position. As shown in Figure 6, the thumb and index finger are at the same position as the baton grip. But, placing the tip of the plunger between the ring finger and lit-

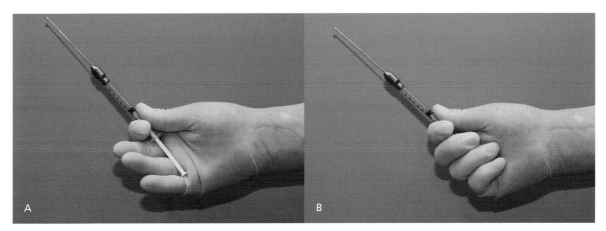

Figure 06 Fundamental positions of the modified baton grip for fat injection (A & B).

tle finger. Pushing the fat while flexing other fingers are in accordance with the motions of baton grip.

2) Methods

Palm faces upward in modified baton grip. Like baton grip, it uses flexion of the thumb and index finger. At the same time, the operator injects fat while drawing back the cannula. However, the method used for drawing back the cannula is different with that of baton grip. See Table 2 for the joint movements associated with modified baton grip.

3) Advantage

Modified baton grip is restrictively used for the ease of operation.

4) Disadvantages

As shown in Table 2, with fixed elbow joint the direction of internal rotation of shoulder joint is different with that of straightly drawing back the cannula. Thus, the operator adducts wrist joint to compensate this. Due to this characteristic of the movement, it results in an unnatural motion. Since the continual motion like baton grip is impossible, it can only be used as a single shot.

Reference

01. Coleman SR. Structural Fat Grafting. Quality Medical Publishing, Inc., St. Louis, Mo. Quality Medical Publishing Inc, St. Louis, Mo. 2004;P 58.

02. Yang DB. Atlas of skill aesthetic plastic surgery of Masarini Ichida, Shinheung Med Science, Inc. Seoul, Republic of Korea,2005;106-107. ISBN-13 : 9788990933454.

03. Amar RE's DVD of FAMI technique.

04. Lam SM. Complementtary fat grafting. Philadelphia, Lippincott Williams and Wilkins 2007.

05. Kim YK. The javelin grip for botulinum toxin injection. Director of 5050 clinic. Bucheon, Republic of Korea. Personal communication. 2006.

a novel facial fat grafting technique with a concept of volumetric lifting

Facial liposuction as a complementary procedure to fat grafting

■1 Introduction

Facial liposuction is often combined with fat grafting in the elderly (Especially, there are many cases of liposuction simultaneously with facial fat grafting to the elders), because this combination procedure brings out natural look and is also very efficient to prevent drooping caused by the weight of injected fat or the relaxation of the liposuctioned area. However, in severe case of skin laxity, additional surgical face lift should always be considered. These two procedures are complimentary to each other because the facial liposuction (or lipolysis) is a very useful procedure for correction of fat grafting–induced complications such as asymmetry, lumpiness, irregularities, fibrosis, hyper-correction, and vice versa.

■2 Possible areas and Kinds of suction

1) Possible areas and safety

Subcutaneous fat layer occupies a significant portion of facial soft tissues and plays an important role in the formation and maintenance of facial contour. This is why facial liposuction is still being used for improvement of facial contour in the field of cosmetic surgery. Possible areas of facial liposuction are shown in Figure 1 below. The most concerned point during liposuction at these regions

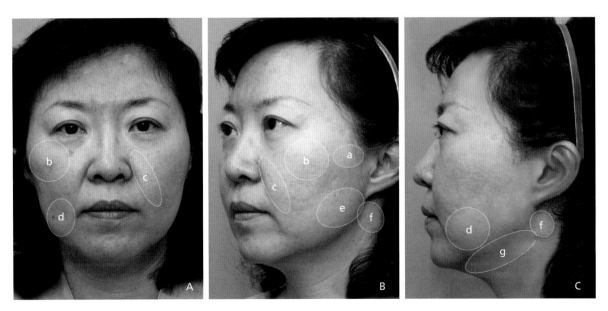

Figure 01 Possible areas for liposuction in the face and neck.

a,b: zygomatic body and arch, d: nasolabial folds, d: jowl, e: lateral cheek area, f: infra-lobular area, and g: submental and submandibular area. The frontal view (A), The oblique view (B), and the lateral view (C).

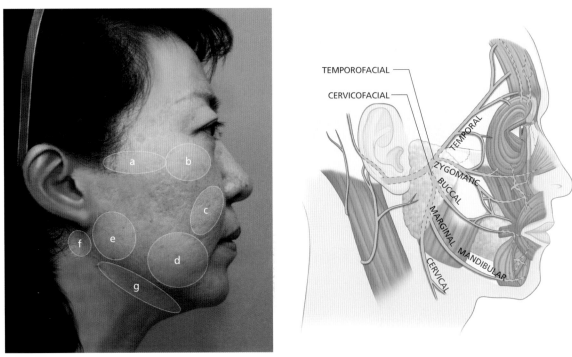

Figure 02 Dangerous areas and their neurologic sequelae associated with liposuction in face and neck. Area a: brow ptosis due to the damage of frontal branch, area b and c: droopy appearance of mid-cheek and upper lip due to the damage of zygomatic and buccal branch, area e and d: lower lip deformity due to the damage of marginal branch, and area f and g: sensory loss due to the damage of greater auricular nerve.

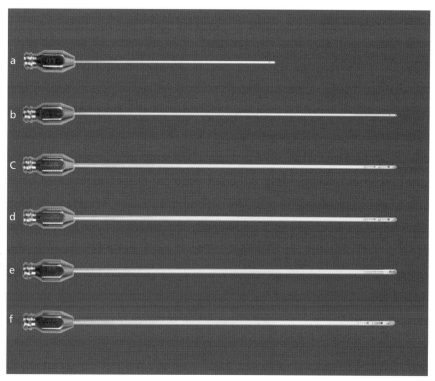

Figure 03 Instruments for suction assisted liposuction.
    a: Tumescent infiltrator, 1.0 mm diameter X 9.0 cm length
    b: Tumescent infiltrator, 1.0 mm diameter X 15.0 cm length
    c: Round-tip with two holes standard liposuction cannula, 1.6 mm diameter X 15.0 cm
    d: Round-tip with two holes standard liposuction cannula, 1.8 mm diameter X 15.0 cm
    e: Spatular liposuction cannula, 2.0 mm diameter X 15.0 cm length
    f: Finness liposuction cannula, 2.0 mm diameter X 15.0 cm length

is the damage of facial nerves as shown in Figure 2. In particular, extreme care should be taken to prevent damage to end branches (frontal and marginal branch). However, in fact, facial nerves are not present in superficial fat layer. This fact becomes the basis of confidence to perform facial liposuction.

2) Kinds of liposuction

Machines and instruments according to the suction type are as follows.

(1) Syringe–assisted liposuction

When performing facial liposuction, I always use a 10ml disposable Luer-lok syringe connected with suction cannula as seen in Figure 3. In particular, I love to use 2 kinds of modified suction cannula. The spatula cannula is designed for prevention of facial nerve damage and the finness cannula is used for avoiding damage to dermis of skin.

(2) Lipolysis-assisted liposuction

When performing facial liposuction, ultrasound, laser, and radiofrequency devices can be used as shown in Table 1.

Table 01 Various machines for lipolysis or lipolysis-assisted liposuction in Korea.

	Accusculpt II®	Bellody II®	Liposound®	Apolex®
Energy source	Pulsed Nd:YAG (1440nm)	Diode Laser 1470nm (980nm,1064nm)	Ultrasound cavitation	Monopolar radio-frequency
Thickness of fiber / probe / cannula	0.3Φ x 4m optic fiber and cannula set	Φ1.6 (9.0cm, 1.0cm) triple type diode module	1.9Φ, 2.9Φ, 3.7Φ titanium	1.0-4.0 Φ titanium insulated probe and cannula
Action mechanism	Laser-lipolysis (Burnning)	Laser-lipolysis (Burnning)	Emulsification	Thermal shrinkage
Suction	NO	NO	NO	YES
Level of energy (power)	Up to 12W	980nm:6W, 1064nm:6W, 1470nm:6W/Steps 100mW.	35kHz-40kKz 0-90W	$20,000 \sim 30,000J$ $/400cm^2$
Control of energy	Max 300mJ (energy) Pulse width 0.1ms/rate 5-40Hz	Yes	Possible	Yes
Control of temperature	No	No	No	Yes
Company	Lutronic Corporation Ltd.	Pibunara Co. Ltd.	Newpong Co .Ltd	Chungwoo Medical Co., Ltd.
Homepage	http://www.korea.lutronic.com/	www.pibunara.com	www.newpong.com	www.mycw.co.kr
Reference	1	-	-	-

3 Methods

1) Posture of patient

Posture of patient is very important in determining a surgeon's successful performance for liposuction in the face and neck. The best posture is hyperextension of neck. It is more helpful to place a silicone block or pillow under the shoulder of patient as shown in Figure 4. During the procedure, the change of soft tissue contour should be often checked from flexed neck posture (as if the patient is standing) since the soft tissues of the face are moved upward and backward when lying. To achieve this, it is convenient to use a surgical table that can put the patient's neck in the state of flexion and extension in lying posture.

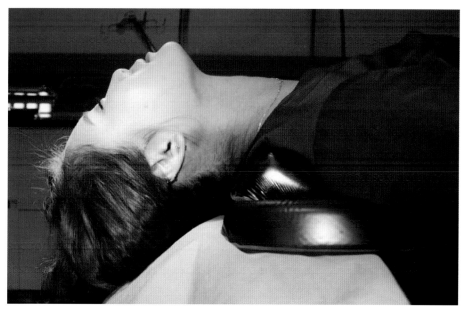

Figure 04 Hyperextension of neck is the best posture for facial liposuction. Various shapes of silicone block or pillows can be used to support the shoulder of patient for extension.

2) Anesthesia

General anesthesia or local infiltration can be applied in facial liposuction. Adits for liposuction are infiltrated with mixture of 1 % lidocaine and epinephrine (1:100,000). It is strongly recommended to infiltrate tumescent anesthetic solution regardless of the anesthetic method selected, and composition of tumescent solution for liposuction is shown in Table 1 of Chapter 6.

The amount of infiltrating tumescent solution should not be more than twice of the amount of fat that can be suctioned. Need to wait at least 10-20 minutes after infiltration of the tumescent. It is strongly recommended to infiltrate tumescent solution only into the superficial fat layer.

If the tumescent is only or more infiltrated into deep fat layer, not only the superficial liposuction cannot be performed properly but risks of bleeding, muscle injury, and nerve damage can also be increased. Hence, for proper infiltration, tumescent should be injected into subdermal layer first, followed by middle and deep part of superficial fat layer. Also, tumescent should be placed evenly under low pressure. The surgeon should bear in mind that the most fundamental and important procedure to prevent complication and to achieve great result from facial liposuction is the optimal placement of tumescent solution.

3) Practice of lipolysis and liposuction

When using lipolysis device, the ending point of lipolysis is when you feel no resistance from the tip of probe. However, it needs to be applied differently according to the characteristics of each device because action mechanism of each device is not same.

Generally, I start liposuction right after lipolysis followed by squeeze. The advantages of lipolysis prior to liposuction are reduced bleeding, ease of suction, and fine suction in peripheral area. However, during the lipolysis-assisted suction, the suction pressure should be reduced compared to that of liposuction without precedent lipolysis. Sequence of facial liposuction from 1 to 7 of Figure 5A is opposite to the sequence of fat grafting. Especially, in the area of jowl and lateral cheek which are easy to sag, the area can be divided into 2-3 subareas and liposuction is performed sequentially from lower to upper subarea as shown in Figure 5A.

During liposuction, it is very important to maintain a constant intraluminal pressure of the 10 ml Luer-Lok syringe (about 2 cm-5 cm of negative pressure). Facial fat must be treated gently and careful because it is quite different from body fat. The suction should be conducted slowly and evenly with small pressure, and it is recommended to use more than one adit for cross suction (Figure 5B).

4 Effects of liposuction combined with SAFI method

If patient undergoes liposuction and fat grafting simultaneously, liposuction prior to fat grafting is the reasonable sequence to prevent sagging after the procedure. Additionally, surgical lifting or thread lifting can be performed after the procedure for better lifting result. In the case of performing liposuction, fat grafting and thread lifting simultaneously, it is recommended to carry out thread lifting lastly.

1) Case I

Patient in Figure 6A came to hospital due to her cheek drooping and rectangular face. After per-

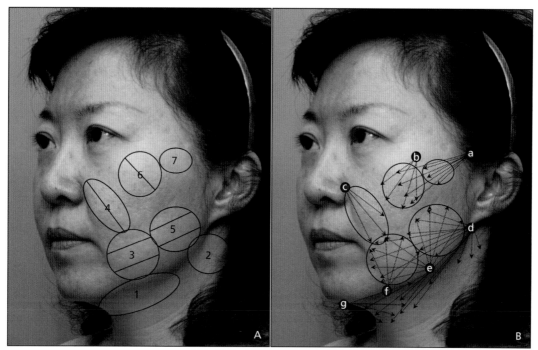

Figure 05 Sequential liposuction of face and neck from area 1 to 7. Each area can be divided into 2 or 3 subareas (lower, middle, and upper). Within one subarea, liposuction should be sequentially performed from lower to upper subarea (A). Possible adits (a~g) for liposuction and directions of suction (a is located at side burn area, b is located at lateral aspect of frontal process of zygomatic body, c is located at upper most part of nasolabial fold, d is located at infralobular area, e is located just above mandibular notch, f is located at the lower most part of marionette line, and g is located at the submental crease) (B).

forming ultrasound assited-lipolysis and syringe liposuction on jowl, about 40 ml of autologous fat was sequentially grafted into temple, preauricular area, lateral cheek depression, malar eminence, infraorbital hollowness, tear trough deformity, mid-cheek furrow, submalar hollow, nasolabial and labiomandibular fold, and prejowl sulcus. The patient's facial contour has changed from pentagonal to triangular shape after undergone SAFI fat grafting. The outcome also shows improved volume of face and naturally lifted-looking face (Figure 6B~6E).

18 months after the procedure, the patient came to my clinic with 7 kg of weight loss (Figure 6F). Comparing Figure 6E and 6F, there was only a slight decline of grafted fat by considering weight loss, no significant drooping, and similar facial contour as before weight loss. However, the patient requested for additional facial lifting to treat drooping due to weight loss. No additional operation was done after the first procedure for 18 months. Figure 6F shows that the effect still maintains after 18 months of follow up study.

2) Case II

A 46 year-old woman with severe lateral cheek depression after botulinum toxin injection to both

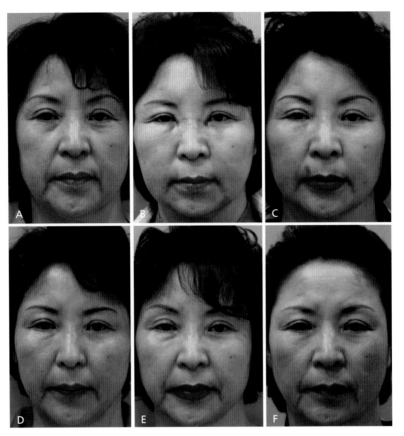

Figure 06 SAFI and lipolysis-assisted jowls liposuction using ultrasound device for the correction of facial soft tissue contouring were performed on a 56 year-old woman. Before (A), 4 days after (B), 10 days after (C), 1 month after (D), 2 months after (E), and 18 months after (F).

masseter muscles came to improve volume restoration with natural facial contour. About 35 ml of fat grafting with ultrasound-assisted syringe liposuction were performed simultaneously. No additional treatment was performed until 5 months after the first procedure.

Figure 7A, 7B, 7C, 7E and 7G shows the deep temporal hollow and badly depressed lateral cheek. It disrupts the natural frame or silhouette of the face, and also exposes the supraorbital ridge, zygomatic arch and malar eminence. Flat and depressed lateral cheeks due to atrophy of masseter muscles are seen, which contribute to formation of sagging jowls and deep labiomandibular folds.

Ultrasound-assisted liposuction was performed at zagomatic arches, malar eminences and jolws. And then, autologous fat harvested from lateral thigh was injected into temple, temporal hollow, whole lateral cheek, anterior part of malar eminence, lateral cheek and submalar hollow, trough deformity, mid-cheek depression, submalar hollow, and nasolabial fold through SAFI method.

5 months postoperative views show a lot of synergic effect between the fat grafting and liposuction. It provides a smooth transition from the temple to the lateral cheek. However, lateral contour of lower face looks wider than that of before because the atrophied masseter muscle was completely recovered.

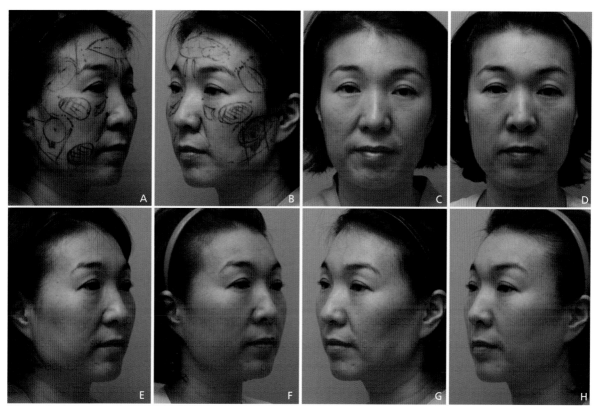

Figure 07 The synergic effect of combination with SAFI and ultrasound-assisted syringe liposuction. Preoperative markings (A and B), preoperative views (C,E, and G), and 5 months postoperative views (D,F,and H).

Malar eminence looks more protruded. It is caused by volume reduction in zygomatic arch and lateral part of the malar eminence together with volume restoration in anterior part of the malar eminence. Mid-cheek furrow, infraorbital hollowness, and orbital fat protrusion were significantly improved and deep nasolabial fold was also softened. In spite of significant volume reduction of jowls by liposuction, there is no obvious skin laxity and gravitational descent. It is mainly prevented by sufficient volume restoration of the lateral cheek and spontaneous volume recovery of masseter muscle.

3) Case II

Figure 8 shows the result of fat grafting, liposuction and thread lifting that were performed at the same time.

A 63-year-old female visited to improve her wide-looking and sagging face. Small chin, well developed jowl, submental and submandibular fat, and blurred demarcation between face and neck are observed. Liposuction, SAFI, modified contouring thread lift (EZ lift®)[2], and chin augmentation were performed in sequence, as shown in Figure 8. Fat was harvested from lateral thigh and about 40 ml was injected into the face. However, aspirated fat from face and neck were not used for grafting. Total

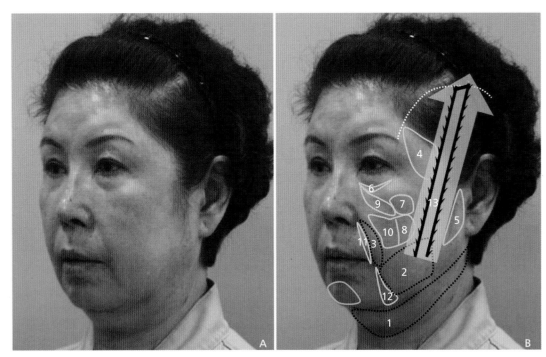

Figure 08 Preoperative plans and sequence of procedures. Syringe-assisted liposuction of submental, submandicular, and nasolabial folds areas (area from 1 to 3) were performed first and SAFI (from area 4 to 12) was done for fat rebalancing. Thirdly, 4 U-shaped bidirectional cogged threads were inserted for tightening (EZ lift, 13). Allograft silicone implant was inserted to chin for strong skeletal support. White dotted line indicates the superior temporal line, yellow circles are areas for SAFI, black dotted circles are areas for liposuction, and green circle is area for chin implantation. Preoperative view (A), Preoperative markings (B).

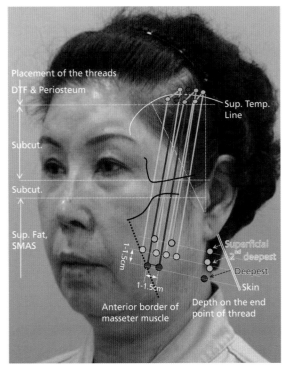

Figure 09 EZ lift® is a modified contouring thread lift without any incision. The EZ lift thread is nearly same dimension with the Contour Thread CT400. The thread is inverted U-shaped with non-absorbable bi-directional cogs, but no cogs in the middle of the thread. Non-incisional fixation is performed at upper part of the temporal area (refer to Figure 26 of Chapter 1) by using a specialized round needle with one hole. Structures for anchoring are the deep temporal fascia and periosteum. The middle, no-cogged part of the thread is used for anchoring. Other part of the bi-directional cogged thread is used for lifting and is placed at the subcutaneous and SMAS layer. My thread lifting method is quite different from the original EZ lift, which is a concept of volumetric lifting by different level of placement of threads and a different anchoring point to reduce postoperative tension headache.

8 permanent non-absorbable threads were used in EZ lift procedure as shown in Figure 9. Silicone implant was used for chin augmentation.

After the procedure, her face became small and naturally lifted with obvious demarcation between face and neck as shown in Figure 10. Successful volume rebalancing with a smooth transition is seen. In addition, no signs of sagging are observed in the postoperative views. Lateral profile was remarkably improved with combination of chin augmentation and neck liposuction. A less protruded mouth with less obtuse labiomental and cervicomental angle is a noteworthy feature.

Sagging as a complication of fat grafting and liposuction needs to be always concerned. To prevent this, I love to perform liposuction first and then fat grafting. It will produce less severe laxity, and sagging after liposuction can be prevented by using volumetric lifting of SAFI method. However, if the patient is aged as shown in Figure 8 or has severe skin laxity or high risk of postoperative sagging, additional lifting procedure is necessary.

From the above results, it is strongly suggested that various and multiple procedures need to be performed simultaneously in aged face and neck in order to achieve the natural look appearance.

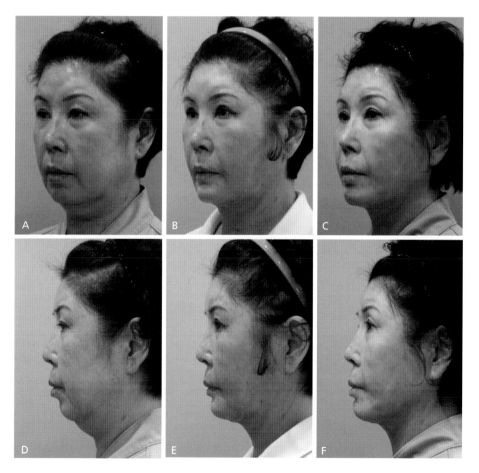

Figure 10   Results of patient in Figure 8 after fat grafting, liposuction, EZ thread lifting, and chin implantation. Preoperative views (A and D), 1 week the procedure (B and E), and 5 months after the procedure (C and F).

5 Complications and treatments

Possible complications induced by liposuction, prevention and treatment are summarized in Table 2.

Table 02 Prevention and treatment of possible liposuction-induced complications.

Complication	Cause	Prevention	Treatment
Edema, bleeding & hematoma	Excessive pre-tunneling	Gentle and elegant cannula movement	Compression and lymphatic drainage
Hyper-correction	Too much liposuction	Always think how much you preserve the fat during the liposuction.	Fat grafting + surgical or minimal invasive face lift
Hypo-correction	Too less liposuction	Exact assessment	Additional fat graft
Irregularities	Uneven liposuction	Careful and elegant liposuction	Fat grafting or skin tightening
Laxity or Sagging	Too much liposuction	Hypercorrection. Patient selection(-) : patient with previous skin laxity	Surgical or minimal invasive lift surgery with/without combining fat graft
Asymmetry	Inappropriate evaluation and hyper or hypo-correction	Close pre-operative evaluation and consultation with patient	Liposuction Additional fat graft
Skin necrosis	Damage to the subdermal vascular plexus	Preserve the subdermal vascular plexus	Prevent infection, Skin protection, ADSCs or PRP, Prostaglandin, Hyperbaric O_2, Skin graft
Depressed scar	Hypercorrection and damage of subdermal layer or fascia of muscle	Preserve minimal subcutaneous fat layer and avoid damage to the subdermal plexus and fascia of mimetic muscle	Subcision and fat graft with PRP or ADSCs Scar revision
Contracture Neck	Too much superficial liposuction Due to damage to platysma muscle and subdermal plexus	Avoid bleeding and muscle damage Preserve the subdermal plexus Should a leave minimal amount of superficial fat	PRP or ADSCs injection Skin care with Ultrasound or high frequency module
Nerve damage	Damage to the marginal mandibular branch or buccal branch	Awareness of the real anatomy (course, level, variations) of facial nerve. exact tumescent anesthesia Fine and elegant liposuction technique.	None Conservative care

Reference

01. CCLMS committe. Laser and light treatment in asian skin. Koonja Publishing, Inc. 2016.Pp.253-273 (ISBN 979-11-5955-017-1)

02. Haearum Co., Lt. (http://ezlift.blogspot.jp), E-mail : exp.ez-lift@gmail.com, Tel +82(2)2058 2230, Fax +82(2)2057 2230.

Results of SAFI

The most significant characteristic of SAFI method compared to other fat grafting is that it makes the face seem to be lifted without sagging despite the sufficient volume restoration.

I do not want to insist that SAFI method with Baton grip is outstanding compared to other methods according to the survival rate or longevity because I does not have enough experiences on performing other methods and no objective data to compare the outcomes with other methods. However, in personal perspective, SAFI method has a significant difference in the basic principle of injection methods to have a concept of volumetric lifting rather than to restore the deficient volume of the face as a simple concept of artificial filler injection.

The result in each picture was relatively explained in detail. And my personal opinion was also added. The content of result was written in the order of face, upper eyelid, and forehead. The results of some cases were compared according to the patients' age and application of CAL(cell-assisted lipotransfer). The result in each picture was relatively explained in detail. And my personal opinion was also added.

Meanwhile, there can be some variations on pre and postoperative views due to different camera-patient distance, patient's conditions (hair style or presence of make-up), or brightness of surrounding. Also, do not correct the ratios of the left-right of the pre and postoperative views to compensate this point. I would like to express my gratitude to patients who approved their pre and postoperative views to be published.

1 SAFI in young woman

1) A young woman without prominent sagging appearance.

A 30-year-old woman visited my clinic to improve her deep lateral cheek, infra-orbital hollowness, and forehead depression. Total 65 cc volume of purified fat was used for volume restoration of the face and forehead. No additional treatment was performed within 6 months. Figure 1-1 and 1-2 show the results of 6 months after the procedure.

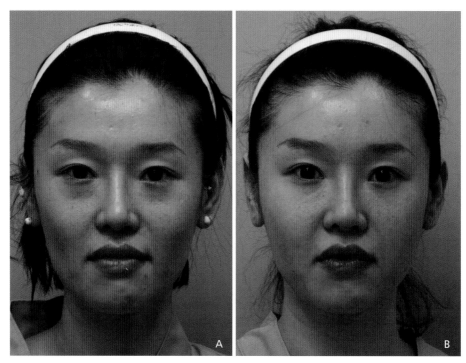

Figure 1-1 Sequential autologous fat injection was performed to restore her facial volume deficiency. Successful volume restoration with feminine appearance can be seen in Figure B. The frontal views, before the procedure (A), and 6 months after the procedure (B) .

The preoperative view (Figure 1-1) shows a rectangular face with disrupted transition of contour, which is caused by volume loss in the areas of lateral forehead, temporal hollows, and lateral cheek. Several depressions are seen in the upper, middle, and supra-brow regions of forehead, which contribute to wide-looking forehead. Temporal hollows are seen and they make the superior-lateral orbital ridge and zygomatic arch look more protruded. Characteristic appearance of mid-facial sagging is caused by volume increase of the hypertrophied nasolabial fat accompanied by volume decrease of the malar eminence, infra-orbital, and upper mid-facial area. A protruded mouth and mild pseudo-ptotic jowls stand out even more because of volume loss in the cheek.

In the postoperative view, the overall facial contour was changed into oval shape with smooth transition. Forehead looks small and round by anterior projection. The medial part of eye brow looks lifted, it is believed to be the result of volumetric lifting. Volume recovery of hollow temple and suprabrow region provide a better overall shape to the upper face and a smooth transition from the periorbital area to the temporal hairline. The palpebromalar groove and tear trough deformity are significantly improved and the lid-cheek length is remarkably shortened and the appearance of dark circle is also considerably reduced (Figure 1-1B and 1-2B, D, F, and H). Volume deficiencies of middle and lower face are also remarkably improved without any sagging, even though large amount of fat was grafted into whole cheek area. This successful volume redistribution makes the face looks lifted very naturally in the postero-superior direction. Full and round cheek tapered the jaw lines smoothly and contributed to less protruded mouth. Prominent nasolabial folds may not look improved much, but look as if there is a significant volume loss of the nasolabal folds (Figure 1-1B). The softening of the folds is mainly achieved through volume reduction of bulging part of the folds by application of volumetric lifting technique, not by direct injection of fat into the depressed part but by injection of fat

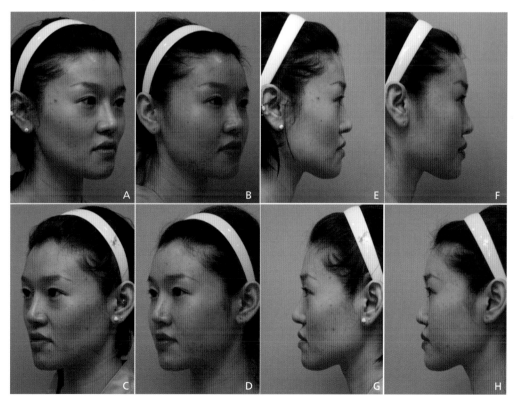

Figure 1-2 The lateral and oblique views from the same patient with Figure 1-1. Volume depletion-induced pseudoptotic face was significantly improved without any sagging appearance. Before the procedure (A, C, E, and G), and 6 months after the procedure (B, D, F and H).

into the malar eminence, infraorbital hollowness, and mid-cheek furrow.

The most remarkable change of the lateral view is the ogee curve in the mid face (Figure 1-2E, F, G and H). The completely isolated ogee curve is connected by the anterior projection through fat grafting (Figure 1-2; F and H). As shown in the above results, successful SAFI effect has lasted up to 6 months. I strongly suggest that SAFI is a reasonable approach for patients who have volume deficiency with present droopy appearance or expected droopy outcome because its volumetric lifting technique can prevent postoperative gravitational descent and increase skeletal support for the surrounding soft tissue.

2) A young woman who has a drooping face

Figure 1-3 and 1-4 are the pre and postoperative views of a 26-year-old woman with dark circle, tear trough deformities, and deep nasolabial folds. Total 45 cc of fat was injected into the whole face through SAFI technique. No additional treatment was performed during 1 year. There were no remarkable changes except 5% increase in her body weight between 6 months and 1 year after the procedure and then return to previous body weight between 1 year and 7 months and 2 years and 10 months.

Figure 1-3 shows the change of face during the 1-year-follow-up. The overall contour has been changed from long and rectangular into oval shape, and the left-right asymmetry is significantly improved in the postoperative views (Figure 1-3, B~D). Dramatic volume rebalancing which is caused by the combination of volume reduction of jowls and nasolabial folds and volume restoration of the temporal hallow and the malar eminence are being observed, which contributes to the appearance of the face looks lifted in postero-superior direction.

The postoperative view of 10 days (Figure 1-3B) shows a dramatic change of the entire facial contour. However, in the view of 3 months (Figure 1-3C), which is thought to be the complete settlement stage of the grafted fat, the facial contour and distribution of volume looked very natural. These results last up to 1 year. Consider that the 1 year after view is taken in a closer distance and the angle is a little towards the bottom compared to the preoperative view. The increased volume of facial soft tissue is seen in 1 year after view due to increased body weight (2.5 kg), but there is no more drooping sign as before (Figure 1-4D).

The characteristics of frontal view taken 3 months after the procedure (Figure 1-3) are described as below. Please consider that the preoperative view (Figure 1-3A) is in un-powered state, and the postoperative view (Figure 1-3C) is in powered state. Also, there are some differences in the brightness and the angle of the face in the pre and postoperative views.

First, the entire face contour became slimmer, and changed to oval shape. The outline became rounder and softer with convex feature. There is a big contrast with the preoperative views in the correction of the asymmetry of face making brighter and stabilized looking face. In spite of the increase of size and convexity of the zygomatic arch and body by fat grafting, the contour of the face is still smooth and looks natural. It is due to the concurrently performed fat grafting to the temporal and lat-

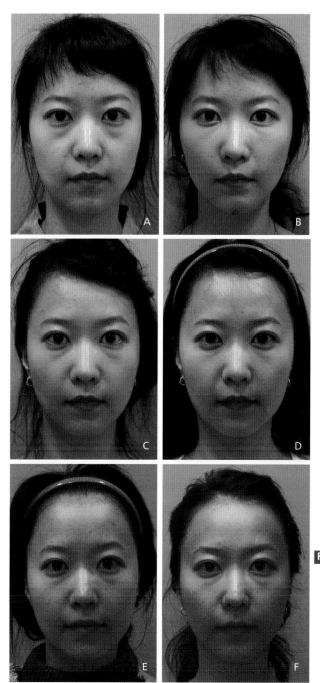

Figure 1-3 Effect of SAFI on sagging face in a young woman. Before the procedure (un-powdered) (A), 10 days after the procedure (un-powdered) (B), 3 months after the procedure (powdered) (C), 1 year after the procedure (powdered) (D). 1 year and 7 months and 7 months after the procedure (powdered) (E), and 2 years 10 months after the procedure (unpowdered) (F).

eral cheek area, which contribute to the countervailing of lateral protrusion. But the patient had complained that her face looks bigger.

Second, the volume deficiency of tear trough deformity and mid-cheek furrow is significantly improved and the orbital fat protrusion is decreased due to the increase of skeletal support by fat grafting.

Third, the nasolabial folds may not look much improved. However, the volume increase of malar eminence, submalar hollow, mid-cheek furrows contribute to the postero-superior displacement of the nasolabial fat as the concept of volumetric lifting, resulting in the volume reduction of nasolabial folds as shown in Figure 1-3 (B and C). This result cannot be achieved by only performing fat grafting to the depressed part of the folds to make it flat. Of course, the fat should also be placed at the depressed part of the folds for flattening. The key point is to decrease the height of the folds by inducing the volumetric lifting and then fat should be injected for flattening the depressed part of the folds. If liposuction is needed for the prominent folds, fat grafting should be followed by liposuction. The result of the natural looking is predominant in the 10 days postoperative views, but the effect maintains over 3 months. Please be reminded that younger looking face can never be achieved by only flattening of the depressed part of nasolabial folds through fat grafting.

Fourth, soft tissue volume of jowls are reduced, and it seemed to be lifted in superolateral direction. It was also caused by the volume increase of malar eminence, lateral cheeks and submalar hollows.

In C and D of Figure 1-4, the effect has been maintained until 1 year and 7 months after, and then the facial contour became slimmed without obvious sagging while she lost body weight. Despite of this

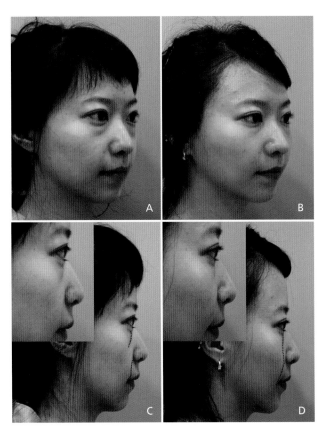

Figure 1-4 The lateral and oblique views of the same patient in Figure 1-3. Right oblique view of before the procedure (A), right oblique view of 3 months after the procedure (B), right lateral view of before the procedure (C), and right lateral view of 3 months after the procedure (D). Black dotted lines express the ogee curves.

change (or fluctuation) of body weight during the long-term follow-up, the final outcome as shown in Figure 1-4D still shows significant improvement.

The comparison between pre and postoperative oblique views are seen in A and B of Figure 1-4. The characteristic of preoperative views from the Figure 1-4 (A and C) is a sagging appearance. It is mainly due to the prominent nasolabial folds and jowls which are accompanied by volume reduction of the temporal hollow, malar eminence, lateral cheek, and submalar areas. The patient looks slightly downwards in the preoperative views. The volume increase in the temporal, zygoma, preauricular area, lateral cheek, tear trough deformity, mid cheek furrow, and submalar depression area, simultaneously, volume reduction in nasolabial folds and jowls are being observed in Figure 1-4B. This is due to successful redistribution of facial soft tissue by SAFI. Eventually, the face looks lifted in postero-superior direction. In spite of considering many factors, nobody can deny the improvement of the drooping or appearance of face-lift as shown in Figure 1-3 and 4B. The most conspicuous change of the lateral view is that of the ogee curve in the mid face (Figure 1-4C and D). The completely isolated ogee curve was connected by the anterior projection.

In conclusion, this effect— the face looks lifted without any drooping despite the volume increases by fat grafting— is the outstanding characteristic of SAFI method.

2 SAFI in middle aged woman

1) A middle aged woman with volume deficiency without sagging

A 47-year-old woman visited my clinic to improve her deep lateral cheek depressions. She had performed SAFI to the whole face (Figure 2-1). Additionally, the fat was only injected into the central region of her forehead for simple augmentation, not by SAFI technique. Botulinum toxin was injected to reduce the wrinkles of crow feet and glabella, and decrease the volume of masseter muscle 2 weeks after the procedure.

The Figure of 2-1 and 2-1 show the change of face during 13 months follow-up.

There was no additional procedure except an injection of hyaluronic acid filler for contouring of pretarsal area at other clinic.

As shown in Figure 2-1B~D, her face has been changed into a smaller, younger, and more feminine appearance with a smooth contour line than before. It was because volume restoration of the temporal hollow and lateral cheek was enough to offset the lateral protrusion of zygomatic arch. Despite of volume increase, gravitational descent is not seen at any of the postoperative views (B~D). Volume reduction of masseter muscle by botulinum toxin lasts up to 5 months but returned to the previous state 13

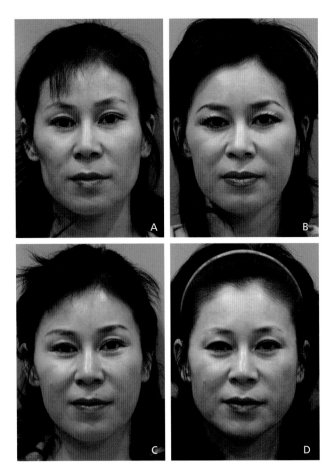

Figure 2-1 Change of facial contour without any sagging. Before the procedure (un-powdered) (A), 2 months after (powdered) (B), 5 months after the procedure (powdered) (C), and 13 months after the procedure (powdered) (D).

months after the procedure.

In Figure 2-2A and D, the body and arch of zygoma looks more outstanding due to the volume loss of the temporal hollows and whole lateral cheeks. The fat grafting was performed with the method of SAFI.

The 5 months and 13 months postoperative views (Figure 2-2B, C, E, and F) show that the volume of survived fat has still maintained. Also, obvious contour change of the jowls and labio-mandibular folds is not seen despite large amount of fat is injected to the whole lateral cheek and submalar hollows. It implies that there was no drooping or downward displacement the grafted fat. The nasolabial fold fat looks a little prominent in the postoperative views (B, C, E and F) because the patient has little smile on her face.

The volume restoration of temporal hollow was almost a failure. It may be caused by hypo-correction with bleeding during the procedure. Additional fat grafting is needed. Forehead depression seems to be improved but not significant, because fat was only injected into the center of forehead.

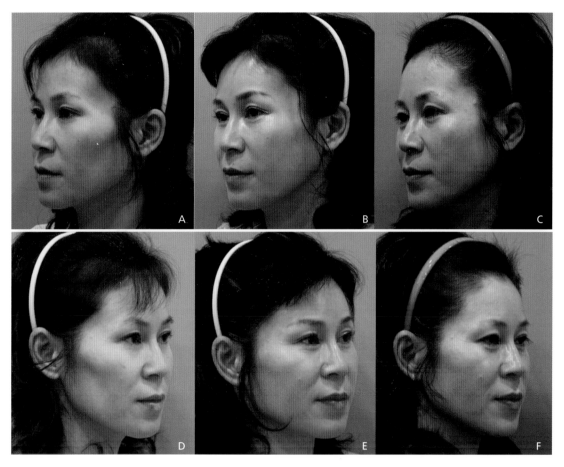

Figure 2-2 The oblique views of the same patient in Figure 2-1. Before the procedure (un-powdered) (A and D), 5 months after the procedure (powdered) (B and E), and 13 months after the procedure (powdered) (C and F).

2) A middle aged woman with 3 sessions of SAFI and a result of long term follow-up.

A 48-year-old woman in Figure 2-3 and 2-4 visited my clinic to improve her deep nasolabial folds, cheek depressions, and perioral wrinkles. Total 3 sessions of SAFI had been performed to the whole face and forehead as described in Figure 2-3. But, 1st and 2nd sessions of forehead fat grafting were not performed by SAFI technique, but only for volume restoration. After 3rd procedure, one procedure of hyaluronic acid filler and botulinum toxin were performed for correction of fine wrinkles in the forehead and perioral region. In all sessions, newly harvested fat was used.

In Figure 2-3A and 2-4AC, the disrupted facial contour is characterized by the deep temporal hollows prominent malar eminances, and lateral cheek depressions which are connected with the area of submalar hollows. This characteristic is the main cause of more prominent malar eminances. In the midface, volume deficiency areas of tear trough deformity and mid-cheek furrow are also being observed.

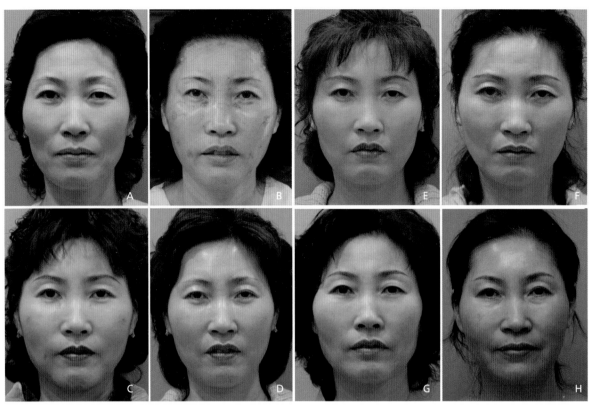

Figure 2-3 Effect of 3 sessions of SAFI on the change of facial contour during 5 years and 3 months follow-up.
Before the 1st procedure (un-powdered face) (A),
1 hour after the procedure (un-powdered face) (B),
5 days after the procedure (powdered face) (C),
1 month after the procedure (powdered face) (D),
3 months after the procedure (powdered face) (E),
10 months after the 1st procedure (before the 2nd procedure) (powdered face) (F),
2 year and 7 months after the 1st procedure (1 year 1 month after the 2nd procedure, before 3rd procedure with blepharoplasty) (un-powdered face) (G), and
5 year and 3 months after the 1st procedure (10 months after the 3rd procedure with blepharoplasty) (powdered face) (H) .

5 days after the procedure, the patient was happy with her postoperative appearance (Figure 2-3C) because she feels that she looks like what she used to be during her high school years. However, she had complained on her relatively large looking malar eminence because I focused on fat grafting to increase the skeletal support rather than the volume increase in cheek areas. Due to this approach, relatively small amount of fat was injected into cheek areas in the first procedure (Figure 2-3C~E). Thus, it was not a surprise that she was not fully satisfied. I explained it to her in detail and she agreed with my suggestion of additional fat grafting.

Postoperative follow-up pictures show considerable changes of facial contour which are achieved by fat grafting of the malar and mid-cheek areas for anterior protrusion despite the prominent malar eminences as shown in Figure 2-3B~F. Interestingly, the actual volume of grafted fat has been gradually decreased since 3 months to 10 months after the 1st procedure. This is a typical finding of fat grafting without application of CAL in the patients of middle and old aged. Generally, 2nd session of fat grafting is most frequently performed around 6 months after the procedure. This, however, is only my personal view. As a final result, the facial contour from Figure 2-3H looks most similar to that of Figure 2-3C. The result of after the 2nd procedure (Figure 2-3G) is most similar to that of 1 month after the procedure (Figure 2-3D).

In the postoperative pictures of Figure 2-4B, D, the facial contour looks smaller and rounder with smooth transition from upper to lower face, the face looks more feminine and also younger than the preoperative 5 years and 3 months before the procedure. In the long term follow-up, the gravitational descent due to the weight of survived fat was not being observed obviously, and still shows successful survival rate and longevity of grafted fat.

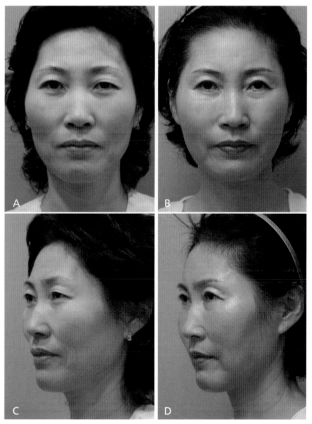

Figure 2-4 The long term follow-up pictures after 3 sessions of SAFI for the correction of facial volume deficiency. Facial volume deficiency was successfully restored and the effect had still maintained after 3 years and 6 months after 3rd procedure.
Before the 1st procedure (un-powdered face) (A and C), and 4 years and 5 months after 1st procedure (2 years and 7 months after 3rd procedure) (powdered face)(B and D).

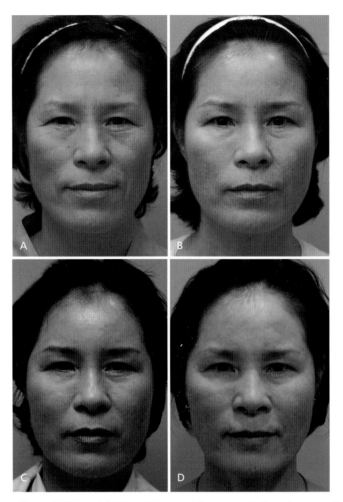

Figure 2-5 Combination effect of SAFI and CAL in a 53-year-old woman. Before the procedure (A), 4 months after the procedure (before the 2nd procedure with remaining frozen fat) (B), 5 months after the 1st procedure (1 month after the 2nd procedure) (C), and 3 years and 6 months after the 1st procedure (3 years and 2 months after the 2nd procedure) (D).

However, need to pay attention that the final result was combined with the effect of Botulinum toxin and hyaluronic acid filler. It was performed to correct the fine wrinkles which were not perfectly improved by 3 sessions of fat grafting. Sometimes, unexpected dissatisfaction would be expressed after the procedure because large numbers of patients have an excessive expectation that all facial wrinkles could be improved only by fat grafting. This reminds us of the importance of preoperative notification. If the liposuction or lipolysis was performed on the zygomatic region to reduce soft tissue volume, the patient would have more natural and smooth facial contour.

3) A middle aged woman performed with combination of SAFI and CAL

A 53-year-old woman has complained about her cheek depressions, deep nasolabial folds, and perioral wrinkles as shown in Figure 2-6. I recommended her to perform a fat grafting with application

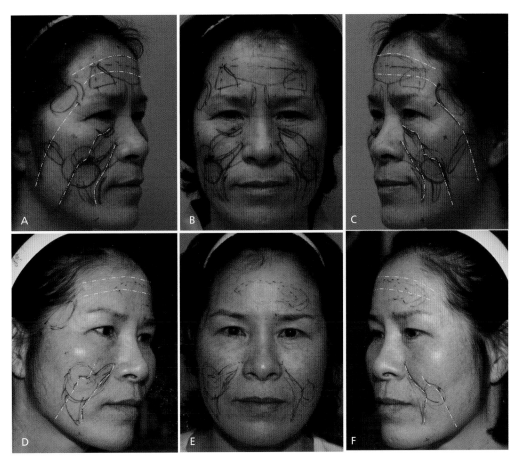

Figure 2-6 Preoperative markings for SAFI of the same patient in Figure 2-5. White dash-dot-dot lines are the SAFI lines. Usually, I do not mark preoperative SAFI lines on forehead because its boundaries are easily distinguished without any marks. In these figures, only volume deficiency areas are marked. Present forehead white lines are imaginary line for reference. Preoperative markings for 1st procedure using fresh fat (A, B, and, C) and 2nd procedure using frozen fat (D, E, and F).

of CAL. Adipose-drived stem cells was purified, total 65 ml of purified fat was injected into face and forehead as shown in Figure 2-6 (A, B and C). After 3 months, about 20 ml of her frozen fat was injected into the areas which the patient wanted to improve more as shown in Figure 2-7. There was no additional fat grafting until 2 years except an intra-dermal injection of hyalruronic acid filler for perioral wrinkles and Botox treatment for forehead wrinkles and crow's feet.

After the fat grafting, the facial contour is changed to oval shape with a smooth transition from upper to lower face as shown in Figure 2-5 and 2-7. The forehead looks more narrow and round due to volume restoration. Volume deficiencies of the tear trough deformity, infraorbiral hollowness and mid-cheek furrow were remarkably improved, but insufficient improvement of lower lid skin laxity and orbital fat protrusion should be corrected by additional blepharoplasty.

Despite her habit of smiling, successful volume restoration of the lateral cheeks, submalar hollows, nasolabial folds, and perioral wrinkles are seen in the postoperative views (Figure 2-5 and 2-7), which also contribute to less protruded mouth and less prominent nose. This collateral effect on contour change of the mouth and nose was due to anterior projection by fat grafting. No sagging appearance is being observed in the postoperative views of Figure 2-7, even though great volume of fat has been injected into the areas of poor soft tissue foundation such as submalar hollow, periorall and superior jowl fat. As shown in Figure 2-5D, present volume deficiency areas such as forehead depressions and deep nasolabial folds are clearly seen. It is suggested that survival rate and longevity is mostly being affected by the activity of facial expression muscles after the fat grafting even though CAL is applied.

It is quite difficult to compare survival rate and longevity of this case with those of previous case (Figure 2-3) objectively. The great effect of frozen fat grafting of Figure 2-5C and Figure 2-7C have been maintained up to 1 year 6 months after the procedure as shown in Figure 2-7D. However, some volume of grafted frozen fat is reduced as shown in Figure 2-5D and 2-7E. It looks similar or a little bit better compared to that of 4 months after the procedure as in Figure 2-5B and 2-7B. Particularly, the volume was continuously maintained during the 3 years and 6 months follow-up period. This is the

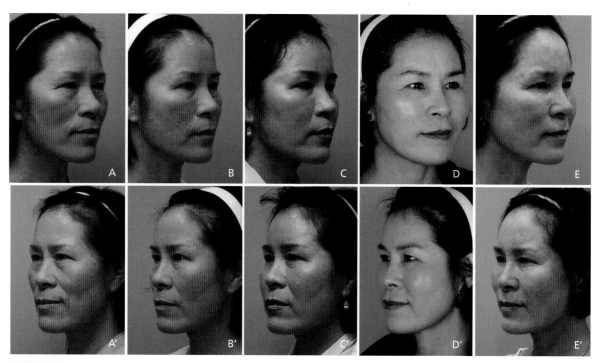

Figure 2-7 Effect of combination of CAL and SAFI on the change of facial contour during 3 years and 6 months follow-up. Both oblique views of the same patient in Figure 2-5.
Before the procedure (A and A'),
4 months after the procedure (before the 2nd procedure with frozen fat) (B and B'),
5 months after the 1st procedure (1 month after the 2nd procedure) (C and C'),
2 years after the 1st procedure (1 year and 6 months after the 2nd procedure) (D and D'), and
3 years and 6 months after the 1st procedure (3 years and 2 months after the 2nd procedure) (E and E').

difference between this case and previous case.

Patient's satisfaction of these two cases was great. Comparing these two cases, I am not sure which approach is more reliable because there are numerous factors such as subject difference of patient's satisfaction, economical factors of the procedure, and patient's sociality and so on which should be considered. However, it would be expected that the application of CAL can reduce the number of additional fat grafting.

■ 3 SAFI in old woman

1) Possibility of SAFI in an old woman

A 64-year-old woman patient (Figure 3-1) who wanted to improve her facial wrinkles visited my clinic. I recommended this patient the combination procedures of surgical face lifting, liposuction, and dermabrasion, but the patient wanted fat grafting procedure with multiple treatments of long-pulsed Nd:YAG laser and fractional laser.

Long-pulse Nd:YAG laser was performed 5 times before fat grafting, and fractional laser was performed 4 times after fat grafting. Total 76 cc of fat was grafted into the entire face and forehead with SAFI method. No additional treatment was performed, and there was no particular signs except 1 kg of weight increase according to the follow-up period of 13 months.

A number of deep facial mimetic wrinkles and a lot of fat accumulation in the jowls and nasolabial folds are being seen in the preoperative views (Figure 3-1 and A, A1, B, and B1 of Figure 3-2). The entire facial contour is close to a bulky pentagonal shape as a typical contour of elder people. And, the relatively small size of zygomatic body and arch, depression of submalar area and lateral cheek, and sagging of jowl are also significantly remarkable.

Noticeable changes right after the procedure in the frontal and oblique views (B and B1 of Figure 3-1) are described below.

First, the entire facial contour is changed from pentagonal to oval shape, and face looks smaller, resulting from the anterior projection due to volume restoration and volume decrease of jowl. But the most noticeable change is that the face looks lifted even though a lot of amount of fat grafting was performed.

Second, the volume of nasolabial fat was decreased and the nasololabial folds were significantly softened. It seems that the nasolabial fat was displaced superolaterally by the concept of volumetric lifting of SAFI.

Third, the size of jowl looks significantly reduced. It is supposed to be the result of liposuction, but

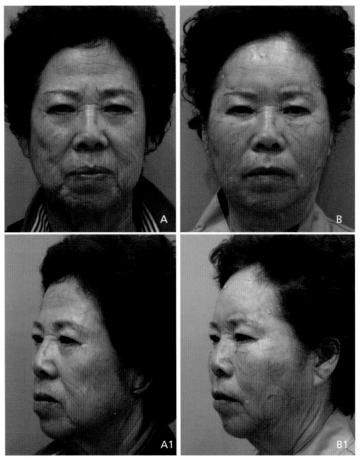

Figure 3-1 Immediate effects of SAFI on volumetric lifting and facial contour in an old woman. Before the procedure (A and A1), and immediately after the procedure (B and B1).

it also seems that the soft tissue of jowl was lifted superolaterally by sequential fat injection to Safi areas 4, 6, 7, 10, 11, and 15 as shown in Figure 14 of Chapter 8.

However, the postoperative dynamic changes as shown in Figure 3-2 provide some interest. The considerably improved nasolabial folds and jowls were returned to almost same state as the preoperative views. It occurred simultaneously with noticeable volume decrease of the malar, submalar, and lateral cheek region. This is just an interesting result fully showing an example of pseudoptosis by volume reduction. Also, it may be same meaning that the supero-laterally lifted soft tissue is drooped antero-inferioly as the volume of fat previously grafted into both malar, submalars, and lateral cheek is decreasing as shown in C, C1, D, D1, E, and E1 of Figure 3-2. It is considered that almost no improvement of nasolabial fold as seen in the 13 months preoperative views (F and F1 of Figure 3-2). However, wrinkles, regional depressions, and skin elasticity and color have considerably improved compared to the preoperative views.

From the above result, it would be quite difficult to get a great expectation and successful survival

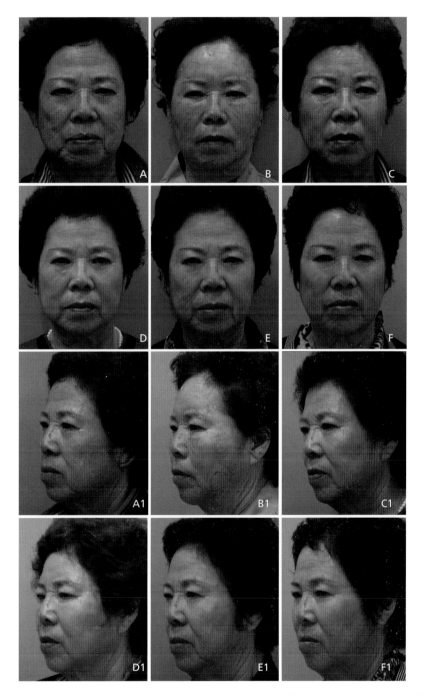

Figure 3-2 Change of deep nasolabial folds and sagging jowls by SAFI technique during 13 months follow-up period. Frontal (A~F) and oblique views (A1~F1).

rate with only one session of fat grafting to elderly patients. But, the patient had great satisfaction with only one session of fat grafting with additional laser therapy since she was happy with her final result compared to her previous appearance.

2) 4 sessions of SAFI with various combination procedures in an old women

A 59-year-old woman visited my clinic to correct orbital protrusion with skin laxity, perioral wrinkles and deep nasolabial folds. She had a bone defect of left frontotemporal region due to brain cancer surgery 12 years ago. As shown in Figure 3-3, fat grafting, incisional lower blepharoplasty, short scar face lift, man-made filler injection, Botulinum toxin injection, and PDO(Polydioxanone) thread insertion had been performed over a period of about 4 years.

Aim of fat grafting, despite her fatty appearance, was to provide volume restoration and treatment of wrinkles. Short scar face lift were performed to improve the laxity of lower face. Additional 3 sessions of fat grafting was being performed by patient's demand. Botulinum toxin and hyaluronic acid filler, and PDO thread were used for further improvement of wrinkles, folds and laxity. Dynamic wrinkles and folds cannot be perfectly corrected only by fat grafting. Even though they are considerably improved after the procedure, it is not caused by the thickening of skin itself but mainly by the

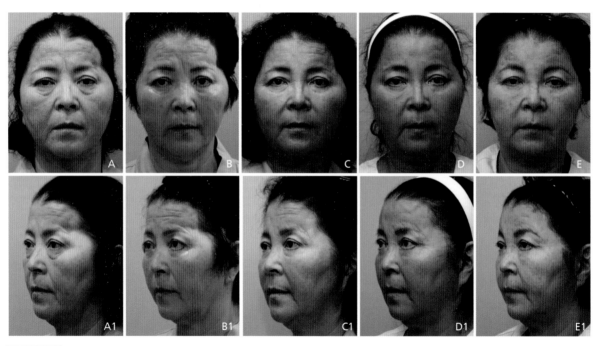

Figure 3-3 Combination effect of 4 sessions of fat grafting and other procedures in an old aged woman
A and A1: before 1st procedure with incisional lower blepharoplasty and short scar face lift(S-lift).
B and B1: 8 months after 1st procedure. Before 2nd procedure, hyaluronic acid filler to glabella, nasolabial folds and marionette line, and Botulinum toxin for corrugator muscle,
C and C1: 2 years and 8 months after 1st procedure (2 years after 2nd procedure). Before 3rd procedure, hyaluronic acid filler to perioral and lip wrinkles, and Botulinum toxin to corrugator muscle,
D and D1: 3 years and 9 months after 1st procedure (1 year and 1 month after 3rd procedure). Before 4th procedure, Botulinum toxin to corrugator and frontalis muscle, and PDO threads insertion for tightening of perioral and marionette lines, and
E and E1: 4 years and 3 months after 1st procedure (4 months after 4th procedure).

tightening of skin due to volume restoration. Also, survival rate of grafted fat into regions of wrinkles and folds would not be good because of active facial expressions in the wrinkled and folded areas. This can help explain the reason why the significantly improved folds are deepened again after immediately after the procedure. It is occurred more frequently in middle and old aged patient. During the follow-up period, combination therapy of intradermal filler injection, botox treatment, and PDO insertion had been performed by the patient's persistent demands for further improvement.

Disrupted facial contour was greatly improved by fat grafting and face lifting as shown in Figure 3-3 and 3-4. In the forehead, severe volume defect of left frontotemporal area was perfectly corrected by fat grafting and transverse and vertical wrinkles and depression were also significantly improved by combination of botulinum toxin, filler and fat grafting. In the mid-face, lower lid skin laxity with protruded orbital fat and infraorbital hollowness were improved by combination of blepharoplasty and fat grafting. The mid-face looked narrow and tightened, the malar eminences looked less prominent, and deep nasolabial folds were also significantly softened. In the lower face, multiple perioral wrinkles and marrionatte lines disappeared, volume deficiency of prejowl sulcus was greatly improved, and jow line was tightened.

This final outcome became possible because of the combination of various procedures that had been performed. It reminds us again that the application of combination procedure is a reliable approach for achieving natural and successful rejuvenation in old aged face. Successful result from the postoperative pictures of Figure 3-3 and 3-4 strongly supports the necessity of combination therapy as a compulsory procedure in elder patients.

4 Forehead fat grafting

In many cases, forehead fat grafting shows unstable outcome of survival rate and longevity compared to that of facial fat grafting. This is largely due to the overuse of mimic muscles and the structural characteristics of the forehead. In spite of using SAFI methods, there was a significant difference in the survival of grafted fat according to the patient's status of facial soft tissue and using of botulinum toxin as described below.

1) In a patient presented with dry and thin skin and overuse of facial expression muscles

Figure 4-1 shows the pre and postoperative views of a 29-year-old woman who had performed 3 sessions of forehead fat grafting. Forehead eminences look prominent because the patient's skin is very

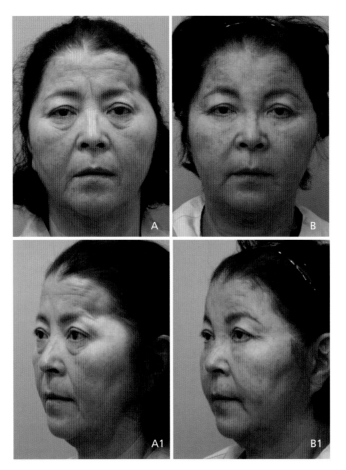

Figure 3-4 Enlarged photographs of the same patient in Figure 3-3. Before the procedure (A and A1) and 4 years and 3 months after the procedure (B and B1).

thin and has very little subcutaneous fat.

The corrugators are always in stressed state as seen in the preoperative views (A and A′ of Figure 4-1). Also, the hypertrophy of the muscle and depressions of the surroundings indicate that the muscle was frequently and habitually used. The suprabrow area and middle of forehead shows overall depression due to active mimetic movement of frontalis and procerous muscle. Typically, the patient's left eyelid has a mild ptosis with a high positioned left eyebrow. As described in Figure 4-1, two sessions of fat grafting (fresh fat first and frozen fat second) were performed during 24 months follow-up period. Botulinum toxin was treated only 10 days before the 3rd procedure.

In the postoperative views of Figure 4-1 (B and B′), the considerably improved forehead depressions are seen except a shallow depression of left suprabrow region as an early sign of low survival of fat. It was caused by compensatory contraction of frontalis muscle to eyelid ptosis.

After 2 months, the patient complained that "Almost all of the grafted fat is lost, and whole forehead is partly bumpy". There was no postoperative weight change. Some uneven and irregularities

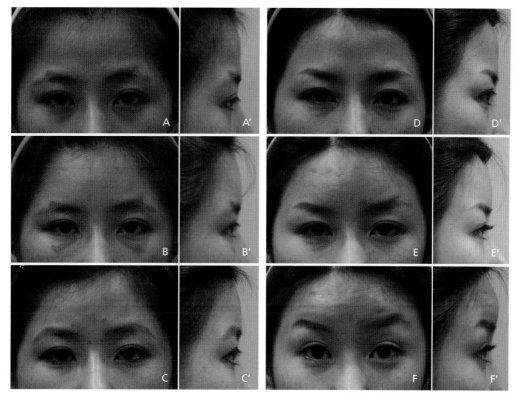

Figure 4-1 Successful result of fat grafting with precedent botulinum toxin followed by unhappy outcome of forehead SAFI without pretreatment of botulinum toxin in a 29-year-old woman.
Before the 1st procedure without pretreatment of botulinum toxin (A and A'),
1 month after the 1st procedure (B and B'),
2 months after 1st procedure and before 2nd procedure with frozen fat (C and C'),
22 months after the 2nd procedure and before 3rd procedure with fresh fat, and 10 days after pretreatment of botulinum toxin to forehead (D and D'),
resting state of 4 months after the 3rd procedure, and 4 months and 10 days after the botulinum treatment (E and E'), and
frontalis muscle-contracted state of 4 months after the 3rd procedure (F and F').

to corresponding to the activity of the facial expression muscles is due to the regional reduction of grafted fat as seen in the postoperative views (C and C' of Figure 4-1). The overall face contour of the lateral view (Figure 10-1, C') looks smoother than that of before. However, the mid-forehead, where active movements of frontalis and procerus muscles exist, shows unsmooth outline due to the regional fat reduction. Despite my detailed explanations of the low survival rate, the patient has declined my recommendation of botulinum toxin treatment. Additional session of fat grafting was performed using her frozen fat without botulinum toxin treatment.

21 months and 20 days after 2nd fat grafting, the patient visited my clinic again for an additional fat grafting for further improvement. In D and D' of Figure 4-1, little volume restoration without activity of forehead expression muscles are being observed. On the other hand, a little more ptotic left eyelid

and same height of both eyebrows are being observed. The 3rd session of fat grafting was performed with freshly harvested fat.

After 4 months after 3rd procedure, the patient had great satisfaction of last session of fat grafting pretreated with botulinum toxin. And, she had required an additional botulinum toxin treatment because she had felt some development of forehead wrinkles for the last few days. As shown in E and E′ of Figure 4-1, volume deficiencies of forehead were significantly improved, and moreover the forehead became more rounded and protruded. It also contributed to the deep-set eyes and lower nasal dorsum of the patient. However, very shallow transverse depressions are being observed in the resting state of Figure 4-1D. It may be caused by the combination of little loss of grafted fat and decreased activity of botulinum toxin. Interestingly, the shallow depressions of forehead in Figure 4-1 (E and E′), are correctly corresponded to the wrinkles activated by contraction of the frontalis muscles as shown in F and F′ of Figure of 4-1.

2) In a patient presented with thick skin and inactive facial expression muscles

Figure 4-2 is the pre and postoperative views of a 24-year-old woman patient performed with SAFI for forehead augmentation. In the preoperative views (A and A′), the mild retrusion of lateral forehead and slightly outstanding forehead eminences due to the entire depression of forehead are seen. And, the hypertrophic mimic muscles are not seen. In two sessions of fat grafting, 18 cc and 10 cc of purified fat was injected respectively. 20 units of Botulinum toxin was injected into the frontalis and corrugator muscle 10 days before the procedure. During the 5 years follow-up, one or two treatments of Botulinum toxin were performed every year.

The postoperative views from Figure 4-2 (C and C′) show great outcome of fat grafting 5 months after the procedure. Compared with the preoperative views, the lateral profile of the entire forehead connecting hair line to the eyebrows was fully projected and smoothly connected as shown in Figure 4-2C′. In the frontal view (Figure 4-2C′), the natural and harmonized contour of forehead with a smooth transition from upper to middle face is seen. It is due to successful volume restoration of lateral forehead. Despite the lateral expansion of forehead, the reason that the forehead looks round and short is due to the effect of anterior projection by successful fat grafting.

Patient's satisfaction was very high after the 1st procedure, but she still wants a more protruded forehead. We can see the restored volume of grafted fat have maintained up to 5 years after the procedure. She visited my clinic 2 times for treatment of mild acneform eruption on her forehead skin as shown in Figure 4-2. Her condition was improved by anti-acne drug and recommendation of changing facial cleanser to powder type. Comparing the two cases described above, it is suggested that the characteristics of recipient area, such as thickness of soft tissue and activity of mimic muscle deeply affect the survival rate of the grafted fat. The results of both two cases were wonderful. However, I am not sure whether the application of SAFI technique for forehead volume restoration was worthwhile in

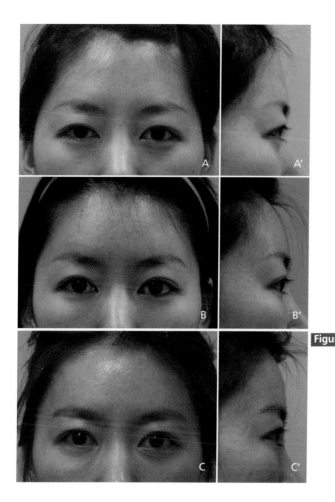

Figure 4-2 Successful forehead fat grafting with pretreatment of botulinum toxin in a young woman who had thick and oily skin. Before the procedure and 2 weeks after the treatment of botulinum toxin (un-powdered state) (A), 5 months after the procedure and just before 2nd procedure (un-powdered state) (B), and 5 years after the 1st procedure and 4 years and 7 months after the 2nd procedure (powdered state) (C).

increasing survival rate of grafted fat, but patients are more satisfied and the overall contour is much improved than only injecting fat into the depressed area of the central forehead.

5 Effect of Baton grip on fat grafting

Baton grip technique was applied to a 34-year-old woman patient who wanted to improve her angular and masculine face using SAFI technique. About 40 cc of purified fat was injected into the upper sunken eyelid, tear trough deformities, mid-cheek furrow, nasolabial fold, temporal hollow, nasal dorsum, sub-malar area, temple and forehead. I did not apply any molding and shaping with finger during the procedure. Figure 5 shows her follow-up pictures.

Irregularity is a common complication during the forehead fat grafting. The surgeon's skilled Baton grip can evenly inject fat into the forehead, and small depressive areas can be corrected by Baton grip

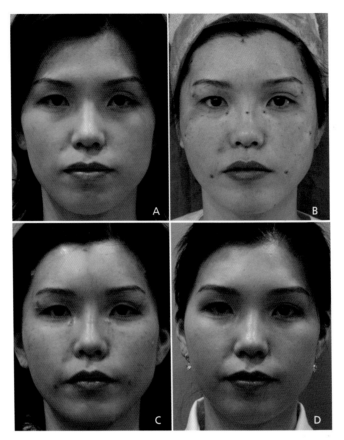

Figure 05 Preventive effect of Baton grip on fat grafting-induced common complications such as bleeding, edema, irregularity and lumpiness. Before the procedure (A), Just after the procedure (B), 2 hours after the procedure (C), and 3 months after the procedure (D).

technique without any molding. Figure 5B and C are the postoperative views of right after the procedure and 3 months after the procedure, showing a smooth forehead surface without any irregularities. Especially, there are tendencies of more serious edema in the forehead compared to other areas. There is a conspicuous difference on edema in postoperative view of right after and 2 hours after the procedure. Generally, patients are highly satisfied in convex forehead due to edema within 2 weeks after the procedure. This also results in the large disappointment after the complete settlement. Thus, it is important to let the patients understand the dramatic change of forehead fat grafting during consultation.

Sunken upper eyelid was more severe on the left side, and a slight hypo-correction of the same side is being seen in the postoperative views (Figure 5B and 5C). Volume restoration was naturally achieved as shown in the 3 months postoperative view (Figure 5D). The height of the double fold in left eyelid became smaller and more natural looking than the preoperative view. Also, no lump and irregularities are being observed. Any restriction of eyelid movement is also not found in Figure 5D.

In the postoperative view of 2 hours after the fat grafting to lower eyelid (Figure 7B), slight bleeding was seen around the entry site lateral to the left eye. Significant improvement of tear trough deformity and mid-cheek furrow without any lump or unevenness is seen in the postoperative view. 3 months postoperative view shows considerable improvement with overall natural looking compared to the preoperative views. These are achieved by fine and elegant injection of Baton grip as well as SAFI technique.

In conclusion, I do not think that my Baton grip is the best injection technique. But, I would like to reemphasize how important is a physician's grip technique for fat grafting.

6 Fat grafting for the upper sunken eye

1) A safe approach for correction of upper sunken eyelid using fat grafting

A 55-year-old woman (Figure 6-1) with sunken upper eyelid visited my clinic to correct her upper sunken eyelids. The symptom was more severe on the left upper eyelid due to her habit of raising the eyelid and dermatochalasia was not found. Her levator function test was estimated as normal range.

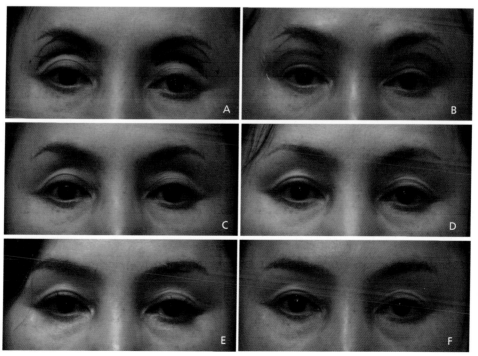

Figure 6-1 A safe result of 1st fat grafting for the correction of upper sunken eyelid. No additional fat grafting was performed until 23 months after the procedure.
Preoperative markings (A), just after (B), before (C), 3 months after (D), 8 months after (E), and 23 months after (F).

Design of upper sunken areas for fat grafting is very important. I divided the sunken area into three portions as marked in Figure 6-1A. Pretarsal portions of the sunken eyes (marked in black); the pre-orbital portion (delineated with black marks in blank); and brow portion (the common area of brow and preorbital portion). About 2.0 cc of fat grafting was performed to each of the sunken eyes. The fat grafting did not have any effect on the upper eyelid movement at all. It is seen in the postoperative view (Figure 6-1B) that the amount of injected fat into the sunken area of left eye is not sufficient.

With only one trial of fat grafting, the upper eyelid sunken seems significantly improved as shown in Figure 6-1D. The preoperative shallow and triple fold line was changed into a more vivid double fold line. However, it is almost certain that the left sunken eye lid is hypo-corrected. I recommended additional fat grafting for better outcome but the patient declined because she was satisfied with her result. It is suggested that the volume restoration effect has maintained over 8 months until 23 months after the procedure (Figure 6-1E and F).

2) Successful correction of sunken eye with unilateral mild ptosis by 2nd sessions of fat grafting

Two months after the procedure, the sunken lids are significantly improved. However, the ptosis of left eyelid slightly got worse than that of before, the left eyebrow is still positioned higher than the right eyebrow, and multiple crease looks more obvious than before as shown in Figure 6-2B. However, fortunately the patient did not have any subjective symptoms of eyelid ptosis.

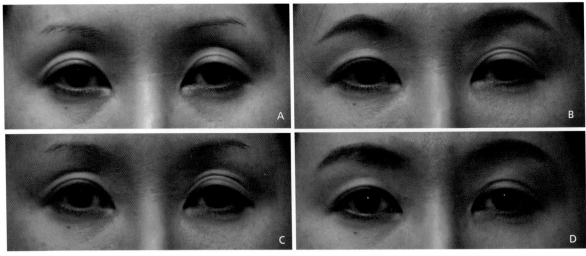

Figure 6-2 Correction of upper sunken eyelids with 2nd session of fat grafting.
Before the procedure (A),
2 months after the procedure (B),
4 months after the 1st session and before 2nd session with frozen fat (C), and
10 months after the 1st session and 6 months after the 2nd session (D) .

4 months after the procedure, the restored volume of the sunken lids is slightly reduced. On the other hand, the ptotic appearance has returned to the preoperative state as shown in Figure 6-2C. Additional fat grafting was performed, 1.0 ml and 1.5 ml of fat was injected into the right and left sunken eyelid respectively.

Six months after the 2nd procedure (Figure 6-2D), the sunken eyelids were much improved, multiple crease is not seen, the ptotic appearance of left eyelid is almost the same as before the procedure. Subjective symptoms of the ptosis such as heaviness or fatigue were not detected, but asymmetry of the eyebrow and folds thickness still being seen, which can be corrected by levator shortening surgery.

In this case, if fat was not placed at the appropriate layer of sunken eyelid or the volume was overcorrected, there would be a high risk of severe complications such as severe ptosis, irregularities, and lumpiness, etc.

3) A case of low survival rate and patient dissatisfaction

A 51-year-old woman patient presented with very thin and dry skin type with low body fat is shown in Figure 6-3.

The function of upper eyelid was normal through preoperative physical examination. She had a habit of raising her eyebrows, but she did not notice it. Excessive loss of soft tissue was concerned as the cause of sunken eyes. About 2.0 ml of autologous fat was placed into each of the preorbiral and pretarsal areas.

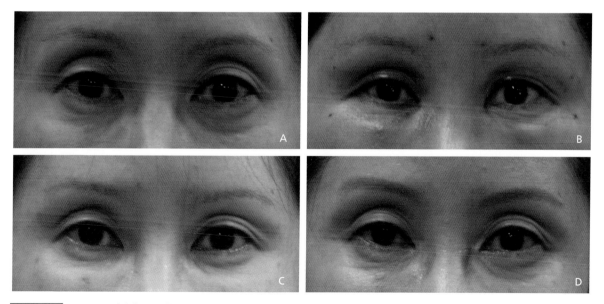

Figure 6-3 Unsuccessful fat grafting for the correction of the sunken eyelid in a 51-year-old woman. Before the procedure (A), immediately after the procedure (B), 2 weeks after the procedure (C), and 3 months after the procedure (D).

Hypocorrection is doubtlessly observed in the view of immediately after the procedure (Figure 6-3B). A slight improvement of volume restoration is seen in the 2 weeks of the postoperative view (Figure 6-3C), but there is almost no effect except for a little bit smoother looking in the 3 months of postoperative view (Figure 6-3D). Patient was also deeply disappointed with the low survival rate.

Hypocorrection is doubtlessly observed in the view of immediately after the procedure (Figure 6-3B). A slight improvement of volume restoration is seen in the 2 weeks postoperative view (Figure 6-3C), but there is almost no effect except for a little bit smoother looking in the 3 months postoperative view (Figure 6-3D). Patient was also deeply disappointed with the low survival rate.

I have regretted for not correcting the hypo-correction immediately after the 1st procedure. I recommended additional fat grafting combined with CAL, but she declined. This was the case that I felt very sorry to the patient.

4) Combination of SAFI and Cell-assisted lipo-transfer(CAL) for the correction of upper sunken eyelid in an old woman

Almost all upper sunken eyelids in elder patients are accompanied by both weakness of levator palpebral muscle and volume loss. A 62-year-old woman (Figure 6-4) had complained about upper sunken eyelid since she had performed removal of upper orbital fat about 20 years ago. CAL was performed without upper blepharoplasty. The fat was injected mainly into the preorbital area and relatively small amount of fat was injected into the preseptal area. The total amount of injected fat into each sunken area was about 2.5 cc.

In the postoperative views (C and D of Figure 6-4), the sunken eyelids are significantly improved, however, the volume still looks somewhat insufficient. Interestingly, the contour of double folds was changed dramatically from shallow and thin shape folds to clear and definite one. The definite folds are formed by descent of excess skin and bulging of pre-orbital and septal area by grafted fat. After the procedure, the patient had pleased with less fatigue of her eye, no tired-looking appearance, and recovery of her previous double folds. Additional fat grafting was done because she wanted more volume restoration on her upper eyelid. Compared with the case of Figure 6-3 which CAL was not applied, the effect of this patient is much better and successful despite her older age. Until now, it seems to be the best approach to increase the survival rate of grafted fat.

In the immediate postoperative views (E and F of Figure 6-4), any limitation signs of eyelid movement are not being observed, however, volume restoration of the preseptal areas looks slightly insufficient

In the long follow up postoperative views (G and H of Figure 6-4), the volume restoration for sunken eye lid is much more improved than that of Figure C and D. The patient had a great satisfaction with her volume recovery without any limitation of eyelid movement. Particularly, she was also so pleased that her eye fatigue symptom had been greatly improved.

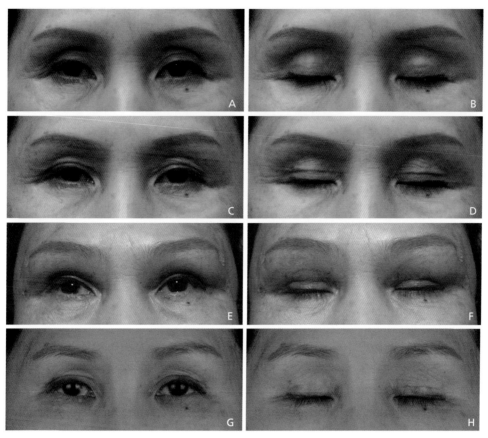

Figure 6-4 Combination effect of CAL and SAFI for the correction of upper sunken eyelid in an old woman patient who had performed blepharoplasty with orbital fat removal about 20 years ago. A and C: before the procedure, B and D: 3 months after the procedure and before the second session of frozen fat grafting , E and F: Just after 2nd session of frozen fat grafting, and G and H: 2 years & 3 months after 2nd session of fat grafting

My principle for safe fat grafting to the sunken eyes is as follows: avoid hypercorrection, and plan an additional procedure by performing hypo-correction (estimated as 100% of volume restoration, regardless of swelling and volume of anesthesia) in the first procedure. Of course, there are cases that showed good improvement only after the first procedure, but the principle is a safer approach in preventing severe complication by unwanted hypercorrection. Also, I would like to recommend 2 suggestions for correction of sunken eyelid with fat grafting. One is to combine with CAL, and the other is to perform it after gaining confidence in performing fat grafting with Baton grip technique to the entire face.

5) Correction of sunken upper eyelids by levator shortening surgery

Figure 6-5 shows a case of a 55-year-old woman patient who wanted correction of upper sunken eyelid using artificial filler injection or autologous fat grafting. Upper lid ptosis, lower eyelid ectropion (complication of previous lower eyelid surgery), and dry eye syndrome were found by the physical

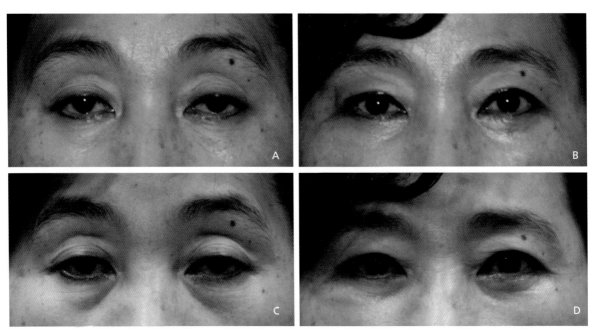

Figure 6-5 Correction of upper sunken eyelids only by levator shortening in a 55-year-old woman. Before (flash photo) (A), 3 months after (flash photo) (B), before (no flash photo) (C), and 3 months after (no flash photo) (D)

examination (Figure 6-5A and C). According to the indirect examination, it was estimated that there was no volume loss of orbital fat. Performing fat grafting for the correction of sunken eyelid is an absolute contraindication in this case.

I explained the pathological co-relationship with upper lid ptosis and sunken eyelid in detail. The levator shortening for the correction of lid ptosis and the revision lower blepharoplasty with canthopexy and SOOF (suborbicularis oculi fat) suspension suture were performed at the same time.

Prominent sunken with severe lid ptosis, and raising of eyebrow due to the compensation of the frontalis muscle are found in the preoperative views (Figure 6-5A and C). Significant improvement of sunken eyes is being seen in the postoperative views (B and D of Figure 6-5). The eyebrows are also normally positioned. This result is accomplished by the recovery of the function of levator muscle by levator shortening. Consequently, there is no need to raise the eyebrows and the orbital fat is being pulled down to its normal position.

However, the unexpected wrinkles of medial part of the eye and the dorsum of nose are found. It can occur to patients with preoperative brow ptosis or the hypercorrection of levator shortening even without previous brow ptosis. Thus, it occurs because there is no need of compensation by raising the eye brow. The side effect should have been explained in advance, especially if the brow ptosis is confirmed before the operation, and the need for eyebrow or forehead lifting should be discussed.

■7 Fat grafting combined with lower blepharoplasty

Lower blepharoplasty can be classified roughly into 2 types, such as surface surgery and volume surgery. Generally, the surface surgery is represented by transcutaneous lower blepharoplasty. Transconjunctival removal of orbital fat (TCR) or fat grafting or fat reposition can be classified as the volume surgery.

Lid-cheek junction is the visible groove to delineate the location where the lid meets the cheek and consists of palpebromalar groove laterally and tear trough medially. With aging, the length between this junction and lower lid margin is increased and the volume of the junction is also changed remarkably. These morphological changes on the junction imply many complicated signs of aging related with lower lid and mid-face. I measured the changes of volume and lid-cheek length on a line dropped from the mid-pupil to evaluate the effects of various kinds of blepharoplasties on rejuvenation of lower lid and mid-cheek according to the classification in Table 1.

Table 01 Various procedures and possible combinations for lower lid rejuvenation

Case 1	Transconjunctival removal of orbital fat (TCR)
Case 2	TCR +fat graft
Case 3	Transcutaneous lower blepharoplasty (TLB)
Case 4	TLB+ mid-face lifting
Case 5	TLB+ fat graft
Case 6	TLB+ mid-face lifting+ fat graft
Case 7	Only fat graft

1) Effect of transconjuctival orbiral fat removal (TCR) on lower lid rejuvenation

TCR is most commonly performed to correct orbital fat protrusion and dark circle in young woman as shown in Figure 7-1A. After TCR, protruded orbital fat was not seen. However, the dark circle becomes darker and the infraorbital hollowness also becomes more extended than that of before the procedure as shown in Figure 7-1B. These unfavorable outcomes are more frequently occurred in patients who have protruded eyeball with poor skeletal support of lower orbital rim. TCR did not show any effect on the lid-cheek length. But, it is the best procedure for correction of protruded orbital fat in young patients.

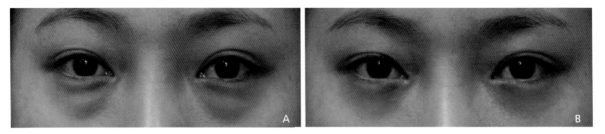

Figure 7-1 Effect of TCR (Transconjunctival removal of orbital fat) on length of the lid-cheek junction and infraorbital hollowness. Before the procedure (A), 1 month after the procedure (B).

2) Combination of Transconjunctival orbital fat removal and fat grafting

Figure 7-2 shows the combined effects of TCR and fat grafting for improvement of aged lower lid in a woman patient in her 30s. Fat grafting was followed by TCR. The fat was injected transcutaneously. The postoperative views (B and D of Figure 7-2) show shortening of the lid-cheek length, improvement of dark circle, and volume restoration of tear trough and palpebromalar groove. When compared to the result of Figure 7-1, it is strongly suggested that this combination procedure provides better and natural rejuvenation effect.

3) Transcutaneous lower blepharoplasty (TLB) without orbital fat reposition.

TLB is the most commonly performed procedure for correction of aging lower lid in middle or old aged patients. It is the surface surgery that serves removal of excess skin, muscle, and orbital septum with protruded fat. The postoperative view (Figure 7-3) shows remarkable improvement of these aging

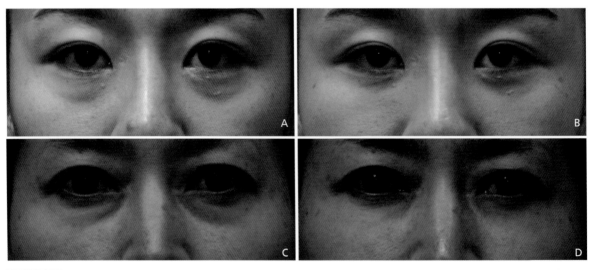

Figure 7-2 Results of combination procedure of TCR (transconjunctival removal of orbital fat) and fat grafting for the correction of aging lower lid in 34-year-old (A and B) and 36-year-old (C and D) woman. Before the procedure (A and C), 3 months after the procedure (B and D).

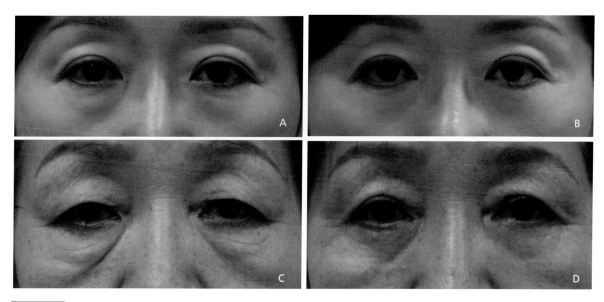

Figure 7-3 Effects of transcutaneous lower blepharoplasty on aging lower lid in middle aged and old woman. Before and 10 months after the procedure in middle-aged lady (A and B), before and 7 months after the procedure in old-aged lady (C and D).

signs such as excess skin, wrinkles, and protruded orbital fat. But, not only the lid-cheek length is not changed but also the infraorbital hollowness is still not improved. To achieve better harmonized result, additional volume surgery is absolutely necessary.

4) Transcutaneous lower blepharoplasty with mid-face lift

Mid-face lift is often performed in combination with lower blepharoplasty in old patient who has moderate or severe laxity of lower lid. The postoperative view (Figure 7-4) shows a successful result of the combination procedure of TLB and mid-face lifting in an old woman. The lid-cheek length was greatly shortened, the skin laxity and protruded orbital volume was also remarkably improved as well. Interestingly, the infraorbital hollowness was noticeably improved by displacement of soft tissue of the mid-face lift, but typical features of the tear trough deformity and mid-cheek furrow are still be-

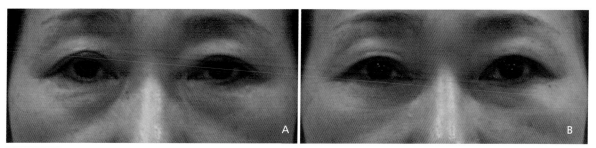

Figure 7-4 Combination effect of transcutaneous lower blepharoplasty and mid-face lift on the correction of aging lower lid in an old woman. Before (A), 6 months after the procedure (B).

ing observed as shown in Figure 7-4B. If the patient is not satisfied, additional volume surgery will be needed.

5) Combination of transcutaneous lower blepharoplasty and fat grafting

I love to perform fat grafting to reinforce the limitation of TLB, which could not restore the volume deficiency as shown in Figure 7-3.

In both cases in Figure 7-5, fat grafting was followed by TLB. Aim of fat grafting was to restore the volume deficiencies and increase skeletal supports of the lower orbital rim. Fat is injected transcutaneously. The postoperative pictures (B and D of Figure 7-5) show significantly shortened lid-cheek length, with removal of wrinkles and protruded orbital fats, with volume restoration of infraorbiral hollownesses and mid-cheek furrows, and with reinforcement of skeletal support to the zygoamtic and maxillar bone. Compare with the effect of TLB as shown in Figure 7-3, this combination procedure showed more natural and perfect outcome.

Mid-face lift was performed only to the patient of Figure 7-5C, because she had suffered from dry eyelid syndrome since her previous TLB. Lid ectropion with lid laxity is obviously seen in Figure 7-5C. In the postoperative view (Figure 7-5D), this iatrogenic complication is almost improved and her mid-face looks more lifted and tightened than that of Figure 7-5B.

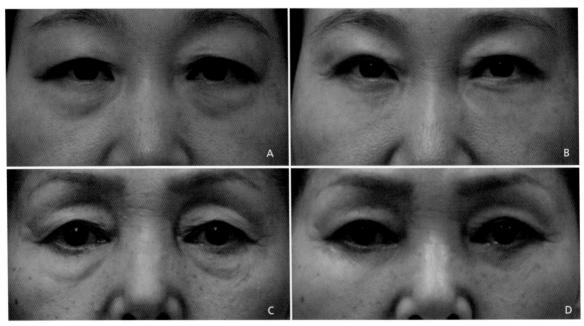

Figure 7-5 Combination effect of transcutaneous lower blepharoplasty and fat grafting. Before and 8 months after the TLB and fat grafting without mid-face lifting in a 50-year-old lady (A and B). Before and 4 months after the fat grafting and revision TLB with mid-face lifting in a 57-year-old lady (C and D). Incisional upper blepharoplasty was performed in these two cases simultaneously.

From the above results, it is strongly suggested that combination procedure should be performed to achieve natural and harmonized rejuvenation effect. "The more procedures are combined, the better is the outcome."

6) Fat grafting as a single procedure

When I perform fat grafting, I prefer to apply it not only as a simple concept for volume augmentation, but for volumetric lifting using my SAFI technique.

These 4 woman in Figure 7-6 had protrusion of orbital fat which is mainly caused by poor skeletal support of medial part of infraorbital rim. Also, with aging, the laxity of skin, muscle and orbital septum affect the development of the orbital fat protrusion. Fat grafting was performed to these 4 patients who had no experience of lower lid rejuvenation procedure. Figure 7-6 shows the outcomes of rejuve-

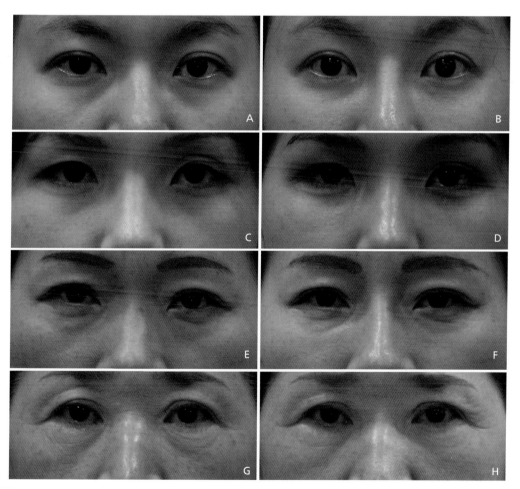

Figure 7-6 Effects of fat grafting as a single procedure on the aged lower lid of a 24-year-old woman (A and B), a 34-year-old woman (C and D), a 45-year-old lady (E and F), and a 55-year-old woman (G and H). Before the procedure (A, C, E, and G) and 6 months, 3 months, 4 months, and 5 months after the procedure (B, D, F, and H).

nation achieved only by fat grafting.

The effect of fat grafting on two patients in their 20s and 30s from Figure A and C is actually fantastic because the protruded orbital fats were dramatically disappeared and the infraorbital hollowness is also perfectly improved. It is because the protruded orbital fat is pushed back into the orbit by the increased skeletal support. Eventually, the lid-cheek length was remarkably shortened and dark circle is also significantly improved. This concept of fat grafting will be helpful to prevent acceleration of aging process in the lid-cheek junction over the next few years.

However, the results of fat grafting on the other two patients in their 40s and 50s from E and F of Figure 7-6 show limitation of the fat grafting. I advised a 45-year-old woman (Figure 7-6E) to do TLB, but she refused and only wanted non-incisional fat grafting and simple augmentation of nasal dorsum.

In the postoperative view (Figure 7-6F), volume deficiencies of the mid-cheek furrow and tear trough deformity were significantly restored and the lid-cheek length was also shortened as well. But the protruded orbital fat and laxity of skin were not improved sufficiently. Even though the effect of fat grafting in this patient is not bad, there is definitely limitation of fat grafting on successful rejuvenation of aged lower lid.

Moreover, in the preoperative view (Figure 7-6G), the patient had severe protrusion of orbital fats with laxity of the whole layer in the lower lid, tear trough deformity with poor skeletal support, and deep and wide mid-cheek furrow. In the postoperative view (Figure 7-6H), skin of the lower lid looks tightened and brightened. However, except of insufficient volume restoration in the tear trough deformity and mid-cheek furrow, there were no significant anti-aging effects such as shortening of the lid-cheek length and loss of orbital fat protrusion. Practically, it is not useful to perform fat grafting to this type of old aged patient.

From the above results, I would like to emphasize that either the surface or volume surgery have their obvious limitations on successful rejuvenation with natural harmony in aged patient. As we all know, because aging is always accompanied with volume deficiency and sagging, therefore, the ideal approach for rejuvenation of aging lower lid should be a combination procedure using both the surface and the volume surgery.

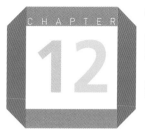

a novel facial fat grafting technique with a concept of volumetric lifting

Pre-and post-operative patient management

1 Preoperative management

Preoperative management is not very different from that of other cosmetic surgery. However, if the patient has overly expressive face, it is suggested to do botulinum toxin injection 2 weeks before or at least 2-3 days before the procedure because reduction of facial animation by botulinum toxin increases the survival rate of grafted fat.

2 Postoperative management

The purpose of postoperative management is to increase wound healing and to prevent decrease of survival rate.

1) Patient management and care up to 3 days after the procedure

(1) Cold compress or ice pack

2-3 days after the procedure is the peak period of edema. Ice pack is the best management during this period to decrease edema or inflammation. Apply cold pack at 30 minutes interval rather than continuously. However, patient should be aware that strong pressure with hard cold packs can change the contour of the face.

(2) Wearing the facial band or elastic compression garments

① Facial area

After fat grafting or facial liposuction, patient should be fixed with tapping (Figure 1) or put on a facial band (Figure 2)[1], to minimize facial movement, migration of infiltrated fat, edema, and bleeding after procedure. Avoid excessive strong pressure on the infiltrated area during taping and leave the taping in place for 3 days. Put on the facial band for at least 2 weeks.

② Body area

On the following day, remove the Reston® foam used for compression of the liposuctioned area. Put on elastic compression garments as seen in Figure 3 designed to suit patient's body to eliminate edema, bleeding and postoperative drooping of the area[1]. The area of liposuction for fat grafting is not large. Thus, patients do not have to wear it for a long time. However, if there is severe skin drooping or relaxation in abdomen, the physician would recommend wearing the garments for 2-3 months.

(3) Limit usage of facial mimic muscles

For limit usage of facial mimic muscle, it is recommended to take liquid form food, such as porridge during this period.

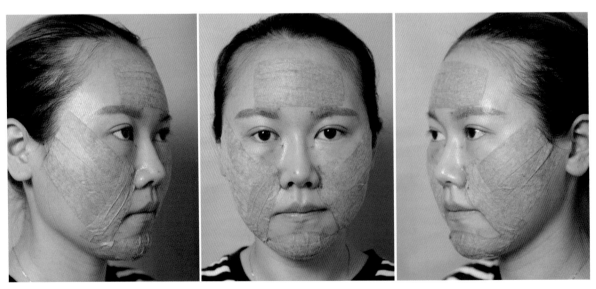

Figure 01 Facial tapping for fixation.

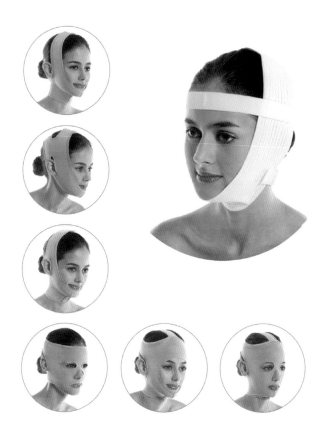

Figure 02 Various kinds of facial compression garments.

(4) Daily activities and sleeping posture

Oversleeping or continuously laying down for a long time after the procedure can worsen edema. Therefore, it is recommended to maintain daily activities without touching or pressing the infiltrated area. Particular attention must be taken not to be under pressure on the infiltrated area during sleeping. Patients should keep their face above their heart during sleeping.

(5) Stitch removal

3 days after procedure, remove the suture of entry site, and then apply Steri-strip® for 2 days.

2) Postoperative management 4 days after the procedure

(1) Limit usage of mimic muscles

4 days after the procedure, facial expressive movement starts to increase due to the reduction of edema. Therefore, patients should be instructed not to overuse the facial muscles.

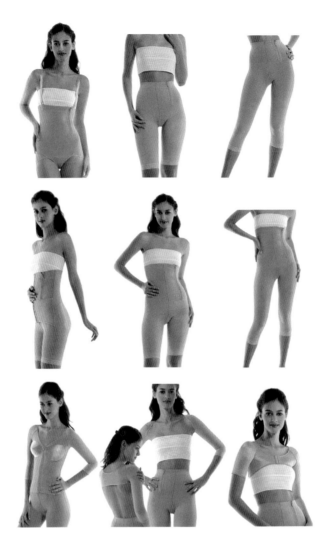

Figure 03 Various kinds of elastic compression garments.

(2) Hot pack

Stop application of ice packs from 4 days after procedure. After this period, application of hot packs may eliminate edema. But, it needs to be careful in avoiding burn since the face is less sensitive to temperature after the procedure. The physician must inform the patient in advance that continuous application of ice packs after 4 days of procedure can make edema last longer.

(3) Management of bruise and edema

Various maneuvers such as hand massage, high radiofrequency, or ultrasonic wave can be used to facilitate lymphatic drainage to eliminate severe postoperative bruise and edema. But, perform it on the surroundings and not on the infiltrated or suctioned area.

3) Other pre and postoperative management

(1) Drinking and smoking

Stress that the benefits and out the principle of quitting smoking: more than 8 weeks before and 12 weeks after the procedure. However, it is realistically impossible for heavy smokers to quit smoking according to this principle. Thus, ask them to reduce smoking as much as possible and educate them to stop smoking at least 2 weeks before and after the procedure. Especially, in concerns of bleeding or anesthesia, patient must stop smoking at least 12 hours before the procedure. Also, remind the patient about the possibility of lower survival rate due to smoking and suggest to stop or to reduce smoking at least 1 month to 3 months after the procedure to alleviate the problem.

(2) Daily activities

Patients tend to touch and massage when they feel the infiltrated area is over-injected. Warn the patients not to touch or press the infiltrated area by themselves or other people after the procedure. Recommend to sleep in supine position until 3 months after the procedure. Taking shower is fine, but avoid going for a sauna for at least 1 month.

(3) Exercise and weight management

Do not exercise too much within 1 month. 4~5km/hour mild walking is recommended during this period. Swimming is permissible 1 month after the procedure. Violent exercise negatively impacts on the survival rate and final outcome, caused by frequent fatigue combined with increased plasma lactate concentration, movement of facial mimic muscles, and decreased body weight. It is recommended to maintain body weight 6 months after the procedure.

(4) Optimum time for other aesthetic procedures

It is appropriate to inject Botulinum toxin at least 2 weeks after the procedure. The physician has to be cautious in injecting botulinum toxin after the procedure because the positions of subcutaneous structures have been changed due to the injected fat and edema. Also, the physician and the patient have to be cautious about the onset of inflammation.

IPL or laser toning can be applied 1 month after the procedure. High frequency, long- pulsed Nd:YAG laser, and fractional laser for skin tightening are allowed after 3 months.

Prohibit from moving skin physically even if it is only for washing face within 4 days after the procedure. Generally, acupressure massage for aesthetics is not recommended until 6 months after the procedure. However, like cleansing, skin massage without physical stimulation and pressure on skin is permissible.

(5) Additional fat grafting

Additional fat grafting can be performed always. I suggest that the optimal time for additional procedure is at least 3 months after the 1st fat grafting. However, if the patient demands strongly, it may be performed at least 1 month after the procedure using fresh or frozen fat. Frozen fat stored over 3 months must not be used. If the frozen fat is used inevitably, the physician has to be careful to prevent inflammation.

Reference

01. C&C medical Co., Ltd. (www.cncmedi.co.kr) E-mail : bbom0310@naver.com, Tel: +82-2-515-8264, Fax: +82-2-515-9687.

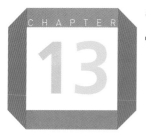

The complications

1 Complications of recipient area

1) Migration of grafted fat

The grafted fat can migrate to the surroundings during or immediately after the procedure.

This is mainly caused by direct pressure to the infiltrated site or active movements of the mimic muscle. Migration caused by overusing the mimic muscle frequently occurs in the forehead, periorbital, and perioral areas. Also, intraoperative pressing and touching by the doctor's hand and postoperative deep pressure or purposeful manipulation by patient are the causes for early migration and abnormal distribution of fat. Pressure caused by bad sleeping posture is another important cause for early migration. The migration might be improved by molding with gentle digital pressure or can be prevented by pretreatment of botulinum toxin.

Patients sometimes complain about migration of fat after a considerable time passed, which mostly occurs at regions such as nasolabial folds, cheeks, and jowls. However, in the area of cheeks and jowls, it is caused by gravitational descent due to the weight of injected fat. In case of nasolabial folds with a lot of facial movement, it is caused by lower survival rate in the depressed part of the folds and relatively high survival rate in the lateral part of the folds which look larger than before the surgery. As the above cases, the patients may feel like "migrated" or "accidentally injected".

The migration can be mostly corrected with additional SAFI method combined with adequate liposuction.

2) Gravitational descent

Gravitational descent may occur after fat grafting. It varies according to the location of injection, depth and amount of injected fat, and the patient's degree of aging.

Patients occasionally use the word "migration" to explain this. It is more likely to occur in the elders. The facial soft tissues descend to the antero-inferior direction because of aging. It often happens when the physician inject the fat into the depressed area focusing on the volume restoration only, without understanding or considering the aging of the surrounding areas. For example, Figure 1 is a case with gravitational descent caused by fat grafting into the face. Autologous fat was injected only into the antero-medial cheek of the right face for correction of depression. After injection, the lower cheek and jowl area look droopy and the volume of the submalar and midcheek areas is significantly decreased. This phenomenon is thought to be caused by soft tissue sagging due to the weight of the grafted fat and postoperative swelling. Particularly, this phenomenon may occur much more outstanding in patients with hypercorrection.

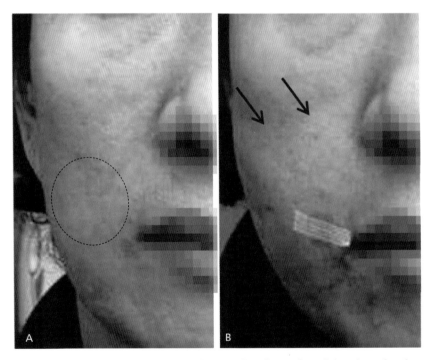

Figure 01 A case of the gravitational descent by fat grafting. Before fat grafting (A), 5 days after fat grafting (B). Black dotted circle means the area of fat injection and two black arrows means depressed areas of submalar and midface, and a whitish Steri-strip® (B) is for the wound closure of the entry site.

Almost all of the descent due to fat grafting needs overall approach because it changes the contour of surrounding face. The principle of correction is to do proper liposuction of the descent area first and then fat grafting into the depressed area, then sagging appearance is improved and natural contour of surroundings can be made. Especially, more caution should be taken on patients with low elasticity of skin and subcutaneous tissue. Additionally face lifting is recommended for severe and complicated cases which cannot be corrected perfectly by combination of liposuction and SAFI.

3) Edema

Edema or persistent edema after fat grafting may occur by the tissue damage during pretunneling and injection, the hypo-osmolarity due to the tumescent fluid for local anesthesia and the lipoaspitated fat itself, and several other systemic diseases.

It commonly occurs immediately after the procedure, peaks at 2-3 days, and disappears within 2 weeks. But, concerning about individual variations, there are patients who suffer more than 10 weeks. Preoperative inspections on the presence of zygomatic edema and its connection with systemic diseases should be evaluated.

Prolonged edema which does not subside after 2 weeks of fat grafting should be differentiated from hyper-correction, hematoma, inflammation, and factors due to systemic disease. Generally, medical devices using radiofrequency or ultrasound which accelerates lymphatic circulation might be helpful to reduce it. Steroid injection can also be recommended.

4) Bruising or hematoma

Bruising or hematoma in company with edema is the most common factors that make patients uncomfortable during recovery period. The major causes are vascular or muscular damage caused by cannula stimuli. Bleeding is frequently occurred in the area of forehead, temporal, perioral, and periorbital region.

Figure 2 is a case of mild bruising in medial canthal and prejowl sulcus area after fat grafting. It mainly occurs if the entry site for injection is positioned right above tear trough. To prevent bruise in medial canthal area , set the entry site between SAFI areas 13 and 14. In general, bruising will be fully disappeared by 2 weeks. Especially, persisting bruise on orbital or periorbital area should be completely blocked from sun light because previous pigmentation might worsen or hyperpigmentation might occur.

Figure 3 is a case with severe bleeding in lower eyelid after fat grafting. When accompanied by severe bleeding, grafted fat's survival rate is decreased and the patient may have side effects such as fibrosis or lumpiness. Subconjunctival hemorrhage after fat grafting is due to the rupture of blood vessel in the orbicularis oculi muscle, orbital septum, and orbital fat. Mostly, it lasts up to 2 weeks, but it may lasts up to 1 month in severe cases (Figure 3B, C). It is a self-limiting condition that requires no treatment infection or significant trauma. Conservative approaches such as administration of artificial tears or ophthalmic topical drops containing antibiotics, wearing of protective spectacles with sunscreen function, and application of hot packs can be recommended.

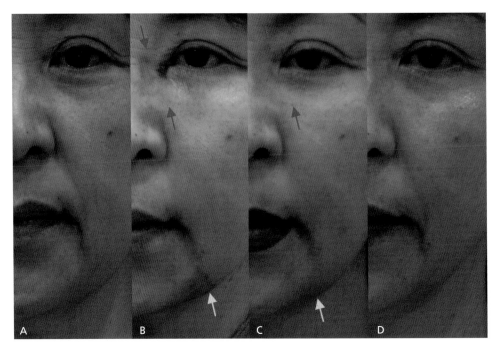

Figure 02 A case of mild bruising after fat grafting. Before (A), 4 days after (B), 10 days after (C), and 4 weeks after (D).

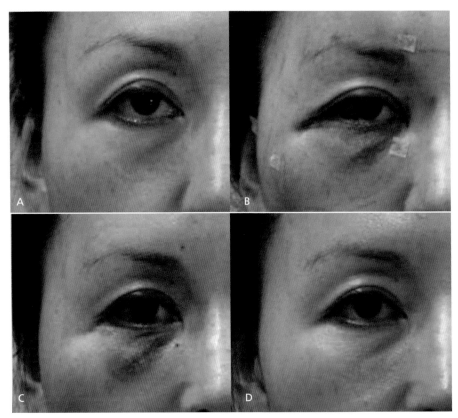

Figure 03 A case of severe bleeding and bruising in the right lower lid after fat grafting. Conjunctival hemorrhage is also combined. Before (A), 1 day after (B), 6 days after (C), and 4 months after (D).

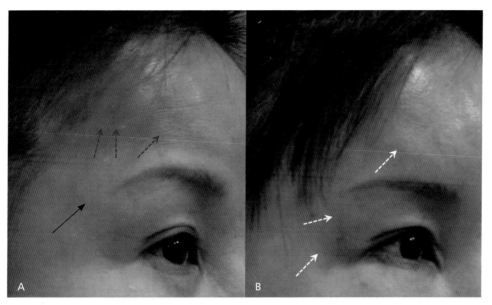

Figure 04 A case of hematoma and bruising in fronto-temporal area. The blue dotted arrows indicate the branches of the superficial temporal veins which can be seen easily through the skin (A). The white dotted arrows indicate the suprabrow swelling (hematoma) suspected to be a bleeding focus and the upper eyelid ecchymosis which is migrated from the suprabrow area (B). The black arrow indicates the location of sentinel vein. Before the fat grafting (A, and 6 days after (B).

In Figure 4A, relatively large superficial veins are easily seen around superior temporal line. These veins are frequently ruptured during injection because of thin skin and week subcutaneous fat. On a sudden swelling during fat grafting, it is strongly assumed that there is bleeding. Figure 4B is 6 days of postoperative view with bruise formed by gravitational migration of bleeding from forehead to eyelid. Especially, when fat is injected into temporal hollow, attention should be paid to avoid rupture of this vein because the vein is an important landmark for the frontal branches of facial nerve. Preoperative markings of the course of these vessels are helpful to prevent this problem.

Using blunt cannula significantly reduce the occurrence of bleeding and hematoma compared to using sharp needle. But, we are still not completely free from bleeding the excessive pretunneling or aggressive use of cannula. Press immediately for 2-3 minutes if bleeding occurs during the procedure. Then, cautiously start again. Sometimes, hematoma is developed intra or postoperatively. Therefore, check the occurrence of further bleeding or hematoma before allowing the patient to go home.

5) Irregularity, lump, and bump

The occurrence of irregularity, lump, and bump usually depends on the physician's grip technique, experience, and aesthetic sense. Especially, elegant grip technique and determination of optimum layer and amount of fat to be placed are essential for consistent and smooth placement.

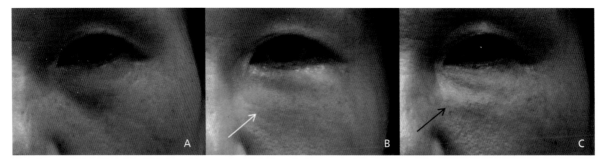

Figure 05 A case of fibrotic lump in tear trough after combination procedure of fat grafting and transcutaneous lower blepharoplasty. White and black arrows mean a fibrotic lump. Before (A), 1 month after (B), and 2 years and 6 months after (C).

During or immediately after the procedure, if lump is seen or touched, remove it properly by using liposuction cannula until the lump is disappeared. Also, if any irregularity is seen after removal of the lump, it is suggested to correct immediately with additional grafting.

Figure 5B shows a typical case of fibrotic lumpiness after fat grafting to tear trough and mid-cheek furrow and transcutaneous lower blepharoplasty in a 45 year-old woman. The contour of lump caused by overcorrection is seen in Figure 5B. The protruded movable lump, a hard papable sausage-like mass, is also seen in Figure 5C.

The treatment principle of the lump or bump is removal of it by liposuction or excision as well as making a smooth fullness using liposuction or/and additional fat grafting if needed. In the early stage of development, it might be helpful to improve these complications with injection of catabolic steroid solution or application of ultrasound or radiofrequency-assisted lipolysis. Patient of Figure 6 had performed one fresh fat grafting and two additional frozen-fat grafting with 1 month interval for correction of tear trough deformity and mid-cheek furrow in other clinic. The preoperative view shows a big sausage-shaped bulging (bump) in the tear trough and mid-cheek furrow of ultrasound-midface marked with arrow (Figure 6A). It was movable in front of the infraorbital rim. I attempted to treat this patient with ultrasound-assisted liposuction. Most of the aspirates were composed of fibrotic fat and scar tissue. Figure 6B shows a significant decrease in the size of the bump without any irregularities. However, a small bump was still left. Additional lipolysis or catabolic steroid injection might be helpful to remove this small bump.

The most common site of irregularity, lump, and bump as a complication of fat grafting is the eyelid region. Also, it is very difficult to do successful fat injection into the eyelid because of thin skin of eyelid, active motion of muscle, and dynamic aging process. Therefore, it is essential to have some experience and aesthetic sense on how to decide the optimal layer and volume for prevention of these complications. Additionally, I would like to suggest cosmetic surgeons to use: i) lesser fibrotic fat, ii) combination of CAL method, iii) PRP mixtured fat, iv) good grip technique for smooth placement and less tissue damage, v) fresh fat (not frozen fat), and vi) botulinum toxin.

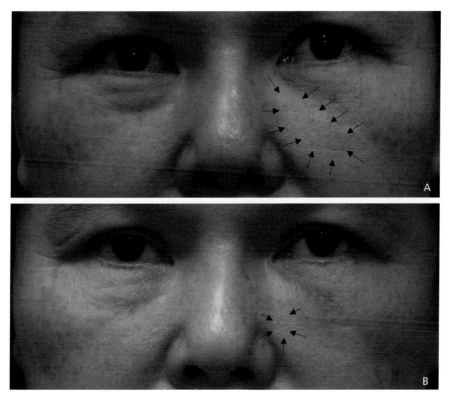

Figure 06 A large sized movable fibrotic bump in the tear trough deformity and mid-cheek furrow was improved by lipolysis-assisted liposuction. Before (A), and 2 months after the procedure (B).

6) Inflammation and infection / abscess formation

I would like to introduce three cases of inflammation after fat grafting.

(1) Infection or abscess formation after forehead fat grafting

The first case is described as below. I would like to express my appreciation to Dr. Kang-Hoon Ko[1] for providing the data and information.

Figure 7 is a case of a 55 year-old woman with a complaint on postoperative irregularity in other clinic. She had first fat grafting on forehead, nasolabial fold, and chin. After 6 weeks, frozen fat was injected into the same areas, and additionally into mid-cheek furrow for second fat grafting. Antibiotic intravenous injection (Cephradine 1g/day) and oral administration were given 3 days after fat grafting.

Figure 7A is the postoperative view of just after the second fat grafting. Figure 7B is the second post-operative view after 1 week. Edematous look and distinctive outline around the injected area are being seen.

About 3 weeks after the procedure, the patient came to the clinic with edematous pain on the center of the forehead (especially in the area marked ② in Figure 7C). However, other infiltrated areas of the

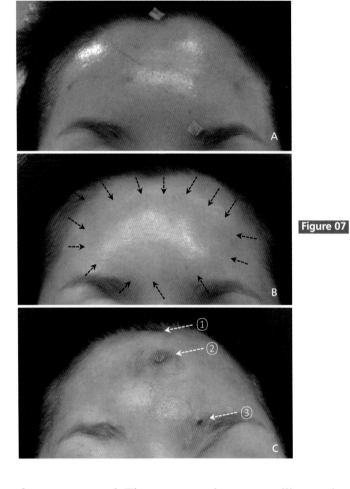

Figure 07 A case of infection and abscess formation of the forehead after second session of fat transfer using frozen fat. There are nothing unusual except the volume augmentation with post-operative swelling in the view of right after the procedure (A). The distinct dermacation with edematous status and different color can be seen prominently between injection and non-injection area in the view of a week after (B). Typical infection are seen in the view of 5 weeks after the fat grafting as the status of 3 weeks after infection occurrences. ① Entry site for the irrigation as the previous fat injection site ② spontaneous skin opening after the needle aspiration ③ Dependent drainage site (C).

face were normal. There were tenderness, swelling, and serous fluid collection on the central part, and no improvement was seen after 1 week of intravenous antibiotic injection (Ceftezol: Ceftezol 1g/day, I.V.). After this, antibiotic treatment with combined cefotaxim sodium and ciprofloxacin was administered for about 2 weeks.

Figure 7C is 5 weeks of second postoperative view. 2 weeks after the procedure, the patient came for bulged central forehead. At this time, infection focus was found at the central forehead, and typical inflammation signs of swelling, overall heating sense, and tenderness were seen in the infiltrated area.

Wound care and irrigation were performed every day. Blood test and antibiotic susceptibility test were also performed. Antibiotics and high concentration of vitamin C were simultaneously administrated. But, the symptoms periodically got improved and worsened, and the necrotized fat dissolved out from the drainage site near left eyebrow. To accelerate the improvement, squeezing was performed and the squeezed area was recovered by delimitating the infected fat. But, nevertheless, the infection spread to nearby area: the boundary of forehead. These treatments were carried out daily for about 3 months until full recovery.

Placing unsanitary and wrong applied hydrocolloid bandage on the area of needle aspiration is considered to be one of the direct causes of inflammation. But postoperative treatment without suturing the injection site cannot be excluded from the direct causes. Also, this patient is a smoker and an animal lover who lives together with many animals. Frequent contacts with animals can be another direct or indirect cause of infectious inflammation. Additionally, sterilization of the surgical instruments used in the fat grafting are judged not to be the cause since the other patient who was operated at the same day had no problem.

(2) Abscess after fat grafting to lateral cheek.

Figure 8 shows a case of abscess formation after combination procedure of fat grafting and non-incisional contouring thread lifting using a barbed, cogged suture (EZ lift) to improve jowl sagging and lateral cheek depression. I would like to thank Dr. Kang-Hoon Ko[1] for providing the data and information.

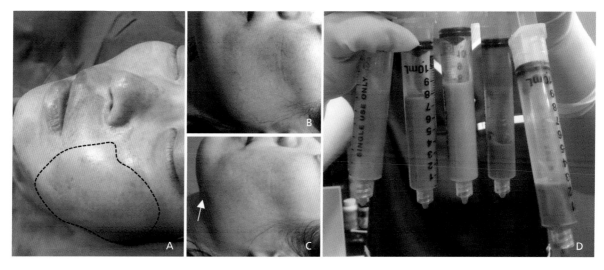

Figure 08 A case of abscess formation. A 43-year-old woman had performed fat grafting and EZ thread lifting. This picture was taken in the operation room 3 weeks after fat grfting and EZ lifting. Huge swelling is seen in the left face indicated by dotted line (A). This picture shows the preoperative status of her left face (B). Fresh fat was re-injected into her lateral cheek for further volume restoration at 6 months after I&D (C). This picture shows the final result of 6 months after the 2nd fat grafting and 1 year after the 1st procedure. The white arrow indicates a linear depressed scar formed by I & D. About 75 cc of bloody and dark yellowish necrotic fat was removed by I & D (D).

Two weeks after the 1st procedure, there was a 3 cm diameter induration at the lateral cheek which had no respond to antibiotic treatment. Needle puncture was performed to remove 3 cc of necrotic tissue, and hematoma occurred.

Symptom of huge swelling with fluctuation was shown as in Figure A. Incision and drainage was performed 3 weeks after 1st fat grafting to remove pus and necrotic tissue but thread was not removed. Inflammation was cured after that. New fat was grafted into lateral cheek after 6 months. Figure C is the photo of 6 months after the 2nd fat graft and showed increased volume at cheek compared to before.

In this situation, because operations for several patients were performed on the same day, the sterilization problems of surgical instruments can be excluded. But contamination during surgery and inappropriate postoperativecare cannot be ruled out. The 3 entry sites used for fat graft for this patient were 1 cm lateral to mouth corner, posterior part of malar area and anterior to side burn. The area where induration first occurred was the entry site which was nearest to mouth corner. In particular, the entry site nearest to mouth corner was the easiest area to have contamination occurring from mouth. Furthermore, sterilization of lips and oral cavity was not carried out for this patient.

Incomplete removal, stimulation of inflamed and surrounding tissue, and bleeding are the reasons of rapidly developed inflammation and abscess, when performing needle aspiration in order to remove induration. Threads, always need to pay attention to the possibility of release of cog and the danger of occurrence of inflammation. In the case of this patient, threads are inserted into the deep fat layer or SMAS and imflammation was seen in superfacial fat layer only.

Author meet cases of combined procedure of fat grafting and thread lifting sometimes. Author do not insert threads into other areas beside areas of liposuction or fat grafting as explained in Figure 8 in Chpater 10. This is because of the foreign body reaction of the inserted threads and occurence of synergistic effect caused by necrosis during survival process of the grafted fat, and inflammation or higher possibility of secondary inflammation.

(3) Inflammation after nasolabial folds fat grafting

I would like to acknowledge Dr. Young-Gun Yoon[3] for the data and information of this case. The 55 year-old woman patient in Figure 9 had performed fat grafting for the correction of nasolabial folds and perioral wrinkles. But, unfortunately, the oral mucosa of the left nasolabial fold was penetrated by the injection cannula during the procedure. Figure 9A is the preoperative view, and Figure 9B is the view of right after the procedure showing a slight hematoma around the infiltrated area. As shown in Figure 9C, the patient had skin erythema, edema, and tenderness 2 days after the procedure. After 4 days, these symptoms got worsened. Especially, severe tenderness below skin erythema with relatively hardened tissue was found.

Drainage was tried after removing the suture of entry site but only serous fluid was extruded. The patient was hospitalized for optimal antibiotic treatment. Since the hardened area became smoother and fluctuated after 2 days of hospitalization, incision and drainage was performed. 4.5g/day of amoxicillin antibiotics was administrated immediately after grafting. Combination of antibiotics was administrated during hospitalization. Antibiotic therapy did not work to eliminate inflammation and the inflammation continued to progress. But, it started to improve after incision and drainage (I & D). The inflammation was completely subsided after 2 weeks of hospitalization.

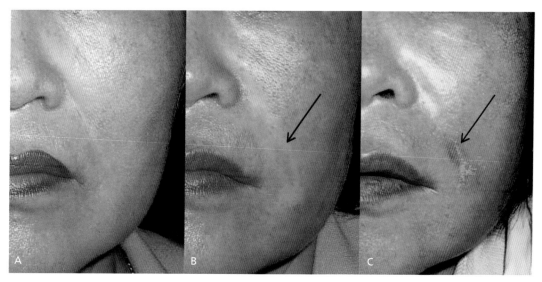

Figure 09 A case of infection and abscess formation of the left nasolabial fold after the fat grafting. Approximately 3 ml of fresh fat was injected into the left nasolabial fold (A), Placement of fat is appeared as a whitish-colored skin area with small amount of the subdermal hemorrhage (white arrow) (B). Typical infection signs of the erythematous the induration, the tenderness and the swelling (black arrow) are seen in the view of 2 days after (C).

The most direct cause was assumed to be the contaminated cannula which was penetrated into the oral cavity during fat injection. However, if the oral cavity was sterilized before the procedure or the physician drew out the cannula after sterilization, the infectious inflammation might be prevented.

From the three cases above, I would like to briefly mention the general matters of inflammation that occurred after fat grafting.

The bacterial infection occurred after fat grafting is accompanied by pain, swelling, and erythematous induration, which last 2-3 days to 1 week after the procedure. Abscess is commonly formed if it was not eliminated at the early stage. If occurred, an obsessive treatment is needed since the infection can spread to the surroundings, causing severe complications such as cellulitis[4].

Main causes of infection are inadequate sterilization of surgical instruments, contamination of fat during harvest and separation, contamination of cannula during the procedure, and infection of skin entry site. Especially, since frozen fat may have higher incidence of infection the physician must be cautious about it. Also, concern about the patient's present or past history since immunocompromised patient or patient with immune diseases have much higher possibility of infection. The bacteria commonly causing infection abscess are staphylococcus[5], streptococcus[6] and mycobacterium[7,8].

There are several precautions. Wash the inside of the cannula thoroughly, and delicately sterilize other surgical instruments. Also, maintain germ-free condition of several fluids and keep the condition while harvesting, isolating, purifying, and recharging the fat. Avoid using perioral or nasal cavity as an entry site of injection, and administrate adequate pre and postoperative antibiotics for prevention and treatment.

Only use frozen fat within 3 months, which is stored at -20°C without cryoprotective agents (CPA) treatment in the freezer. Must be defrosted in the refrigerator and then centrifuge it. Do not use if the color of the centrifuged fat changed. More cautions are needed during the procedure for prevention of infection compared to that of using fresh fat grafting.

The acute inflammation of infiltrated fat is not much different to that of artificial filler injection because the grafted fat is supplied by diffusion without any vascular supply. However, antibiotics should be administered to prevent the spreading of infection and secondary infection. Microbiological study and antimicrobial susceptibility test should be performed.

The basic goal of the treatment is to remove the contaminated soft tissue. Sometimes, early infection can be eliminated by adequate antibiotic treatment. However, reinfection after quitting antibiotics can be subsided only by removal of the contaminated fat and soft tissue. It is not uncommon, so careful treatment and management is needed. Generally, about 2 weeks to more than 3 months is usual time for infection control.

Continuous application of ice packs may prevent spreading of infection and inflammation surroundings at early stage. Sterilize the entry site and protect the skin where inflammation is active. Early antibiotic administration and optimized I & D when induration becomes softened are very important. Also, be cautious of skin damage while squeezing. Besides, once inflammation occurs, try to remove all environmental factors that weaken patient's immune system or worsen inflammation, such as physical or mental fatigue, insomnia, drinking, smoking, contact with pet, etc. But, if rapid spreading of cellulitis is suspected, hospitalization is the best way to prevent further serious complications.

Late complications such as as various type of scar of incision site or inflamed area, and hyperpigmentation may occur. Additional fat grafting is possible at least after 6 months of complete recovery from the inflammation, and only fresh fat should be used.

7) Asymmetry

Occasionally, some patients complain about asymmetry immediately after fat grafting. Edema is the main cause of asymmetry. For example, in the patient has asymmetry of malar, more fat is injected into smaller side. Then, completely reversed asymmetry may occur immediately after the procedure, because the more fat grafted, the more swollen the grafted area will be. In the case of asymmetry due to over-correction or under-correction, it can be improved by adjustment of the volume using liposuction and additional fat grafting at least 1 month after the procedure.

8) Acneiform eruption

There are cases of complaints on acneiform eruption after fat grafting. Generally, the acnelike eruption develop as a result of infections, hormonal or metabolic abnormalities, genetic disorders, and drug reactions. After fat grafting, it can be exacerbated by excessive oil formation from destroyed fat cell.

It maybe frequently developed in patients with oily skin, previous acne, and unclean washing or stress during the recovery period as the patient of Figure 10. Oily effluxion due to destroyed adipocyte on forehead makes a glossy look (Figure 10B) but it improved after administration of antibiotics. However, Figure 10C and D show much worsened acneiform and it still lasts 3 months after the procedure. This frequently occurs at forehead and T-zone.

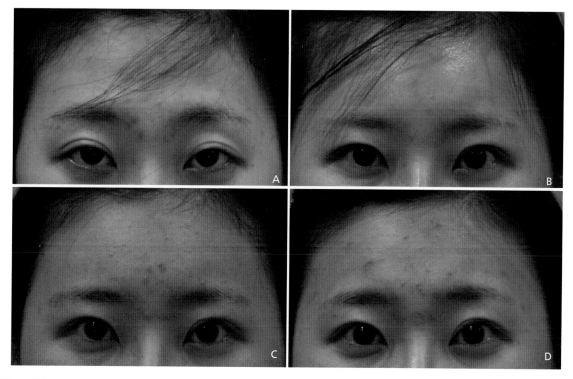

Figure 10 A recurrent of acneiform eruption after forehead autologous fat grafting in a 23 year–old woman with acne vulgaris. Before (A), 8 days after (B), 1 month after (C), and 3 months after (D).

Figure 10D, the 3 months postoperative view, shows an uneven surface of forehead. The depressed area is directly related to the active motion of forehead mimic muscle, not acneiform eruption. Treatment of acneiform eruption varies with the particular disease suspected and consists of a wide range of methods. Acneiform eruption caused by fat grafting is mostly improved by adequately cleansing of face and administration of drug (topical/oral antibiotics or topical/oral retinoids) for about 7 days, usually. But, occasionally it may be developed 2-3 months after the procedure, continuous or intermittently.

9) Hyper-correction

Hyper-correction is mainly caused by the compensation for a concern of the lower survival rate. But, it is very difficult to estimate hypercorrection during or after the procedure because the swelling and survival rate is quite different from patient to patient, from area to area, and even from side to side in the same patient.

If author's baton grip technique is used, hyper-correction found out during or immediately after the procedure can be corrected by gentle squeezing and light liposuction, because the fat is injected as one row and thread like shape. If it is found out within 2 weeks after the procedure, it is best to wait until 1 month, but corticosteroid such as triamcinolone acetonide solution (4-8mg/ml) can be injected primarily for extremely dissatisfied patient for 2 times, with an interval of 10 days between each injection. If it is still judged as hyper-correction after 1 month, wait until 3 months. However, if the patient does not agree, the physician may try lipolysis or lipolysis-assisted liposuction.

If it is developed during the correction of sunken upper lid, the best solution is immediate removal of over-grafted fat with gentle squeezing or suction. Without any limitation of eyelid motion and irregularity, wait until 2 weeks after the procedure. However, when the ptotic appearance or irregularity of eyelid still existed 4 days after the procedure, it is strongly recommended to do immediate postoperative revision for removal of over-injected fat through incisional upper blepharoplasty and/or with the levator shortening surgery for improvement of levator function. Of course, triamcinolone injection can be considered, but more extreme care is needed than other facial areas. This is because if the steroid solution spreads out to the surrounding tissues, it may results in upper lid ptosis and orbital fat herniation by wasting of levator palpebral muscle and weakening of the levator aponeurosis and orbital septum [9].

Ultrasound or radiofrequency or laser-assisted lipolysis is also the possible approaches for the reduction of over-corrected fat without concerns on the side effects of steroid injection and surgical removal. However, particular attention should be paid to avoid damage to fine structure of upper eyelid.

10) Hypo-correction

Hypo-correction is one of the most common complications of fat grafting. It is due to less fullness or low survival rate.

Just before the patient is discharged, the physician should estimate again whether she or he is hypocorrected. If hypo-correction is recognized, even though considering the effect of edema, immediate additional fat grafting can be recommended. Thus, keep the remaining fat in the refrigerator before the patient leaves the clinic, and then move it to deep-freezer. Lower survival rate of grafted fat is the most serious dissatisfaction of patients. It is very difficult to mention one by one because of a lot of environmental and technical factors. However, it could be improved by the application of adipose-derived stem cells, pretreatment of Botulinum toxin, even placement of fat by Baton grip, no smoking, postoperative limitation of facial movement, and 1 or 2 times of additional fat grafting

Figure 11 is a case of hypo-correction, showing changes after forehead fat grafting. Thin skin with less subcutaneous tissue can be seen in the right forehead (Figure 11A). The hypo-corrected area is much in evidence (black arrows of Figure 11B). In the Figure of 11C, the hypo-correction seems to be improved compared to that of 10 days after the procedure.

The optimal time for correction is 3 months after the procedure. However, if the patient strongly demands, or the physician judges that the patient needs an early correction, correction can be performed 1 month after the procedure by using frozen or fresh fat.

11) Hyperpigmentation and scar

Hyperpigmentation is frequently found in the orbital and periorbital area with bruising after fat grafting. Try to help lymphatic system to eliminate swelling, apply sunblock cream, and prescribe 2-4% hydroquinone cream 1-2 times per day if it becomes worse. Safety concerns with hydroquinone consist only of occasional irritation, which can be suppressed with topical steroid, lower concentrated cream or a short drug holiday. Topical bleaching agents remain the gold standard of post-inflammatory hyperpigmentation therapy as they are evidence-based, are cheap, and of equal or greater efficacy compared to lasers. In cases unresponsive to topical therapy, application of appropriate laser such as Q-switch ND Yag-Laser with correct settings might also be helpful.

The damage of approximated epithelium caused by some friction of the cannula is the main cause of scar formation. Because, for facial fat grafting, the incisions closed in a short period of time, almost all incision can be healed with minimal scarring. But in some patients may have a depressed or hypertrophic scar. It is helpful to treat the scar with the application of anti-scar (steroids or certain antihistamine) creams, ointments, or gels, because scars cause itching and are very sensitive. The pressure treatment or silicone gel sheeting to help treat scars or as preventive care is used.Steroid injection to treat keloids or hypertrophic scar and surgical removal or treatment such as skin grafts, excision,

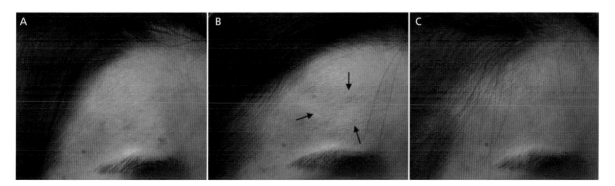

Figure 11 A case of hypo-correction after forehead fat grafting. Before (A), 10 days after (B), 4 months after (C).

dermabrasion, or laser resurfacing are also used under certain conditions. I suggest that the entry site should be made with 18 G needle and sutured after the procedure for prevention of scar and inflammation.

12) Vascular embolization

Incidence of vascular embolization is rare, but if occurs, it can bring severe complications. It has been reported that vascular embolization is frequently developed in the facial fat grafting of glabella, nasolabial folds, nose, and temporal area. When the fat is accidently injected into the artery, regional complications, such as skin necrosis and blindness due to occlusion of an end branch or surrounding branches of the artery, can happen. But, if large amount of fat is accidentally injected into the artery with high pressure, the fat can be refluxed into the internal carotid artery and brain. Eventually, brain infarction as a serious complication occurs. On the other hand, if the fat is injected into the vein, it goes through the heart and then obstructs the pulmonary artery. Finally, pulmonary embolism is developed and its typical symptom is quite different from that of arteria embolization.

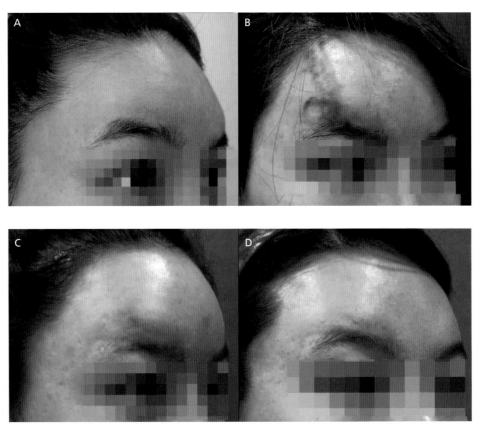

Figure 12 A complete recovery case without any specific sequale after arterial occlusion. Before the frozen fat grafting (A), 3 days after the procedure (B), 18 days after the procedure (C), and 3 months after the procedure (D).

(1) Skin necrosis due to the occlusion of terminal artery

The incidence of arterial occlusion from fat grafting has significantly decreased by using blunt cannulas. However, it still occurs during the procedure even though blunt cannula is used. The two cases of arterial occlusion were developed in the frontal branch of superficial temporal artery. I would like to thank Dr. Dong-Young Yang[10] for providing the data and information.

First Case: A recovery case without any complications after arterial occlusion in a 29 year-old woman who had performed 3rd fat grafting with frozen fat (Fresh and frozen fat was used for her first and second procedure separately) is described in Figure 12.

Figure 12A shows a case of arterial occlusion in 29 year-old woman who had performed 3rd fat grafting with frozen fat. Fresh and frozen fat was used for her first and second procedure separately. Temporal hollow is seen in Figure 12A. During the procedure, the patient had a severe headache and focal redness was founded near the temporal ligament adhesion (TAL) one day after the procedure. In Figure 12B, necrotic finding of the purplish colored linear expansions, which are considered the distribution of the frontal branch of the superficial temporal artery, was seen. And she still complained of her headache.

Immediately, antibiotics (first generation movement with gentamycin), blood circulation enhancer (Tanamin[®])[12], vitaminine B, and analgesics were administered. The wound was cleaned with saline and then Episurge[®][13] was applied every day. Occlusive dressing was performed with hydrocolloid dressing, Duoderm[®]. This treatment was continued for about 15 days, and the lesion got much improved as shown in Figure 10C. Complete recovery status without any sequale is seen in Figure 10D.

Second Case: A case of permanent depressed scar formation after arterial occlusion is described in

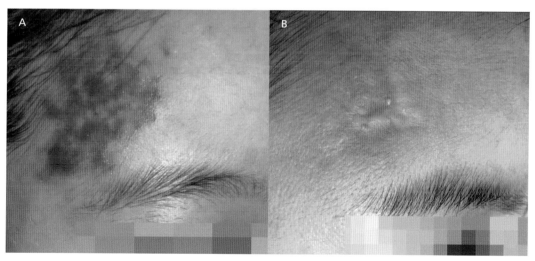

Figure 13　A case of permanent scar formation after arterial occlusion after fresh autologous fat injection. 3 days after the procedure, shows skin ulcer with acute suppurative inflammation and hemorrhage (A), and 4 months after the procedure, shows fibrotic depressed scar (B).

Figure 13.

The patient of Figure 13 had performed second fat grafting using fresh fat. There was a sudden and severe pain following fat injection, and the typical skin lesion of vascular occlusion accompanied with inflammation (Figure 11A). Immediate and appropriate treatment was not performed at all since the patient was uncooperative and eventually refused it. The permanent depressed scar due to skin necrosis is seen in Figure 4B.

Third and Fouth Case: Two cases of nasal alar necrosis after fat grafting are described in Figure 14 and 15.

I would like to express my gratitude to Dr. Dong-Hak Jung from Shimmian Clinic, Seoul for providing the information of these two cases.

The patient in Figure 14 received fat graft to improve deep nasolabial folds. Two months later, sec-

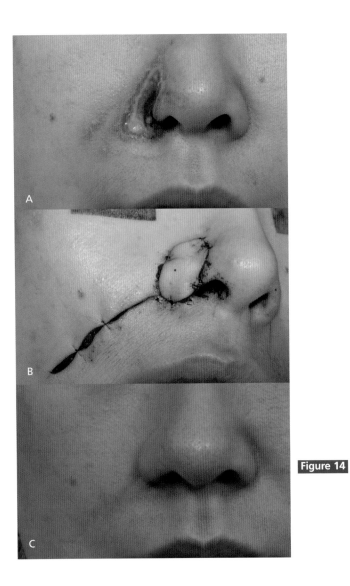

Figure 14 First case of nasal alar necrosis by fat grafting for improvement of deep nasolabial folds. Total thickness of nasal alar was disappeared by necrosis (A), The picture was taken during nasolabial flap surgery for reconstruction of lower lateral cartilage using ear cartilage (B), and 6 months after the surgery (C).

ond fat grafting using frozen fat was performed and her right nasal alar had necrotic changes as shown in Figure 14A. The branches of angular artery, lateral nasal artery and nasal alar artery are fully damaged. Hyperbaric oxygen therapy was performed and one month after the occurence of necrosis, lower lateral cartilage was restored using ear cartilage and nasal alar was restored by nasolabial flap surgery as it is highly possible that the cannula might be located inside the vascular lumen and moved forward within the vessel during the injection. It means high probability of intravascular fat injection in Figure 14B. Figure 14C shows that the nasal alar is restored to almost, even though there is a light scar formed after the the surgeries.

The patient in Figure 15 had necrosis at her right nasal alar after fat graft into whole face as shown in Figure 15A. Lateral nasal artery, the branch of angular artery, is damaged. 3 days later, adipose-derived stem cell was injected into the area of necrosis. Starting from 4 days later, hyperbaric oxygen therapy was performed. 20 days after necrosis, forehead flap surgery, lower lateral cartilage reconstruction surgery using rib cartilage, and tip rhinoplasty are performed at the same time as shown in Figure 15B.

The common important informations alluded from the above terminal artery occlusion cases are summarized below.

First, vessel occlusion occurred at the 2nd session and 3rd session in 3 cases and 1 case occurred at 1st session in 1 case. This means that vessel occlusion can happen at anytime.

Second, the blunt cannula was used in all cases. In first and second cases, the fat was injected not

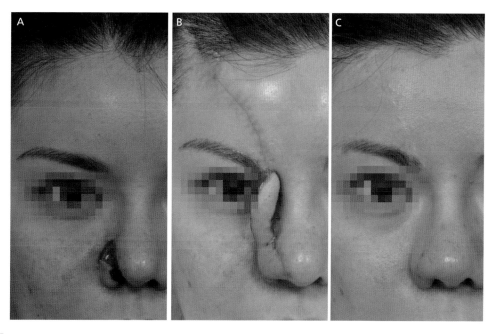

Figure 15 Second case of nasal alar necrosis by fat grafting. Partial necrosis of nasal alar is seen (A). The picture was taken after 1st forehead flap surgery (B). 6 months after the surgery (C).

only when it was drawing back, but also during advancing towards the target area. Direction of injecting was not identified in two cases of nasal necrosis.

Third, arterial occlusion occured when using both frozen fat and fresh fat in the second of the 1st and 2nd cases.

Fourth, the patients in all cases complained of severe pain during and immediately after the injection.

I would like to describe my personal opinions about the possible factors which increase the incidence of arterial occlusion in the cases described above.

Firstly, it is suggested that the mobility of subcutaneous tissue, especially, the vessels, in the infiltrated area was significantly reduced after 1stsession due to fibrosis and fullness. And then, when the fat is re-injected into the previous infiltrated area, the vessels may have much higher possibility of being penetrated by the cannula in spite of using blunt cannula compared to that of 1st session. Meanwhile, even though at the 1st session, the fullness due to overcorrection of fat may reduce the mobility of the vessels.

There is no doubt that fibrosis occurs more frequently when fronzen fat is used for fat grafting compared to fresh fat. But, in second case, arterial occlusion was developed in spite of only fresh fat was used for 2 sessions of fat grafting. It means that another important factor should be considered

Second, in the first and second cases, the fat was injected while the cannula was pushed ahead. Suppose if the vessel have been already penetrated by the blunt cannula, it is highly possible that the cannula might be located inside the vascular lumen and moved forward within the vessel during the injection. It means high probability of intravascular fat injection. On the other hand, if the fat is injected while the cannula drawn back. The cannula may immediately get out from the vessel and a little or no fat will be injected into vessel. Because of all of these reasons, I strongly suggest that the fat must be injected only during the cannula is drawing back. Even though it is not confirmed, application of push ahead fat injection is suspected in the 3rd and 4th cases.

(2) Blindness and infarction caused by arterial emboli

I would like to introduce some examples of serious complications, such as blindness and brain infarction due to facial fat grafting, on the basis of reference literature.

Firstly, there are 3 cases of only blindness resulted from glabella fat grafting[15,17,18];

Secondly, there are 3 cases of only brain stroke resulted from facial fat grafting; One case of aphasia and hemiparesis for 10 months after fat grafting to nasolabial fold, lip, and chin, another case of confusion, hypertonia, and hypertension occurred immediately after the fat injection into left temporal hollow, eyelid, and glabella, which was due to embolism of anterior cerebral artery [19], and other case of critical stroke after fat grafting into only glabella[20].

Thirdly, there are 2 cases of both blindness and brain infarction resulted from fat grafting; One case of blindness, hemiplegia, global aphasia after fat grafting into periorbital area, which was due to embolism of both central retinal artery and cerebral artery[15,16] ,and another case of a sudden right eye pain, blindness, conjunctival injection, and left hemiplegia as a symptoms of frontal and parietal stroke occurred during the glabella fat grafting. These symptoms were result from embolism of choroidal and retinal artery, and middle cerebral artery [16].

Fourthly, there are several cases of skin necrosis, blindness and brain infarction; In one case of blindness, language attrition, and right hemiplegia occurred while losing a sense of direction after feeling pain on the eyes and the head after 10 minutes of the 0.5ml, 3ml, and 3ml of fresh fat injected into the left bridge of the nose, nasolabial fold, and upper and lower lip. Skin necrosis occurred in the infiltrated area on the bridge of the nose within 5 days. It was suggested that the branches of the left middle cerebral artery and the opthalmic artery were obstructed[21]. Blindness is thought to be related to supratrochlear artery because it generally occurs during the correction of glabella frown line with fat grafting. Especially, the fat injected into the supratrochlear artery refluxed into the central retinal artery through ophthalmic artery. On the other hand, embolism is caused by the obstruction of anterior or middle cerebral artery following injection of fat into the opthalmic artery and then reflux into internal carotid artery. Blindness occurs concurrently with a sudden orbital or periorbital pain during or immediately after fat grafting. There is no restoration case of eyesight after fat grafting-induced blindness, but, symptoms of brain infarction are partly recovered in a few cases as time passed.

(3) Pulmonary embolism due to venous emboli

Temporal hollow is a very popular recipient site for fat grafting. Recently, it is reported that non-thrombotic pulmonary embolism occurred immediately after fat grafting for temporal hollow[22]. The fat injected into middle temporal vein might be migrated to lung via retromandibular vein and external jugular vein. Suddenly, clinical manifestations such as sweating, dyspnea, tachypnea, and cardiac respiratory arrest occurred to the two patients during fat grafting under local anesthesia and they were recovered immediately by CPR. However, another patient who had performed fat grafting under general anesthesia died despite CPR was performed. I recommend using blunt cannula, injecting the fat little by little while drawing back the cannula, and using multiple injection sites to prevent this complication. When any abnormal and unaccountable manifestation occurs, discontinue the procedure, and begin emergency treatment (eg, close monitoring of heart rate, blood pressure, arterial blood gas level, and respiration via electrocardiogram) and symptomatic treatment (eg, administration of therapy to lower blood pressure, analgesics, and oxygen inhalation) to minimize the hazard.

2 Complications of donor site

Severe complications from liposuction rarely occur since only relatively small amount of fat is needed for fat grafting. However, the possibility of occurrence of complications always exists. Complications caused by liposuction are briefly described below.

1) Depression or irregularity

The complications such as unsmooth outline, depression, or irregularity between the regionally liposuctioned area and the surroundings — frequently occur in small amount of liposuction for fat grafting. However, patients usually generous for these complications of compared to that of conventional liposuction; but you need to be careful since there is always an exception.

If depressed or sunken area happen while liposuction, it is good to fat graft in that area immediately. Perform fat grafting after 6 months if the sunken area appears as time passes, or correct by using lipo-shifting methods: molding and moving the fat of surroundings towards the sunken area[23].

2) Bleeding and hematoma

Prevent bleeding and hematoma by wearing compression garments, using elastic tape or foam dressings after procedure. Distinguish the bruise and hematoma caused by bleeding. For bruise, enhancing natural excretion is recommended, and for hematoma, squeezing or is needed. Hematoma may be tiny but it can be large and cause significant inflammation. Hematoma, which is formed by neglected mass without treatment, forms seroma. Needle aspiration is used to distinguish hematoma and seroma.

3) Fibrosis

The hematoma and seroma caused by liposuction appears as subcutaneous nodule though fibrous inflammation. Especially, mass is formed when infection is accompanied. Also, the mass caused by wound in the surgical site becomes smooth within 6 months to 1 year, unless there are inflammations.

For regional abdominal liposuction, fibrosis rarely occurs, but can occur because of the wrinkles of compression garments. Thus, in the next day of the procedure, prevent regional pressing by the garments.

Once fibrosis develops it should be cured immediately. Administrate methylprednisolone (Medrol Dos Pak) for 7 days. Then, administrate nonsteroidal anti-inflammatory drugs for at least 8 weeks. Care with ultrasound devices after 3 weeks of the procedure. If there is no effect after 8 weeks of the treatment, inject 1ml of lidocaine (0.5%, mixed with diluted epinephrine) mixed with 1ml of 5-fluo-rouracil (50mg), triamcinolone 20mg of triamcinolone (40mg/ml) until the mass dissociates. When performing the treatment, it is very important to make sure that the injection does not leak out from the mass. If it had leaked out, inject 10 times of the expected drained amount of normal saline to the surroundings to dilute. Surgical dissection must be considered as the last means.

4) Hyperpigmentation

Liposuction caused hyperpigmentation can occur in the outlet or suctioned area with bleeding. Blocking sunlight is very important, and the treatment is same as that of hyperpigmentation of recipient area.

5) Paresthesia and pain

Hemianesthesia or anesthesia can occur as paresthesia, but most of them are temporary symptoms which are naturally recovered. They are accompanied by pains caused by small neuroma but usually by damages on subfascia or muscle (Weird). The pain can be relieved by local anesthetic that can be performed in several times. The neuroma is recovered by surgical excision. The chronic pain due to the scar formation between subcutaneous, or skin, and fascia, is treated by scar dissection.

6) Infection

Early diagnosis or active treatment of postoperative infection is important to prevent severe complications like necrosis, sepsis or toxic shock. Inflammation or infection should be suspected for noticeable erythema. Blebbing should be observed and treated thoroughly since it is suspected as a sign of necrosis.

Infection usually occurs between 10 days and 6 weeks after the procedure. Suspect mycobacteria for erythema with lump. Mycobacteria is hard to diagnose with culture test even though suppurative secretion exists. Administrate 2-3 times of 600mg rifampin with isoniazide, pyrazinamide, and ethambutol per week, or streptomycin up to 6 months.

The cause of blister on skin should be distinguished since it can also be caused by the pressure and friction of tape pasting to the skin, Reston foam, and elastic bandage.

If postoperative infection signs such as fever, skin necrosis, no response to early antibiotics treatment, etc., are appear, moving the patient to a bigger hospital for a quick diagnosis, optimal treatment, and prevention of critical complications are recommended.

7) Seroma

The flap damage, formation of dead space, and hematoma caused by bleeding from hyper-liposuction on a single area is replaced by serosanguineous fluid forming seroma.

Extract serous fluid and perform compression dressing for continuous postoperative seroma. Needle aspiration and compression dressing repeated with a few days interval, or injecting drain to the well drained area among the liposuctioned sites. Drain should be replaced every 2-3 days and perform the antibiotics treatment. Seroma generally disappears within 1 week, but the treatment must be repeated until it is completely vanished. For seroma lasting more than 1 month, inject the same amount of indoor air after serous aspiration and also perform compression dressing.

If erythema and tenderness occur with inflammation sign, suspect abscess formation and perform suction together with microbiological study and antimicrobial susceptibility test. Optimal antibiotic treatment should be performed, but incision and drainage are recommended when big abscess shows slow response to antibiotics.

If an infection is confirmed, primary physicians should consider the interfacility transfer of the patient to a large hospital for optimal treatment and prevention of severe complications.

8) Scar

The scar in liposuction site can be a problem even with morsel liposuction. To minimize the friction of cannula, move cannula by slightly raising up or using a plastic plug (skn protector). Apply steroid cream if erythema outbreaks. Perform general scar treatment if scar is formed. For large scar or keloid, combined injection of steroid and 5-fluorouracil, re-dissection, silicon gel sheet pressure, or radiation therapy can be performed. Large scars get improved naturally within 2-3 years, but permanent recovery is impossible for keloid and it always reoccurs.

The scar caused by skin necrosis mostly brings serious outcomes, transfer to experienced doctor would be better.

9) Necrosis

Even though only small amount of fat is suctioned using sharp-ended cannula, approaching the cannula too close to the skin, or aspiration with the hole of cannula facing hypodermatic area, can cause skin necrosis by destroying subdermal plexus.

Also, the onset of necrotizing fascitis is reported to be caused by the thrombosis of subcutaneous blood vessel, gangrene of subcutaneous layer and surrounding tissues from the infection of subcutaneous tissue, and deep fascia infection (caused by combination of fulminant streptococcus A, and anaerobic bacteria)[24,25].

Recommended treatments are excisional biopsy, administration of antibiotics, platelet rich plasma, fat derived stem cell therapy, or hyperbaric oxygenation. In addition, consider interfacility transfer to a specialized hospital. Heavy smokers who do not quit smoking before and after the procedure have higher incidence rate of necrosis.

10) Severe complications

As widely known, the life-threatening critical complications caused by liposuction are fat embolism[26,27], thromboembolism[28], toxic shock syndrome[29,30], etc.

However, there are almost no cases reported on causing severe complications because liposuction for fat grafting is performed minimumly on partial areas only. Nonetheless, it does not mean that it is free from anaphylactic shock by added preservative or lidocaine, perforation in abdominal wall or thoracic wall during abdominal liposuction, thromboembolism in high-risk patients, spreading into systemic infection due to early treatment and toxic shock syndrome.

The most important factors in preventing these severe complications and performing optimal treatments are to practice a quick diagnosis, prompt treatments, and decision of the time for interfacility transfer to larger hospital.

11) Complications caused by anesthesia

There is almost no severe accident caused by anesthesia when performing liposuction for fat grafting as well as fat injection under local anesthesia. However, conscious sedation is generally used nowadays, so we cannot ingnore the complications caused by anesthesia. For anesthetic accidents, prevention is the first priority rather than treatment. Details are covered in the anesthesia chapter (Chapter 7).

Especially, there is almost no toxic effect of lidocaine itself since only small amount of liposuction is performed. However, there are cases reporting deaths due to allergy reaction caused by antiseptic (methylparaben) included in local anesthetic, lidocaine[31]. Also, there is a report about anaphylatic shock caused by lidocaine. With the onset of acute allergy reaction, rapid injection of normal saline, ephedrine (5-10mg intravenous injection), oxygenation, and intubation for bronchoconstriction should be performed in advance[32,33].

Reference

01. Ko KH. Director of Co & You cosmetic surgery clinic. Seoul Korea. Personal communication,2011.

02. Lee Po. La reine aesthetic clinic, Seoul, Korea, Personal communication,2015

03. Yoon YG. Director of Ran cometic surgery clinic. Bupyeong Korea. Personal communication,2011.

04. Gutowski KA. ASPS Fat Graft Task Force: Current applications and safety of autologous fat grafts: a report of the ASPS fat graft task force. Plast Reconstr Surg. 2009;124(1):272-280. Comment in: Plast Reconstr Surg. 2010 Feb;125(2):758-9; author reply 759.

05. Niechajev I: Lip enhancement: Surgical alternatives and histologic aspects. Plast Reconstr Surg. 2000 ;105(3): 1173-1183; discussion 1184-1187.

06. Beeson WH, Slama TJ, Beeler RT, Rachel JD, Pierno NA. Groop A streptoccoccal fasciitis after submental tumescent liposuction. Arch Facial Plast Surg. 2001:3:277-279.

07. Galea LA. Nicklin S. Mycobacterium abscessus infection complicating hand rejuvenation with structural fat grafting. .J Plast Reconstr Aesthet Surg. 2009;62(2):e15-6.

08. Yang HJ, Yim HW, Lee MY, Ko KS, Yoon HJ. Mycobacterium conceptionense infection complicating face rejuvenation with fat grafting. J Med Microbiol. 2011;60(3):371-374. Epub 2010 Nov 4.

09. Dal Canto AJ, Downs-Kelly E, Perry JD. Ptosis and orbital fat prolapse after posterior sub-Tenon's capsule triamcinolone injection. Ophthalmology 2005;112(6):1092-1097. Comment in: Ophthalmology. 2006 ;113(3):504-5; author reply 505.

10. Ersek RA, Chang P, Salisbury MA. Lipo layering of autologous fat: an improved technique with promising results. Plast Reconstr Surg. 1998;101(3):820-826.

11. Yang DY. Director of DoDo cosmetic clinic. Suwon Korea. Personal communication,2011.

12. Tanamin®.http://www.pharmacyhealth.net/d/tanamin-1702.htm

13. Kuroyanagi Y. The front line of regenerative medicine, Episurge®; Establishment of banking system with cultured dermis. Regenerative Therapy. 2006, 5 (1):119-126. 5 (1):119-126,2006.

14. Jung DH, Shimmian Rhinoplastic Clinic, Seoul, Korea, Personal commumication,2015.

15. Dreizen NG, Framm L. Sudden unilateral visual loss after autologous fat injection into the glabellar area. Am J Ophthalmol. 1989;15;107(1):85-87.

16 Feinendegen DL, Baumgartner RW, Vuadens P, Schroth G, Mattle HP, Regli F, Tschopp H. Autologous fat injection for soft tissue augmentation in the face: a safe procedure? Aesthetic Plast Surg 1998;22(3):163-167.

17. Egido JA, Arroyo R, Marcos A, Jiménez-Alfaro I. Middle cerebral artery embolism and unilateral visual loss after autologous fat injection into the glabellar area. Stroke 1993;24(4):615-616.

18. Teimourian B. Blindness following fat injections. Plast Reconstr Surg. 1988;82(2):361.

19. Thaunat O, Thaler F, Loirat P, Decroix JP, Boulin A. Cerebral fat embolism induced by facial fat injection. Plast Reconstr Surg. 2004;113(7) 2235-2236.

20. Yoon SS, Chang DI, Chung KC. Acute fatal stroke immediately following autologous fat injection into the face. Neurology 2003;61(8):1151-1152.

21. Danesh-Meyer HV, Savino PJ, Sergott RC. Case reports and small case series: ocular and cerebral ischemia following facial injection of autologous fat. 2001 May;119(5):777-778.

22. Jiang X, Liu DL, Chen B. ;Middle temporal vein. a fatal hazard in injection cosmetic surgery for temple augmentation. JAMA Facial Plast Surg. 2014 May-Jun;16(3):227-9.

23. Saylan Z. Liposhifting: Treatment of post liposuction irregularities. Int J Cosm Surg. 1999;7(1):71-73.

24. Gibbons MD, Lim RB, Carter PL. Necrotizing fasciitis after tumescent liposuction. Am Surg. 1998;64 (5):458-460.

25. Heitmann C, Czermak C, Germann G. Rapidly fatal necrotizing fasciitis after aesthetic liposuction. Aesthetic Plast Surg. 2000;24(5):344-347.

26. Laub DR Jr, Laub DR. Fat embolism syndrome after liposuction: a case report and review of the literature. Ann Plast Surg. 1990;25(1):48-52.

27. Scroggins C, Barson PK. Fat embolism syndrome in a case of abdominal lipectomy with liposuction. Md Med J 1999;48(3):116-118.

28. Grazer FM, de Jong RH. Fatal outcomes from liposuction: census survey of cosmetic surgeons. Plast Reconstr Surg. 2000;105(1):436-46; discussion 447-448. Comment in: Plast Reconstr Surg. 2000;106(3): 740-741. Plast Reconstr Surg. 2000;106(5):1211-1212.

29. Rhee CA, Smith RJ, Jackson IT. Toxic shock syndrome associated with suction-assisted lipectomy. Aesthetic Plast Surg. 1994;18(2):161-163.

30. Umeda T, Ohara H, Hayashi O, Ueki M, Hata Y. Toxic shock syndrome after liposuction suction and lipectomy. Plast Reconstr Surg. 2000;106(1):204-207.

31. Kim Y, Hirota Y, Shibutani T, Sakiyama, K, Okimura, M, Matsuura H. A case of anaphylactoid reaction due to methyl-paraben during induction of general anesthesia. J Jpn Dent Soc Anesthesiol. 1994;22(3):491-500.

32. Bircher AJ, Surber C. Anaphylactic reaction to lidocaine. Aust Dent J. 1999 Mar;44(1):64. Comment on: Aust Dent J 1998;43(3):170-171.

33. Zimmerman J, Rachmilewitz D Systemic anaphylactic reaction following lidocaine administration. Gastrointest Endosc. 1985;31(6):404-405.

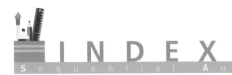

INDEX
Sequential Autologous Fat Injection